The Nutrient-Dense Eating Plan

A Lifetime Eating Guide to Exceptional Foods for Super Health

Douglas L. Margel, D.C.

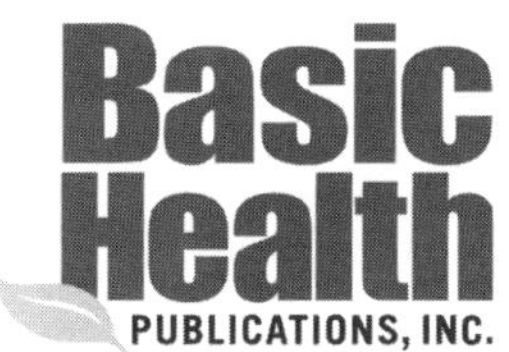

The information contained in this book is based upon the research and personal and professional experiences of the author. It is not intended as a substitute for consulting with your physician or other healthcare provider. Any attempt to diagnose and treat an illness should be done under the direction of a healthcare professional.

The publisher does not advocate the use of any particular healthcare protocol but believes the information in this book should be available to the public. The publisher and author are not responsible for any adverse effects or consequences resulting from the use of the suggestions, preparations, or procedures discussed in this book. Should the reader have any questions concerning the appropriateness of any procedures or preparation mentioned, the author and the publisher strongly suggest consulting a professional healthcare advisor.

Basic Health Publications, Inc.
28812 Top of the World Drive
Laguna Beach, CA 92651
949-715-7327

Library of Congress Cataloging-in-Publication Data

Margel, Douglas L.
The nutrient-dense eating plan : a lifetime eating guide to exceptional foods for super health / Douglas L. Margel.
p. cm.
Includes bibliographical references and index.
ISBN 1-59120-091-1
1. Nutrition. 2. Food—Composition. I. Title.

RA784.M2963 2005
613.2—dc22

2005001823

Editor: Roberta W. Waddell
Typesetting/Book design: Gary A. Rosenberg
Cover design: Mike Stromberg

Printed in the United States of America

10 9 8 7 6 5 4 3 2 1

Contents

PART 3 • Applying Nutrient Density in Daily Life

PART 4 • Nutrient-Dense Recipes

Appendices

For my mother

Foreword

Is it possible that nutrition is the highly coveted, yet extremely ignored x-factor of health? Although Hippocrates, the father of medicine, reminds us that food should be our medicine and medicine our food, his wise words are too often lost in today's cacophony of technological hype and mass consumer marketing. Unlike any other period in history, today we face innumerable threats to our food supply—genetically engineered foods (GMOs), trans-fatty acids, synthetic herbicides, fungicides, pesticides, fertilizers, preservatives, additives, and artificial sweeteners, among others—all developed in the name of prolonged shelf life and corporate profits, and all wreaking havoc on our physiology.

It is not an overstatement to say that nutrition is *the* health issue of the times. Cancer, coronary heart diseases, obesity, osteoarthritis, and osteoporosis are just some of the many chronic health issues confronting a severely unhealthy population. The American Cancer Society states that 60 percent of all cancer could be eliminated if people simply ate healthily, and the same can probably be said for the other chronic conditions as well.

From autumn 1994 through spring 2003, I taught a course in nutrition, health, and performance at the University of Colorado. To give the students a good perspective on what is considered a controversial topic, I invited a number of health professionals, including Dr. Doug Margel, to come share their knowledge and experience as guest speakers. Without exception, the students found Doug extremely knowledgeable and highly engaging. He encouraged them to think deeply about the quality of the food they were putting into their bodies every day, and urged them to question the profit-driven motives of the multinational food corporations. Doug was so popular that I invited him back every semester for the entire decade of my tenure.

While the outlook for the food industry may look bleak to some, Doug is optimistic about our future nutritional habits. In *The Nutrient-Dense Eating Plan,* he helps the reader shift from an adversarial approach to food to a joyous, collaborative celebration of it through his sage advice, his insights, and his delicious recipes, which empower the reader to attain and maintain optimal health.

This book, which fully captures Doug's passion and inspiration, contains the same timeless and time-tested information he shared with my students over the years, and just as they did, you will find him highly informative and engaging. Doug has the unique ability to exclaim that the emperors of the food industry are indeed wearing no clothes. The question is, will you have the courage to listen and act on his clear vision?

Brian Luke Seaward, Ph.D.
Author, *Stressed Is Desserts Spelled Backwards*
and *Quiet Mind, Fearless Heart*

Preface

The Nutrient-Dense Eating Plan seeks to broadly articulate the big picture of nutrition by focusing on foods of the highest quality. It presents a return-to-basics approach to nutrition by emphasizing an appreciation for exemplary food, and importantly, a personal and participatory relationship with food through knowledge and self-empowerment.

The Nutrient-Dense Eating Plan sets forth the profound concept of nutrient density to give you a practical handle on your food and dietary choices. The nutrient density of food describes a continuum of quality, utilizing a combination of science, common sense, ancestral wisdom, and cultural diversity.

This eating plan confronts the dominant eating disorder of our culture, which I consider to be an ambivalent and often adversarial relationship with food. In doing so, it cuts through narrow agendas and specific or rigid diets and replaces them with a sense of the goodness of good food. *Nutrient density* is a term that has resonant power. Whenever I teach or explain nutrient density, people invariably have an *Aha*! experience. They easily connect with this term because it does not intimidate or threaten, but instead reassures by presenting, in simple terms, an overwhelmingly positive image of real food.

Regaining the knowledge and means to properly nourish your body is both empowering and enlightening. The elegant simplicity, ease of applicability, and intuitive correctness of nutrient density is profoundly refreshing and appealing. It is also vitally important in terms of healing much of what has already been damaged if your existing relationship with food is unhealthy.

This book is divided into four parts, with follow-up appendices and a bibliography at the end. Part 1 defines nutrient density and elaborates on how and why it is the best way to eat. In it, I introduce the concept of nutrient density, and explore the dietary landscape of the past. Next, I discuss the perennial philosophy of food (*see* Chapter 6), contrasting it with the overall status of food in America, and much of the world, today. I also take a look at the denigration of food, its reduction to mere entertainment (the happy-meal mentality), and other ways in which our culture tends to devalue or underappreciate food. I then examine the philosophy and importance behind nutrient density as a commonsense approach to healthy eating, and finally conclude that this core set of values, which *celebrates* the goodness of good food, can help heal today's cultural eating disorders.

Part 2 examines many individual foods considered nutrient dense. Most of these foods will be familiar to you. This section will reacquaint you with many old friends (and some new ones), and give you a fresh sense of appreciation for the wide range of wonderful, nutrient-dense foods available.

Part 3 outlines the tier system I have devised to help you phase into eating the nutrient-dense foods that will deliver maximum benefits for your health and happiness. Part 4 lists recipes that can help you implement this plan for eating nutrient-dense foods.

The wisdom of nutrient density lies in knowing what is wholesome, healthy, and safe, a simple message that is highly relevant to these times. Similar to other aspects of life today, how people eat is undergoing a revolution, and *The Nutrient-Dense Eating Plan* promises to be an integral part of this process.

Acknowledgments

The journey of publishing a book such as this extends far back in time and encompasses myriads of influences. Many people have contributed to this book, and many people in my life have contributed to my journey of nutritional awareness. I am deeply grateful to them all. One thing I have learned is that eating is truly an activity that heals, and unites like nothing else.

First I would like to thank my literary agent, Joelle Delbourgo, who had the open mind and courage to take a chance on a new author. Her wisdom and experience were, and continue to be, highly prized. Similarly, my publisher, Norman Goldfind, a genuinely nice guy, believed in this book and made it possible. Bobby Waddell was invaluable as editor—her pruning and clipping kept my words from taking over. Leigh Jude also provided key editorial help, along with generous amounts of encouragement and patience.

Chauntelle Eckhaus, Vanessa Pierce, and Birgit Phillips each gave crucial support at critical junctures in preparation of the manuscript. Chauntelle in particular gave generously of her time, despite being very pregnant—for her grace under pressure I will always be deeply appreciative. Joy Rosenberg also kindly donated time to help with research. My sincere gratitude for the advice and wise counsel of Brian Luke Seward, author, educator, and friend par excellence.

Ellen Friedlander kindly opened her home, kitchen, and computer to me at a time when I needed all three. Similarly, Aki and Melinda Friedman and Kearns and Valerie Kelly also generously provided me with the nicest of writing and living arrangements. To all I am deeply grateful.

For the fantastic recipes contributed by two true kitchen alchemists, Amalia Friedman and Garima Fairfax, deep bows and everlasting gratitude.

The best of friends kept me nourished on many levels throughout the entire process of writing this book. For sharing and caring, deepest thanks and love to Scott and Elizabeth Groginsky, Anne McNamera and Ricky Rakestraw, Patricia Bukur, Kristin Cook, Felicia Trevor Gallo, Charlie and Betsy Liggett, Maggie McVoy, Jeff Pincus, and Carol Warner. Without the unconditional love and support of Pam

Parrott, this book would probably never have been written. Special thanks to Sarah Aley for artistry inside and outside the kitchen.

Finally, a big thank you to all the teachers and students who have helped me along this journey of discovery and learning.

Introduction

Why Nutrient Density?

The Nutrient-Dense Eating Plan is a commonsense approach to food and the ways people choose to eat. Nutrient density is easy to understand—it evaluates food according to its quality, or denseness. A food's denseness is what tells you if your choices are providing you with desired nutrients, or merely empty calories.

The Nutrient-Dense Eating Plan simplifies the quest for a healthier diet by providing you with a yardstick you can use to evaluate the nutritional quality of foods. It shows you how to easily apply this understanding to navigate in the real world as you improve your way of eating. Above all, *The Nutrient-Dense Eating Plan* is a practical approach based on simplicity, the integrity of real food, and the very real needs of your body based on biology, evolutionary consistency, and common sense.

Nutrition is not rocket science. *The Nutrient-Dense Eating Plan* is about real food for real people. It is about treating your body with respect, and about creating a healthy relationship with genuine, good food. *The Nutrient-Dense Eating Plan* is not a quick fix approach to nutrition, nor is it just another fad diet. Instead, it is a plan that reacquaints you with the food of your ancestors, connecting you with the whole world and with what is natural, wholesome, and appropriate. Its approach incorporates common sense and dignity, and is the cornerstone of what it means to build and sustain your health from the ground up.

Above all, *The Nutrient-Dense Eating Plan* restores health through the principle of wholeness. Contemporary food production, driven by agribusiness and chemical-dependent agriculture, fragments the environment, the food itself, and ultimately, you, the consumer. This style of agriculture, where food is more manufactured than grown, cheapens everything food stands for—historically, culturally, and environmentally. It also shortchanges you nutritionally. Real food, on the other hand, connects you to the web of life, and helps restore wholeness to both ecosystems and your own body. Foods that are nutritionally whole and dense are the manna that sustains, both physically and spiritually.

The Nutrient-Dense Eating Plan is not some new-age fantasy or posthippie dream. Instead, it is food as it *always was,* pure and simple. This simplicity, common sense, and intuitive rightness reveals the Tao (way) of food.

In my many years of counseling, teaching, and healing, I have repeatedly seen the frustration that people experience over health issues. People are literally sick and tired of being sick and tired—fed up with being poorly fed and with feeding themselves poorly. Many people are also waking up to the poignant fact that trusting as fundamental a human need as nutrition to distant, faceless, and unaccountable corporations often results in a loss of control and power. This book is all about reclaiming your power and control—eating as if it mattered *is* empowering, and more and more people are making this powerful statement about their lives. Reclaiming your dignity and good health go hand in hand.

The Nutrient-Dense Eating Plan is a lifetime guide to such a reclamation project. Like a road map, it facilitates this process by pointing out where you are right now and where you want to go. One of the principal ways it does this is by prioritizing the steps necessary to increase the denseness of your diet. Instead of guilt-tripping you into trying to be perfect all at once, the plan shows you how to take your current diet and begin the process in manageable steps. This approach allows you to go at your own pace, and encourages you to work within your individual comfort levels and needs. It also helps you gradually process your relationship with food, allowing you to more deeply assimilate these changes. This, in turn, inevitably leads to long-lasting results.

Ideally, no one should need books such as this. Good nutrition is really your birthright, and should be well within the reach of all. However, contradicting information, confusing claims, and aggressive and misleading advertising have led many to question what is correct, true, and right. So, even though I feel that nutrition is mostly common sense, my work as a doctor and educator has taught me that many people need both reassurance and guidance; I hope this book provides both.

Since your potential as a human being is enormous, my primary impetus for writing *The Nutrient-Dense Eating Plan* is to help you regain your confidence and sense of control over your life, especially as your decisions relate to health, well-being, and nourishment. You should feel capable, empowered, and good about your life and the choices you make. I wrote this book because I love good food and want to share, as widely as possible, the joy and pleasure that comes from connecting with, and appreciating, good foods.

EMBRACING CHANGE—THE PSYCHOLOGY OF NUTRIENT DENSITY

As you will see, adopting a nutrient-dense diet essentially means developing an entirely new approach to food. Yet, for many, this is not as difficult as it might seem, because basically, it is a return to our roots. Something in us actually resonates with good, wholesome food, because it speaks to the indigenous wisdom that resides in our DNA. Since nutrient-dense foods are deeply natural to our bodies, we can even find relief in this transition.

Nonetheless, for most people, change is rarely easy. If you grow up with certain beliefs, values, and habits, giving these up can seem scary and intimidating. What will take the place of the familiar, and the safe? What if it is not as fulfilling? What if I have made a mistake? Have I burned my bridges? And perhaps most important, if I adopt new habits and patterns, what will become of the old me? What kind of person will I become? Giving up safe and familiar assumptions for new ground is not something many people are comfortable with. Yet, being willing to move forward and experience the unknown and untried is the way we grow.

It is important to respect this resistance to change. People are, after all, creatures of habit who get very comfortable with what seems to work. Why rock the boat? The problem, of course, is that the diet of most Americans, known as the Standard American Diet (SAD) is not really working very well. This food is abundant, relatively cheap, and tastes good. But the bottom line is that very few people on the SAD diet feel really healthy. Statistics show startling trends: More Americans are overweight than at any time in history; cancer and heart disease strike down younger and younger victims; and super bugs and viruses threaten to overwhelm immune systems as never before. At the same time, untold millions believe it is somehow normal to live with chronic headaches, joint pains, and digestive problems. Their energy is not what it should be. Sleep disorders plague tens of millions, and people's sex lives are too often unfulfilling. On top of all that, people suffer in unprecedented numbers from depression and anxiety. And children are no better off. More children today are beginning their formative years with psychoactive medications than would ever have been deemed imaginable. If the old saying, you are what you eat, is true, then it would seem that the diet of the vast majority of Americans is indeed unhealthy.

In my many years of working to improve the health of my clients, I have found that making consistent changes in the diet is the most profound and lasting way to build health and catalyze deep changes in their lives. Yet, for many, these changes do not come easy. Change pushes everyone's buttons in many ways, and brings resistance and fears to the surface. For each person, change is a process that is always personal, sometimes emotionally charged, and highly unique to the individual circumstances. We bring hopes and fears, anxieties and past triumphs—all our past stuff—to the present moment. Here is where everything converges. If eating is life, then how you eat is truly a reflection of how you are choosing to live your life.

My arrangement of the transition to a more nutrient-dense diet reflects a respect for the individual's personal comfort levels. The tiers are designed to offer stepwise guidelines in order to simplify the process. Please realize that they are not etched in stone. It is my hope that you will use them as you would any map—they can be very helpful if you are lost. If you feel confident that you know the way, however, a map may only serve to verify what you already know.

When you are actually ready for change, it is up to you alone to do it. Friends, companions, teachers, coaches, and authors can be there for you, but ultimately, it is you, yourself, who plunges into this change.

What I have done with these tiers is to make a list of priorities and suggestions. This approach easily maps out the journey by identifying the major milestones, or quantum leaps, you may encounter along the way. I have found that previewing the road ahead removes some of the fear of the unknown from the picture. Clearly identifying these landmarks gives newcomers a sense of understanding and comfort. It also respects the need some people have to go a bit slower with the steps I propose in the nutrient-dense tier system (see Part 3, Chapters 41–43), allowing space for digesting changes in manageable bits. In this way, anyone can test the waters before moving forward into new territory. Looking too far down the road toward the finish line might make the goal appear too daunting. A stepwise approach, however, builds confidence because you can always take the next step.

Incorporating nutrient-dense principles into your life means a willingness to think outside the cultural box of prepackaged, highly processed, or synthesized foods, and begin to learn how to directly experience simple, unadulterated, nutritionally intact foods. It is my hope you will come away from this book inspired to know these foods much better, and empowered to make them an integral part of your own eating plan.

PART 1

The Nutrient-Dense Eating Plan

CHAPTER 1

What Is Nutrient Density?

Nutrient density refers to the nutritional quality of any given food. The concentration or denseness of nutrients that a food contains describes the overall quality of that food. *Foods that are very nutrient dense are the most concentrated sources of vitally important nutrients.* These foods support and build super health because they are exceptional sources of all the building blocks necessary for our bodies to function optimally. In essence, nutrient-rich foods are the opposite of empty-calorie junk foods.

Berries, blackstrap molasses, eggs, fish, gourmet mushrooms, green tea, most nuts, organic meats, sea vegetables, whole grains, and many fruits and vegetables, especially dark leafy greens, all qualify as nutritionally dense foods. Other items often found in health food stores, such as flaxseed oil, fresh carrot and wheatgrass juices, legumes, many herbal teas, nutritional yeast, and wheat germ, also belong in this category. Surprisingly, dark chocolate, microbrew beers, and red wines also qualify as dense sources of important nutrients for specific reasons that I will explore later.

Typically, specific foods are dense for particular nutrients. As an example, eggs contain large amounts of lecithin, proteins, and vitamin A, and are therefore considered to be highly nutrient dense in these nutrients. But it would not be accurate to say that eggs are a dense source of fiber or vitamin C.

Fresh, raw sugar cane (and the molasses that is pressed from it) contains large amounts of minerals, such as calcium, chromium, iron, and potassium, and can be considered nutrient dense. Once refined, however, the end product—white cane sugar—contains virtually none of these nutrients, and is considered very poor in nutritive value. Similarly, although commercial beers contain many additives and few actual nutrients, unfiltered microbrew or homemade beers usually contain relatively large amounts of B vitamins and certain minerals due to the molasses, yeast, and other ingredients used as raw materials.

Nutrient density also teaches us how to look at the nutritional value of food in new and fresh ways. For example, people have traditionally been taught that nutrients are confined to measurable vitamins and minerals. In recent years, however, science has found that numerous other compounds found in nature exhibit health-enhancing properties. Blackberries, blueberries, raspberries, and other brightly colored fruits, for example, have abundant levels of colorful pigments, which act as potent antioxidants. Berries, therefore, are particularly dense sources of important antioxidants. To date, scientists have not put specific values or numbers on how much of these compounds to ingest for optimal health, and there is not yet any consensus on how essential these molecules are. Nonetheless, the plan proposed here ensures that you will get generous amounts of such accessory nutrients.

Similarly, such vegetables as broccoli, cabbage, and onions provide valuable sulfur-containing compounds to aid your immune system and facilitate detoxification by the liver, so these foods are therefore nutrient dense for the essential mineral, sulfur, and its compounds. Another example of a nutrient-dense food would be sushi, which capably supplies beneficial oils, protein, and trace minerals from the seas. These and many other nutrient-dense foods ultimately provide all the amino acids, fatty acids, minerals, phytonutrients, vitamins, and other compounds necessary for disease resistance and the optimal functioning of your mind and body.

Eating with a nutrient-dense sensibility is not an exotic new trend. Whole unprocessed foods that have been human mainstays for centuries are often considered nutrient dense. As you will see, many ethnic cuisines, such as curries and hummus, are dense sources of important nutrients, as are many condiments, spices, and herbs.

How food is grown and cooked can dramatically affect its nutritional quality. Organic foods are generally denser in vitamins and minerals than their conventionally grown counterparts, which contain agricultural chemicals, residues of pesticides, and synthetic fertilizers. In cooking eggs, poaching or boiling them may preserve and protect their vital nutrients, while frying or scrambling, which exposes them to higher temperatures, may destroy sensitive molecules.

A NUTRIENT-DENSE ANALOGY

Food can be thought of as fuel for the metabolic fires burning within each of your cells. Like coal shoveled into a locomotive furnace, the nutrients in food stoke these fires, causing them to run hotter or more efficiently.

Nutrient-dense foods are similar to hardwoods that burn stronger, hotter, and cleaner. On the other hand, nutrient-poor junk foods, such as overprocessed, chemical-filled foods so typical of the Standard American Diet (SAD), are akin to soft woods, which do not burn as hot or efficiently as hardwoods. Research supports the idea that a consistently poor diet, low in nutrients and high in toxic substances, is a major contributor to the poor health and performance of so many Americans today. Eating foods that are low in nutrient density is like driving your car with an octane rating that is too low for your engine. Your body deserves the best fuel possible, and will operate most efficiently when given it.

The Nutrient-Dense Eating Plan is based on the ancient commonsense principle that you are what you eat. Similar to a computer with more memory capability, nutritionally denser foods allow your body the freedom to repair, regenerate, and combat infections and stress by providing all of the necessary building blocks in abundance. Specific nutrients are like bytes of information; the denser the food, the more information and support it conveys to you.

Some nutrients are stored in the body and kept in reserve for later use. Other nutrients are only available on an on-call basis. Still others can occasionally fill in or substitute for other nutrients. For example, there is an enormous range of food-derived compounds that provide antioxidant capabilities. Eating a diverse, nutrient-dense diet is therefore important and helpful in ensuring that you have an inner environment where different types of these nutrients will be optimally available. As it is virtually impossible to eat a diet that consistently supplies you with all of these, it is reassuring to know that, by grazing through a variety of foods, you can bathe your body tissues in varying combinations of these antioxidant molecules, knowing that the protection these antioxidants provide is available when you need it.

Nutrients are classified as either essential (needed to sustain life) or nonessential; nutrient-dense foods are notable in that they can generously provide both. Nonessential nutrients, such as phytonutrients, may not be indispensable, but are important because they contribute to the overall *quality* of your health. These so-called accessory nutrients may improve your health by strengthening your endocrine and immune systems, your vitality, and your overall sense of well-being.

CALORIES—EMPTY AND DENSE

Calories were once thought to be pretty much the same. A calorie is defined as a unit of metabolic heat or energy derived from food that is used to run the body's cellular machinery. While it was understood that different food sources yielded different concentrations of calories (per unit of weight, fat contains more than twice the calories of protein or carbohydrates), calories got little attention, aside from being blamed for weight gain and related problems.

In this climate, the notion of the empty calorie was largely overlooked. An empty calorie implies that the contribution of the food in question lies in its ability to supply energy while not contributing any accompanying nutrients. Thus, empty calories became generally associated with processed junk foods, and in particular, with foods comprised primarily of white sugar or white flour, both famous for supplying very few nutrients of value, yet supplying calories in abundance.

The empty calorie is a good starting point for a discussion of nutrient density, as it represents the polar opposite of nutrient-dense foods. An empty calorie is not, as was once thought, a neutral energy source, but is actually a *negative* source, as the body requires nutrients in order to metabolize a calorie to generate heat. By contributing nothing of nutritional value while using up nutrients that are present in the body, empty calories actually end up robbing, or depleting, the body of nutrients. The long-term consequence of relying on a diet that is heavy in empty calories is nutritional depletion, resulting in low-level reserves of vitamins, minerals, and other vital nutrients.

A calorie is not, therefore, an isolated entity. Rather, its importance lies in whether or not it is accompanied by specific nutrients. From this perspective, it would be wisest to select a diet in which most caloric contributions are accompanied by the nutrients needed for the body to rebuild, repair, and maintain tissue and overall health. In the language of *The Nutrient-Dense Eating Plan,* such a diet would principally contain dense, as opposed to empty, calories.

CHAPTER 2

Celebrating Exceptional Foods

The heart of *The Nutrient-Dense Eating Plan* is its celebratory approach to food. This novel point of view paves the way to a truly healthy relationship with food because, instead of seeing food as the problem, the plan sees food—good food—as the solution. Such food is the central focus of a truly healthy dietary lifestyle, and celebrates these delicious and satisfying foods by acknowledging and honoring them for their exceptional ability to support, nourish, and delight.

Recognizing and celebrating exceptional foods alters your relationship with food in fundamental and profound ways, and is an important stepping-stone toward reconnecting with the *fun* of food. Whether discussing ripe luscious blueberries (which recent research has shown can actually reverse signs of aging in test animals), rich dark chocolate, liquid golden flax oil, succulent sushi, rich buffalo steaks, or a myriad of other nutrient-dense foods, the appreciation of such food marks an important step in the evolution of people's ability to nourish themselves.

Most diet books today focus on the negative. Food is too often portrayed as the enemy, or as a problem to be solved. The society we live in seems to have developed an adversarial relationship with food. According to many diet experts, food makes you fat, zaps your energy, clogs your arteries, and gives you allergies, digestive problems, and headaches. But, what about the other side of the coin? Food also nourishes you, keeps you alive, and gives you great satisfaction and culinary pleasure. Food also brings people together, and provides a focal point as well as a cultural identity; it links countless generations of people who, in their time, also farmed, cooked, ate, and loved. Creating an enemy out of one of the most central and basic aspects of life is crazy, yet the current dietary landscape is so out of balance that it makes this unprecedented negative relationship with food seem normal.

Fortunately, there is a better way to relate to food. When you give up trying to eat in unnatural ways, you can begin to relax, reexamine your relationship with food, and start cultivating a healthy relationship with genuine good food. Celebrating the *goodness* of good food is not difficult because it is quite natural. Embracing the ancient awareness that food should nourish, support, and strengthen can come as a refreshing surprise. It is actually a relief to discover that you can *appreciate* truly good food, instead of dreading it.

Celebrating good food is natural and normal. Fearing it as something dangerous is unnatural and, historically speaking, unprecedented. It is also unnecessary. Of course, you need to be aware of which foods to avoid, but you need to balance that awareness with an adequate knowledge of the many safe, healthy, and desirable foods available to you. Once you make this basic distinction, you can safely embark on a lifetime journey of healthy eating.

Wonderfully delicious, nutrient-dense foods are easy to incorporate into your diet. Celebrating these foods simply means appreciating them for what they are. Cinnamon not only tastes wonderful, but helps to metabolize and regulate blood sugar. Olive oil helps keep arteries pliable and open. Luscious blueberries and other berries help keep nervous systems strong and youthful because they contribute an important class of antioxidants. Seaweeds offer a storehouse of trace minerals from the world's oceans. Healthful teas give a myriad of plant-based molecules, and nuts give essential oils, protein, and other important compounds. Cocoa solids, present in dark chocolate, contain potent flavonoid antioxidants, while organic eggs and healthy meats give amino acids, fats, iron, zinc, and other vital nutrients.

It is important to *like food*. While working throughout the years as a nutritional consultant, coach, and doctor, I have been amazed by the many people who have expressed fear about food. And often, shame or embarrassment is mixed with their fear, a sad, unnecessary state of affairs. Yet, I have also witnessed people's ability to heal these feelings and come to a healthy appreciation of food and its place in their lives. I have seen the joy and relief that accompanies the healing of such a fractured relationship with diet.

Celebrating food is the heart of cultivating a healthy relationship with it. As with people, each food is unique, individual. At its best, a good meal should be able to shock with its freshness, boldness, or even its simplicity. Nutrient-dense meals can be elaborate or simple, humble, and wholesome, or complex and exotic. The piquant spiciness of a perfect pomegranate, the satisfying texture and crunch of fresh walnut meat, a perfectly balanced salad, or the shape and fragrance of a piece of seaweed in a soup or stir-fry engages your senses, alerting you to the satisfaction and excitement good nourishment can accomplish.

Many people seem to find reassurance in the consistency and predictability of food purchased from chains, big-name brands, and fast-food outlets. I, however, find boredom in boxes. Although nutrient-dense foods can be obtained from commercial outlets, restaurants, and name-brand companies, the celebration of food I am referring to is more concerned with an appreciation for the individual elements so often missed when food comes in a prepackaged or premade form. It is the beauty of an individual carrot, the freshness of a bright red pepper or the crispness of a bunch of fresh spinach that can reconnect you in an instant with the bounty and goodness of the earth.

Food should never be taken for granted. Thankfully, you do not have to worry about the availability of food the way your ancestors might have. Like many people, you may not be directly involved in growing, raising, hunting, or foraging for your food. But, does this mean it is all right to undervalue it? I believe that this lack of appreciation for food is the underlying cultural eating disorder of our time, and may be partly responsible for many of the other neurotic or maladaptive attitudes toward food that are so pervasive in society today.

Celebrating good food really means trusting it. It also means trusting yourself and your innate ability to sort out what is good, and not good, for you. Trusting yourself with food also means you can begin to relax and enjoy it in a more guilt-free way. For some, this is truly difficult because the thought of food can carry a charge that makes many people deeply uncomfortable. Issues of worthiness, or body image, are feelings that can signify a deep lack of trust in food, in ourselves, and in the world itself. As a result of this relationship with food, many develop a deep ambivalence toward the ways in which they get nourished.

Personally, I love food. I enjoy shopping for it, cooking it, eating it, even growing it. As a consequence, food rarely bores or disappoints me. I think this is important, and I know it is partially responsible for the fact that I never feel I am wasting my time when preparing a meal or a snack. Celebrating food in this way also means that food can become a constant source of delight, and that it is rarely boring or perfunctory. Resenting the time food takes (shopping, cooking, eating) indicates a life that is possibly out of balance, and may also be a telling statement about a person's basic priorities.

It is a good idea to examine how you react around food. In teaching and sharing, I have discovered that many people really do have a problem with food. Everyone knows people who never cook, always eat the same food, buy the same few brands, or repetitiously eat at the same restaurants. Although this familiarity might bring comfort and predictability, the lack of trust it signifies can be quite limiting. Sometimes growth comes best with experimentation and a willingness to take a chance on something new.

I rarely use a recipe when I cook, but I know people who would never consider cooking without one. I find this fascinating. To these people, the idea of getting a meal "wrong" is scary, and deeply threatening. Yet, the truth of high-quality nutrient-dense foods is that they are very forgiving. In fact, their very quality gives the cook a wider latitude. In other words, good food allows for experimentation, and in fact, often seems to ask for it. This playfulness is the essence of what I mean by celebrating good food.

Nutrient-dense foods are not only good or nutritious. They are, by their very nature, fun. They call to you, seduce you with their beauty, and request you to participate with them in a mutual dance of life.

Nutrient-dense eating, then, is about diving deeper into life. Nutrient-dense foods can be friends, inspirations, or lovers, teaching and helping to dispel some of the fears or insecurities people may harbor about their lives. They can also be a portal to a deeper knowing of the world, and ourselves.

CHAPTER 3

High-Quality Nutrient-Dense Foods

As a nutritionist, probably the most common question put to me is, "What can I eat?" When told I am writing a new book on nutrition, the question becomes, "In your diet, what can I eat?" My simple answer is, of course, "lots of things," because nutrient-dense eating is more about expanding your options and awareness of what you can eat than about limiting them too severely. Since nutrient density is about celebrating exceptional foods, my focus here is on uncovering all the good things about good foods. Once you understand the basic guidelines of healthfulness and naturalness, the poor quality of many foods becomes rather obvious as well.

We have grown up in a culture that promotes fast foods and convenience over wholesomeness, and holds up artificial ingredients, preservatives, and heavy processing as normal and acceptable. Reconnecting with natural, wholesome foods does take a little time and effort. However, like most skills, once you get familiar with the basics, recognizing these foods becomes second nature. You *can* develop a sixth sense, and begin to trust your instincts. All you really need, in the beginning, is a little direction, and a little encouragement.

What follows is a list of foods that reasserts the goodness of good food. It covers many common nutrient-dense foods and, while not meant to be exhaustive, it is intended to act as an introduction to the variety and breadth of nutrient-dense foods that are readily available. Many foods are listed because they make unique contributions of specific or hard-to-get nutrients. Of course, they may be lacking in several other key nutrients because no one food is nutrient dense for all known nutrients. Rather, the point of adopting a nutrient-dense eating plan is to learn how to selectively graze across a broad diversity of these foods.

Because people's tastes differ dramatically, a wide range of options are found in this list. Learning to stock your kitchen is an art, and should change with the seasons, your moods and cravings, your lifestyle, the availability of foods, and other factors.

You should be in control of your diet and pleasures, not the other way around. Instead of feeling intimidated by the large number of nutrient-dense foods available, realize that you have innumerable options, so you can relax and appreciate the diverse array of nutrient-dense foods you have to choose from.

There are many regional foods available that I do not mention, either because I am not familiar with them, or I do not ordinarily use them. However, just because a food is not on the list, please do not think it cannot be nutrient dense. On the contrary, if a food fits the basic criteria for nutrient density, and is not highly processed or adulterated in some way, it stands a good chance of being nutrient dense for at least some of the nutrients discussed.

Also, even if a food is on the list, cooking or preparation techniques can affect the nutrient quality of the finished product. For example, potatoes are listed, but there is a big difference between a baked or boiled potato with skin, which is nutrient dense, and a French fry or a potato chip, which is not. Also, please realize that, although every food on this list is nutrient dense to some extent, that does not mean all foods listed here are appropriate for every tier level. (The tier system, as outlined in Part 3, Chapters 41–43, is a method I have devised to help ease your transition into nutrient-dense eating.) As you will see later, depending upon your personal needs, each tier has specific guidelines for what is appropriate.

THE LIST

- **Alliums:** Garlic, leeks, onions, shallots
- **Beverages:** Fresh juices, microbrew beers, red wines (organic), spring water, herbal teas
- **Breads:** See Chapter 21, Grains, for the best breads to buy
- **Butters:** Almond, pumpkin seed, sunflower seed, tahini (sesame-seed butter)
- **Canned foods:** Sardines, tomatoes, tomato or pasta sauce (in jars)
- **Dairy:** Fresh, raw (upasteurized and unhomogenized) milk (especially goat); certified raw milk cheeses, nonhomogenized milk and yogurts, organic butter
- **Eggs:** Deviled, egg salad, hard-boiled, poached, soft-boiled (do not overcook or brown them, never use powdered, always organic)
- **Fish:** Albacore, flounder, haddock, halibut, mackerel, salmon (wild), sardines, trout (except for trout, avoid freshwater species; beware of fish farming, avoid unsustainable and declining species, such as orange roughy, shark, or swordfish; be aware of mercury toxicity advisories for canned white albacore tuna and others)
- **Fresh fruits:** Numerous, including all berries, apples, bananas, cherries, citrus, guava, kiwi, mango, melons, papaya, peaches, pears (organic, whenever possible).

- **Fresh vegetables:** A partial list includes asparagus, avocados, beets (roots and tops), bok choy, broccoli, Brussels sprouts, cabbage, carrots, cauliflower, chard, collards, green beans, kale, leeks, mustard greens, onions, peas, peppers, potatoes, spinach, squashes, tomatoes, yams.
- **Herbs and spices:** All, including basil, cinnamon, cumin, curries, dill, ginger root, oregano, pepper, rosemary, saffron, thyme, turmeric (seek out nonirradiated forms)
- **Legumes:** Beans, lentils, split peas
- **Meats:** Any certified hormone-free meats, buffalo, elk, lamb, venison; organ meats, such as liver, are particularly nutrient dense
- **Miscellany:** Brewer's yeast, cod-liver oil, gomasio, hummus, olives, salsas, sea salt (unrefined), umeboshi plums (paste, vinegar)
- **Mushrooms:** Chanterelles, morels, portobello, shiitake, wild edible, commercially available exotics (avoid button-type mushrooms)
- **Nuts and seeds:** Almonds, Brazil nuts, cashews, hazelnuts (aka filberts), peanuts, pine nuts, sesame seeds, sunflower seeds, walnuts
- **Oils:** Coconut, cold-pressed blends, extra-virgin olive, flaxseed
- **Sea vegetables:** Alaria, arame, bladderwrack, dulse, hijiki, kelp, kombu, laver, nori, wakame
- **Soy products:** Miso soup, tempeh, tofu (small quantities)
- **Sushi and sashimi:** Best varieties are albacore, fatty tuna, mackerel, salmon, wild yellowtail, (avoid freshwater eel, other freshwater sushi; use MSG-containing soy sauce sparingly)
- **Sweets and sweeteners:** Blackstrap molasses, carob powder, honey, organic dark chocolate, stevia
- **Teas:** Black, green, herbal, maté, rooibos tea (South African red bush tea)
- **Whole grains:** Amaranth, brown rice, millet, quinoa, teff
- **Wild edibles:** Locally foraged wild vegetables, including burdock root, chickweed, dandelion greens, edible flowers (such as nasturtium), fresh nettles, lamb's-quarter, purslane (ask your local herbalist)

This list is far from exhaustive. For example, relatively nutrient-dense sweets, such as candied ginger and natural licorice, are not listed.

More notable, however, is what is *not* on this list: Baked goods, candy, chips, crackers, commercial dairy products (such as cream cheese, ice cream, milk, and sour cream), margarine, muffins, pasta, and soda. There is also no mention of the many convenience foods that have become standard fare, particularly breakfast foods. Most households rely on toaster/microwave breakfast pastries, pancakes, waffles, and other empty-calorie carbohydrates. These foods simply do not fit in with nutrient-dense guidelines, as they typically contain hydrogenated oils, refined flour, and a host of additives, flavorings, preservatives, and other chemicals.

Remember, the important thing is to appreciate and identify what I call the exceptional foods—those foods of high quality with known nutritional benefits. With such foods at hand, you cannot go wrong.

CHAPTER 4

Best of the Best: The Highest-Quality Nutrient-Dense Super Foods

In the previous section, I listed a number of foods that qualify as nutrient dense. All of them are high-quality foods known to make strong contributions to your diet. Each has one or more strengths, contributing specific antioxidants, essential fats, minerals, phytonutrients, protein, vitamins, or other nutritionally important factors. Such a list shows the breadth, diversity, and availability of such good foods, and it is also supremely practical because it tells you how to think about, and shop for, specific foods. This is particularly important during the crucial time when you may be transitioning away from the Standard American Diet (SAD) toward a denser, more nutritionally potent one.

But what if you want to be more specific? The list in Chapter 3 is fairly comprehensive, and for some, perhaps a bit overwhelming. Clearly stating the very best, most nutrient-dense foods, might be a more practical approach, so the following list identifies those few super foods at the top of the heap. Although many excellent foods are not listed because I want to keep this short and simple, the ones I have included will give you a clearer idea of how I prioritize the very best of the best. (*See also* Table 4 in Appendix G for the nutrient content of exceptional foods.)

THE BEST OF THE BEST

- Beet greens, chard, collards, kale
- Berries
- Blackstrap molasses
- Broccoli, cabbage
- Buffalo liver
- Eggs
- Flaxseed oil, cod-liver oil
- Garlic
- Halibut, wild salmon
- Nutritional yeast
- Red meat, organic (beef, buffalo, elk, lamb, venison)
- Sea vegetables
- Sunflower seeds
- Wheatgrass juice (fresh)

HONORABLE MENTION

- Amaranth, millet, quinoa, teff
- Beans, lentils, split peas
- Beets
- Cinnamon
- Chlorella/spirulina
- Coconut butter
- Dairy products, raw (cow and goat)
- Ginger root
- Green and herbal teas (various)
- Herbs and spices (various)
- Kiwi fruit
- Spinach
- Tomatoes
- Turmeric

CHAPTER 5

Nutrient Density in Your Life

For many, relating to food is a task that quite literally consumes their lives. Some base their dietary choices on the latest fads or proclamations from experts, and when new studies come out, they test the findings on themselves. Religious or ethical beliefs often influence food choices too. At other times, motivation for dietary change comes from an illness, a diagnosis, or a feared disease. Diet is often a key component of a person's self-identity, and what you eat literally defines who you are. It is no wonder, then, that along with dietary confusion comes a lack of direction, and even confidence, about how to conduct your life.

I strongly believe you can eat in a way that will nourish all the layers of your life. From the standpoint of nutrient density, eating healthy is neither a fad nor a style of food consumption based on the latest research, but is rather what I call a common sense way of eating. Nutrient density is about nourishing yourself with high-quality foods that are usually left close to the way they come from nature. These are often simple, nutritionally supportive, minimally processed foods that retain ample quantities of the essential amino and fatty acids, fiber, minerals, pigments, phytonutrients, vitamins, and other essential building blocks of health.

An important aspect of nutrient density's widespread appeal is its simplicity and ease of applicability. You can easily identify nutrient-dense foods by recognizing their wholesome, nourishing qualities. *The Nutrient Dense Eating Plan* is accessible because it quickly becomes intuitively obvious. Once you grasp the basic principles of nutrient density, putting them into practice becomes incredibly easy. Healthy eating, using nutrient-dense criteria, is effortless and natural, like a rock falling down a cliff. On the other hand, unhealthy eating is like fighting gravity. It is unnatural and often dangerous.

Healthy eating boils down to making conscious choices based on what you know, or intuit, will be good for you. However, for most, eating healthily means first overcoming some obstacles. Explore with me a few of the ways in which your selection of truly healthy foods could be compromised.

OBSTACLES TO HEALTHY EATING

According to the principles of nutrient density, there are two primary causes that lead to nutritionally poor food choices. The first is societal, or cultural, inertia. The second is your personal inertia.

Cultural Inertia—The First Obstacle

What I call *cultural inertia* is the unquestioning acceptance by society that low-quality or mediocre food is okay. The first, most obvious, hurdle to healthy eating is the abundance of inexpensive and widely available low-quality food. I call this a cultural factor because our cultural environment defines what is an acceptable, or normal, way of eating. Vending machines, fast-food restaurants, gas stations, and quick-stop markets are accepted parts of the cultural culinary landscape. Most of the food choices staring people in the face today are not the most nutrient-dense options. Convenience foods are typically prepackaged, precooked, and ready-to-eat. While convenient, from a nutritional standpoint these fast foods are not usually high caliber. They are often laced with preservatives, artificial flavors, and taste-enhancers, such as hydrogenated oils, MSG, and synthetic dyes, and frequently contain antibiotics, hormones, and pesticides. A majority of fast food is also overcooked, which depletes it of nutrients. Many fast foods rely on refined sugars and flour, notorious sources of empty calories, and they are often heated in microwave ovens, a process suspected of further compromising nutritional value. All too often, a meal becomes an on-the-run snack of sugar-laced pastries or power bars that are little more than carbohydrates or empty calories. And adding synthetic vitamins does little to recoup the real nutrition that has been lost. This is not a pretty picture, but it accurately describes much of the gas-and-go mentality of today's eat-on-the-run lifestyle, one that certainly makes it more challenging to eat healthily.

Additionally, with the onslaught of television, radio, magazine, and billboard advertising telling us what to eat and where to buy it, people are immersed in a sea of messages, all attempting to influence which brands to buy and which restaurants we should patronize. Even more pervasive (and subtle) are the expectations and demands of friends, families, and business associates. Almost everyone assumes you will eat the same food and at the same restaurants that they do. Doesn't everyone eat this way? This background noise is the cultural environment in which daily choices necessary for proper nourishment must be made.

It is important to know it is possible to eat healthily with a full schedule and a busy life in today's world. You just need a clear perspective on your priorities in order to think and act proactively. You have to care enough about your health and the quality of your life in order to make changes. You also need to develop the courage and confidence to pursue this new, and better, vision of healthy food, and then make the connection in your mind between what you eat and how you feel. Once started, you will quickly discover how easy and fun the process can be. Identifying and recognizing cultural inertia is the first step toward developing a new, personalized way of eating.

Confronting Personal Inertia—You Are What You Eat

The overwhelming availability of poor-quality convenience foods (the cultural environment) is the first factor contributing to a low level of nutrient density in people's lives. The second factor is the one that permits these foods into your life. *What* you choose to eat is related to how you view yourself, and is more insidious because it is more subtle. This second factor is related to your expectations of what you think you deserve. I call it personal inertia because these expectations allow you to perpetuate unhealthy patterns and habits of eating. What you feel you deserve ties in with your self-esteem, and what you believe about yourself.

One of the oldest maxims is that you are what you eat. Unfortunately, the timeless wisdom behind this cliché often gets ignored, yet its essential truth is really a cornerstone of nutrient density. It should be obvious that you really are what you eat because it is literally true. Every atom in every cell, and every molecule—antioxidant, carbohydrate, hormone, lipid, neurotransmitter, protein, or vitamin—originates in the raw materials you ingest. Since you are what you eat, it follows that what you put into your body will determine the overall quality of your body in return. Simply said, if you eat junk food, you will end up with a junky body (garbage in, garbage out). If you want a quality body, quality cells, and quality health, then it stands to reason that you should eat quality food. As I said earlier, nutrient density is largely common sense. Unfortunately, common sense is not always that common.

The human body is remarkable, truly a wonder. How much abuse it can take is amazing. Everyone knows people who can go for decades on the strangest foods. Kids and teens seem to eat endless quantities of very questionable foods with little apparent consequence. Like a perpetual motion machine, they seem to keep on going. For most people, though, the consequences of chronic poor nutrition will show up sooner or later. The effects of a suboptimal diet often go unnoticed until the depleted state manifests itself as depression, disease, illness, lack of energy, obesity, or other symptoms. People, as well as their doctors, often fail to make the connection between chronically poor eating habits and poor health. If you fail to take the saying that you are what you eat seriously, sooner or later you *will* pay the price.

You Are What You Eat . . . and You Eat What You (Think You) Are

If you are what you eat, then you also eat what you think you deserve. If your expectation is that of ordinary (mediocre) health, then you are certainly not going to consistently reach for food that can build super health. If, on the other hand, you *expect* to be radiantly healthy and productive, it stands to reason you will seek out foods to help you attain that goal.

Unfortunately, many people do not feel they deserve great health. Again, the media plays on this by saying it is normal to have acid reflux, flu bugs, frequent colds, headaches, high blood pressure, iron poor blood, low energy, and premenstrual syndrome. But do not worry, there is always a drug, nighttime cold remedy, or pill waiting to address these inevitabilities. You can cover up your symptoms, bounce back, and enjoy life again. Of course, in this simplistic business and advertising view, the deeper questions of how to build *real* health, or how to *prevent* colds and other symptoms, are never raised. Cultural inertia and the *illness industry* prefer that mediocre health be considered both normal and acceptable.

So, the questions become, Do I really *want* to be healthy? Do I really believe I *can* be healthy? And, deep down, do I feel I really *deserve* to be healthy? If you are completely honest, you may not be fully prepared to answer *Yes* to these questions. Yet, in order to fully enter the path of nutrient-dense eating, you have to ready yourself by believing that you *do* deserve the best, most nutritious food possible, not the quickest, easiest, or cheapest. You also have to accept that health is something you achieve proactively, and that it is your individual responsibility to maintain and safeguard it appropriately.

CHAPTER 6

Reclaiming Ancestral Wisdom: The Perennial Philosophy of Food

Eating healthily involves a level of personal commitment and responsibility. Nourishing yourself effectively, however, need not be a burden or chore. Many people find a deep sense of satisfaction in having a healthy relationship with wholesome food—it is a great pleasure, a deeply empowering dance, and a refreshing return to the very basics of life. At its best, food can become a true source of connectedness. At its worst, it can increase the fragmentation and alienation from the broader world that marks too much of life today.

When you eat, you incorporate the energy and molecules of the world. Taking food into your body is an intimacy, and this relationship represents the most sacred and universal of partnerships. Every time you eat, you make a statement about yourself, your values and assumptions, even your belief in the sacredness of life.

In today's world of supersized sodas, microwaved instant snacks, happy meals, and vending-machine offerings, people have forgotten the essential truth of food—that when you eat, you consume the body of the universe. Food is a gift from the world for the express purpose of sustaining and perpetuating life.

Tendencies to trivialize food, take it for granted, or view it as a nuisance, are disturbing trends that reflect an increasing alienation from nature and from the common sense of our ancestors. This lack of appreciation is a dangerous precedent, and may be a principal reason behind many of the personal, cultural, and environmental imbalances seen today. But no one has to subscribe to such mediocre standards. We have a saner model of how to relate to food, which I call *the perennial philosophy of food.*

This approach borrows its name from Aldous Huxley's book *The Perennial Philosophy,* which is based on the common thread that runs through the world's great religious, spiritual, and philosophical traditions. *The Perennial Philosophy* built bridges by emphasizing common perspectives, and it revealed the underlying unity behind seemingly different cultures and beliefs. In a similar way, this book also shows how various traditions of eating have always had several basic themes in common. Following these guidelines will lead to saner and denser eating, and provide a road map of commonsense options in an otherwise increasingly risky nutritional landscape.

THE PERENNIAL PHILOSOPHY OF FOOD—PRINCIPLES OF NUTRIENT DENSITY

Following in Huxley's footsteps, take a look at these unifying principles of healthy eating by comparing the common ground within differing healthy diets. Applying these principles, using common sense and modern scientific understanding, will help you see how to better nourish yourself. The perennial philosophy of food offers guidelines for a sensible, historical, science-based approach to eating that could significantly improve the health and nutrition of millions.

People have eaten quite well for countless millennia, and today does not need to be different. Prior to the past few decades, humans never consumed many of the foods and additives eaten now. What is there to learn from our ancestors and from other cultures? What new insights can science offer? How can you take the best from both worlds to arrive at a contemporary style of eating that will offer the greatest nutrition and health benefits in the world today? *The Nutrient-Dense Eating Plan* offers a clear-eyed vision of just how to accomplish these goals.

Ancestral Principles of Diet

First, let me clearly state what traditional ancestral diets were *not.* Our ancestors did not eat foods with antibiotics, artificial dyes, artificially created flavors, hormones, preservatives, synthetic sweeteners, texture enhancers, or a lot of refined carbohydrates (sugars and white flour). And they *never* consumed homogenized milk and dairy products, irradiated foods, partially hydrogenated oils and shortenings, or genetically modified foods created by splicing together genes from widely differing species. But today's culinary landscape is rife with these modifications, and the foods that result are so vastly different from those of our ancestors that we might as well be inhabiting another world.

What this different world looks like to the interior of your body, and to the cells and tissues that must live, grow, divide, and function in this strange new molecular environment, is the story of nutrient density. By nourishing yourself in a way that links you with ancestral patterns, you can return to a saner and more respectful approach to eating.

How Our Ancestors Ate

Our early ancestors predominantly ate locally available foods. Seasonable variations made food supplies uncertain, but by foraging from a wide variety of sources, by utilizing the biodiversity available, and by using appropriate technologies for preserving foods, such as drying, fermenting, pickling, salting, and smoking, a reasonably healthy food supply was ensured. Early people presumably bartered or traded for more exotic items in order to round out their diets. Lean times and hardships certainly existed, but on the whole, resourcefulness and an intimate working knowledge of nature and the seasons allowed the human population to adapt, sustain itself, and even thrive in virtually every climate and ecosystem on the planet.

The point here is not to emulate the diets of the distant past, but instead to acknowledge that indigenous diets were, and usually still are, comprised of fresh, minimally processed, and locally grown foods. While our earliest ancestors probably traveled in bands, sampling a wide variety of animal and vegetable foods, later groups began the process of farming and raising livestock. The emphasis, though, was always on whole foods—edible vegetation, eggs, fish, fruit, herbs, honey, insects, and meat. The evolving human diet was, by and large, omnivorous, and opportunistic—and also incredibly diverse.

The origins of nutrient density can be traced to this time, and today's nutrient-dense foods are much the same as those eaten by your ancient ancestors. It is still quite easy to find an abundance of foods that are minimally processed and present in their whole state (still retaining a large percentage of their original nutrient value). And it is still possible to hunt and gather plenty of wonderful, nutrient-dense foods in health food, ethnic, and conventional grocery stores, farmer's markets, backyard gardens, fields, and woods. The legacy of nutrient-dense foods is alive and thriving, and can nobly reconnect us with many of the nourishing traditions of centuries long past.

In recent years, several books have been written that embrace large segments of the nutrient-dense philosophy while embodying much of the perennial philosophy of food. *The Paleolithic Prescription* by S. Boyd Eaton, Marjorie Shostak, and Melvin Konner, *Nourishing Traditions* by Sally Fallon and Mary Enig, and *Food, Your Miracle Medicine* by Jean Carper are notable for the consistency of their nutrient-dense approaches to eating. There are also numerous books on macrobiotic cuisine, a healthy style and philosophy of food from Japan, that advocates a nutrient-dense approach to food. The *120-Year Diet* by gerontologist Roy Walford also advocates a very nutrient-dense style of eating. Finally, works that explore indigenous and traditional ways of eating, such as Gary Paul Nabhan's *Coming Home to Eat* and *Enduring Seeds,* argue eloquently for the benefits of eating in a manner close to nature, celebrating our indigenous heritages. Other than Fallon's and Walford's books, these books seldom use the actual phrase *nutrient density,* but its basic principles pervade these (and other) authors' ways of thinking.

The concept of nutrient density is not limited to any one style of eating, and this book does not pretend to invent some new fad or diet, but is rather a synthesis of ancient principles that uphold the very best of what the natural world has to offer. Through the years, many authors have addressed nutrient-dense principles. Recognizing the common threads among these culinary thinkers is the perennial philosophy of food in action.

When it comes to eating in a healthy manner, people are often limited by their imaginations. Relying on the nutritionally poor fare offered by global food, pharmaceutical, or chemical companies (increasingly one and the same) is really an abdication of personal responsibility for safe nourishment. Nutrient-dense foods represent a return to the basics of using common sense and self-respect. Nutrient-dense foods are readily recognized by the body, and make sense because they are rooted in the indigenous wisdom of the body. Providing essential nutrients while minimizing man-made toxins makes a powerful statement and affirms the importance of taking good care of your mind and body, and even your own worthiness.

Although *The Nutrient-Dense Eating Plan* recommends eliminating junk food from the diet, it is far from a limited eating plan. Instead, it celebrates the huge diversity of foods provided by nature—humans have always been able to partake in edible and nourishing foods from an astonishing variety of sources. This rich heritage of dietary choices is the perennial philosophy of food. Prior to the invention of happy meals, soft drinks, artificial colors, an endless array of candies and snacks, and countless poorly tested chemicals, people ate from the bounty of nature, celebrated the seasons, learned how to work with the land, and respected and revered the awesome beauty, power, and beneficence of nature.

Nature provided a huge array of nutrient-dense foods for early humanity: Berries and all manner of fruits, edible flowers, eggs, fowl, grains, grasses, herbs, nuts and seeds, meats, plants and salt from the sea, roots and tubers, spices, wild honey, and wild mushrooms and vegetables. As time passed, people began to learn simple technologies, including how to grind grains and seeds into nutritious flours, ways to preserve certain foods, ways of fermenting grains into alcoholic beverages, and the domestication of certain animals and wild plants. Later came further refinements, such as the extraction of oil from seeds and nuts.

All these methods can be considered components of the nutrient-dense perennial philosophy of food, a diet that provides a rich spectrum of amino acids, essential fats, fiber, essential minerals and vitamins, phytonutrients, pigments, and other vital constituents.

Today, few would recommend returning to many of the ways of our distant ancestors who had more than their fair share of disease and other health problems. Hygiene and other basic commonsense advances have led to a dramatic increase in the average life span, a significant reduction in infant and childhood mortality, and the virtual elimination of several diseases that seem to have ravaged people of long ago.

Nonetheless, it is fair to ask if people today are experiencing the vibrant health, mental well-being, and freedom from disease that they should, given these advances. While many of the infectious diseases of the past, such as polio, smallpox, syphilis, and tuberculosis, are no longer the scourges they once were, there are other diseases now—AIDS, attention deficit disorder, cancer, diabetes, chronic depression, heart disease, obesity, and premenstrual syndrome, to name a few—that our ancestors did not have to deal with to any significant degree. These diseases are believed to arise largely as a result of lifestyle, environmental, and nutritional factors. Some might counter that people today are far better nourished than their paleoancestors were, and that cases of beri-beri, goiter, pellagra, rickets, and scurvy (all diseases of vitamin and mineral deficiencies), are rare today. They might point to the fortification of breads, cereals, milk, and salt as the reason for elimination of these deficiencies. But does the absence of a vitamin deficiency mean people are well nourished? What about the various all-too-prevalent modern ailments listed above? Isn't it possible that current nutritional practices could be partially to blame for some of these ailments?

Much can be learned, both good and bad, from traditional (ancestral) diets, and much can be gained from today's scientific wisdom as well. The challenges and opportunities of *The Nutrient-Dense Eating Plan* link the best of the past and present because all the ancestral, reliably nutrient-dense foods discussed in this book are rich in substances that contemporary nutrition considers important to health, well-being, and successful aging. These include antioxidants, essential fatty acids, major minerals, trace elements, and vitamins, among others. This eating plan requires you to take a good hard look at the state of your health. You may not have beriberi, rickets, or scurvy, but do you really have the vibrant health you deserve? Perhaps you experience anxiety, arthritis, excess weight, headaches, high blood pressure, lack of energy, stomach or digestive problems, or any of a number of other conditions? If your health is not as good as you think it could be, then you probably need to acknowledge that your diet may be at fault. Your diet can, after all, hold the key to your health—both good and bad.

CHAPTER 7

Fundamental Concepts of Nutrition

The science of nutrition is surprisingly young. Despite ancient acknowledgment of the role of nutrition in health, such as Hippocrates' famous, "Let food be thy medicine; let medicine be thy food," investigations into the importance of individual nutrients didn't really begin until the British surgeon James Lind's 1753 book, *Treatise of the Scurvy*, showed the value of fresh citrus fruit against this disease. Unfortunately, Lind faced many of the same prejudices then that conventional doctors still hold against nutrition, and his work linking diet and health languished for many years. In fact, vitamins were not discovered until 1911, when the Polish chemist, Casimir Funk, isolated the first, vitamin B_1 (thiamine).

Since those early years, although much has been learned about individual nutrients and their essential role in human health, nutrition is still largely misunderstood by the general population and undervalued by the mainstream medical community. Today, nutritional misconceptions remain the rule, not the exception. Outmoded concepts, such as the food-industry-influenced four food groups, are still promulgated. Industry and agribusiness helped influence the food pyramid, and these vested interests are still largely responsible for governmental food policies. The advertising blitz is still, sadly, the principal way most people get their nutritional information.

Fortunately, you don't need to have a Ph.D. in nutrition in order to understand the basic principles of nutrient density. Selecting the foods that are the richest in nutrients and the most nourishing is actually an intuitive process, and this very simplicity is what lends it universal appeal. Since this way of eating is grounded in your ancestral eating patterns, it makes sense on an historical, even anthropological, level. Discovering that it is okay to eat nourishing foods like eggs, fish, fresh produce, meat, nuts and seeds, and whole grains, comes as a relief to most people. When you realize you can respect the needs of your body and enjoy doing so, the responsibility for nourishing it properly can become a gratifying task rather than a dreaded chore filled with guilt and confusion.

At the core of the eating plan is an appreciation for the wonder that human beings are. When the full complexity of the body is realized, it may be easier to treat it with the respect it deserves, and not fill it up with empty calories, fast foods, and chemical additives. More important, you can begin to regain control of your life, by thinking for yourself, and nourishing yourself based on what you *really* need, as opposed to what advertisers say you need. This could be the most crucial contribution of this eating plan—turning healthy eating into a journey of self-discovery that reestablishes your connection with personal responsibility.

Nutrient density looks at food and nutrients—the basic elements of nutrition—and how they interact with the human body to promote health. Ideally, food should provide pleasure and enjoyment, support the body's manifold functions, and contribute little in the way of toxicities and other burdens. Nonetheless, this is not an ideal world and adjustments must always be made. When all is said and done, nutrition is about real food for real people, and it is at this point that the concept of biochemical individuality comes into play.

BIOCHEMICAL INDIVIDUALITY

The concept of biochemical individuality is central to understanding the best way to nourish yourself. Biochemical individuality does this by acknowledging the obvious and fundamental fact that everyone is different, that each person possesses slight variations in how they function, and that every person has differing biological strengths and weaknesses. These unique and often subtle differences account for the different nutritional needs between people.

This may seem obvious today. However, this insight was far ahead of its time when, in 1956, the renowned chemist, Roger Williams, first proposed that "Nutrition applied with due concern for individual genetic variation, which may be large, offers the solution to many baffling health problems." Williams, a highly respected chemist and nutritionist, was also the discoverer of vitamin B_5 (pantothenic acid) and folic acid.

Biochemical individuality helps explain why certain people get sick when exposed to a virus, while others do not, why some people can drink or smoke and live to a ripe old age, while others succumb to cancer or heart disease, and why two people can eat identical diets and still have varying cholesterol or insulin levels. It also explains why people may have widely varying needs for certain vitamins and minerals.

Biochemical individuality shows there is no one perfect diet for everyone, that what's best for a vegetarian may not be right for a meat eater. Even within a single family, individual reactions to foods, such as dairy or wheat, can also vary widely.

The Chemistry of Biochemical Individuality

Our bodies contain thousands of different enzymes, molecular substances that catalyze and activate *all* the biochemical processes occurring at the cellular level. Yet, because of biochemical individuality (due to genetic variation), everyone has unique enzyme patterns and amounts. As Williams's revolutionary discovery showed, a person can have more or fewer enzymes than his or her neighbors, parents, or siblings.

Nutrients are vital to the proper functioning of enzymes in the cells. Enzymes are manufactured out of the amino acids supplied by dietary proteins. Fats and carbohydrates supply the energy sources for enzymatic reactions to occur, and minerals and vitamins act as their essential cofactors, activating these reactions. But, the picture is even more complicated than that. An individual's reactions to specific compounds in food may further induce or suppress enzymatic activity, with subsequent consequences to health.

This is the nitty-gritty of nutrition. After taste, ingestion, and absorption occur, the complex interaction of nutrients and enzymes is the point at which nutrition can make or break you. Biochemical individuality is the factor that shows why you are what you eat. It also shows why a diet that might appear adequate for one person can be marginal or deficient for another.

Biochemical individuality demolishes the argument for the recommended dietary allowances (RDAs), which attempt to give guidelines for the minimum amounts of vitamins and minerals needed to ward off deficiencies. Unfortunately, they are a very imperfect attempt, as they average the needs of many people but fail to take into account the biochemical uniqueness of those individuals who fall outside of the norm. Consequently, many people fall through the loopholes created by this compromise. This is another example that indicates why nutrition really does need to be about real food for real people. As Dr. Roger Williams astutely said, "Statistical nutrients will never nourish real people."

The key difference between nutrient-dense standards and the RDAs is that the latter are concerned with supplying the *minimal* amounts of nutrients necessary to ward off deficiency states (beriberi, rickets, scurvy, and so on), whereas nutrient-dense principles are more concerned with the larger issues of getting *optimal* amounts of the elements necessary for preventing disease states, realizing peak performance, and enjoying life to the fullest. While most mainstream physicians, food companies, and policymakers seem to be content with ordinary poor health, nutrient-dense principles envision radiance, resistance, and vibrancy, the elements of *true* health.

Nutrition is far from an exact science. It involves a complex mixture of variables, from the biochemical uniqueness of each person to the many subtle nuances that can affect the nutritional quality of food. Further, these nutrients may interact with elements commonly found in the environment, such as tobacco smoke or plastic residues, in ways not fully understood. To be honest, at the present time, nutritional understanding is still in the very early stages. Yet instead of saying it's hopeless—*the experts all disagree, so I might as well eat anything I want*—perennial wisdom counsels that you should err on the side of caution. Because of the complex interplay of factors, it is all the more important to choose wisely what and how you eat.

Approximately fifty nutrients are now considered essential for life. *The Nutrient-Dense Eating Plan* helps you obtain adequate amounts of each by emphasizing diversity and quality of foods. With careful attention to the quality of food, much can be done to optimize health, to build resistance to diseases, to prolong life and to enjoy it to the fullest.

CHAPTER 8

Land, Agriculture, and Nutrient Density: The Green Ceiling

How we treat the land, we treat ourselves.

—CHIEF SEATTLE

It has been said that the story of civilization is the story of land and soil, and that the rise and decline of great civilizations can be traced directly to the productivity and treatment of their land.

Given that Americans today have access to an excess of food, you would think that our agricultural resources and crop-management practices would be second to none. Indeed, America has been called *the breadbasket of the world.* Birthplace of the green revolution of the 1960s, an enduring vision of the American dream has been that of unlimited bounty. Yet today, agriculture finds itself facing a green ceiling as declines in crop productivity, degradation of groundwater supplies, and irreplaceable loss of precious topsoil continue at an alarming and unprecedented rate.

In the decades since World War II, agriculture in America has grown increasingly dependent on chemicals for its productivity. Chemical-based agriculture is so pervasive now that it is synonymous with how food is grown—outside of the organic movement, it is an unquestioned assumption. Yet chemicals are a double-edged sword. While synthetic fertilizers, herbicides, and pesticides can dramatically increase yields *in the short run,* they eventually lead to an inevitable reduction in soil quality and health, the pollution of surface and groundwater, a lessening of biodiversity, and a reduction in the uptake of key trace minerals. In addition, they are now being implicated in increased rates of certain cancers in farmers, their households, and their communities.

Further, the use of agricultural chemicals leads to dependency by the farmer. Once used, these chemicals create soil imbalances that necessitate the further use of even greater quantities in an escalating spiral that resembles true chemical dependency—addiction. Our agricultural system is literally addicted to these drugs. Sociologists endlessly warn of the perils of drug use, but how many grasp that agriculture also has a pervasive deep-rooted dependency on chemicals?

You are what you eat is a saying that has its roots, literally, in the soil. How people treat the land, and what the land is able to return via the plants (and the animals that forage on them) is the story of agriculture. And the story of agriculture—the ability of land to grow and sustain nourishing food—is also the story of life and of the nutrient-dense foods that sustain it. Thus, *The Nutrient-Dense Eating Plan* has its foundation in a balanced ecosystem, with good healthy soil full of minerals and organic matter, on which the farmers and stewards of the land all work together to sustain healthy, nourishing plants and people.

THE ORGANIC ALTERNATIVE

The term *organic* has come to mean the production of food without the use of chemical additives or preservatives. The idea of organic food production is grounded in age-old principles of respect for land, plants, and people. At its heart, organic agriculture involves building and nurturing healthy soil through recycling and restoring optimal levels of organic matter to it, supporting a healthy microclimate rich in normally present bacteria and other soil microorganisms, and avoiding harsh or toxic chemicals.

Although now considered an alternative to conventional agriculture, for the entire span of time that humans have cultivated and grown plants for food (tens of thousands of years), it has been the *only* way people have grown food. Far from being some new-age or health-nut concept, organic, chemical-free agriculture is as ancient as civilization itself. The widespread and indiscriminate use of synthetic chemicals in agriculture, on the other hand, has only been around for the past century.

Whether it is the return of nutrients to the land via composting of animal and human wastes; allowing fields to remain fallow for periods of time; winter cropping by growing nutrient-rich plants; applying seaweeds and other natural fertilizers to the land; or working with natural cycles, such as the flood plains of the Nile; land has been traditionally seen as the source of life, to be treated with respect and even reverence. One symptom of contemporary life is how nature is increasingly seen as being in the way, needing to be overturned, subjugated, or corrected. In fact, it's the unprecedented and shortsighted arrogance of dumping powerful and toxic chemicals onto our crops and soils that is misguided.

This chemical-based agricultural system is a relatively new experiment being conducted on vast numbers of human beings without any real consent, with consumers the unwitting guinea pigs. With artificial dyes and preservatives in foods, hormones in dairy, eggs, and meat, hydrogenated oils, pesticides, synthetic sweeteners, processing technologies, such as homogenization, and new cooking methodologies, such as microwaving, and other so-called breakthroughs, it is vital to acknowledge that today's *approach to food, eating, and self-nourishment is off-target.*

You can, however, look at your current relationship with food and the land it grows on in a fresh way.

Nutrient density is all about taking responsibility for how you eat. Becoming a conscious eater is a big deal, and in order to become empowered in this central aspect of your life, it is helpful to increase your awareness of the routes that your food takes from its time growing on the land until its arrival at your table. You might not always like what you find, and you might not always agree with other people's conclusions, but discovering the truth is, in itself, powerful, dense medicine.

There are several important reasons why organic food is preferable to conventional, processed food. The principal one, of course, is to reduce the load of toxic chemicals in your body and in the environment. Many of the synthetic herbicides, hormones, and pesticides used in agriculture are known or suspected carcinogens. Over time these toxic materials build up in tissues, increasing the *body burden*, especially in fat cells and such vital organs as the liver. Some chemicals, including certain pesticides, can directly affect the nervous system. Others affect cell division and growth by interfering with DNA or protein synthesis. Many of these chemicals are fat soluble and are stored for long periods of time in fatty tissues, such as the brain and breast. And, it is well known that some chemical residues are passed from mother to child, in utero, and during breast-feeding.

This negative picture aside, there is a much more positive reason for choosing organic foods—they are simply more nutritious. Organic advocates have claimed this for years, despite scientists with ties to the chemical and fertilizer industries who say there is no evidence that organic produce is nutritionally superior. That all changed recently, however, when several key studies demonstrated convincing evidence that organic produce is, in fact, higher in nutrients.

NEW STUDIES

Several recent studies of a broad range of nutrients have demonstrated that there are higher levels of nutrients in organically raised produce. Soil scientists have known for decades that healthy, living soil is crucial for the optimal absorption of nutrients, especially minerals, by actively growing rootlets. As might be expected, minerals were markedly higher in the organic produce, as were several vitamins, most notably vitamin C (ascorbic acid). But a new and really interesting find is that *secondary plant metabolites*, nonessential nutritive substances, were also consistently and dramatically higher in organic food. Secondary plant metabolites include such substances as phenolics and other bioflavonoid compounds with biologically active functions that can enhance or protect health. Many of these substances are active antioxidants, and include anthocyanins (colorful pigments found in many fruits) and lycopene (a red pigment found in tomatoes and watermelons).

One such study, conducted by researchers at the University of California, Davis (UCD) and published in the prestigious *Journal of Agricultural Food Chemistry*, compared the levels of certain phenolic compounds, as well as vitamin levels, in organic and conventionally grown corn, marionberries, and strawberries. The organic strawberries had more than 20 percent higher ascorbic-acid levels than conventional strawberries, while the sustainably grown corn had ascorbic-acid levels approximately 67 percent higher than conventional corn. The level of total phenolic compounds in the organic marionberries was also more than 50 percent higher than the levels in conventional marionberries. The phenolics in organically raised strawberries were 19 percent higher and more than 50 percent higher in the chemical-free corn.

Similar results were found in a 2002 Italian study on fruits. There were measurably higher levels of healthy polyphenols in organic pears and peaches, and an approximately 8 percent superiority in ascorbic-acid levels over conventional, nonorganic pears and peaches. Another European study, also published in 2002, found higher levels of the naturally occurring, aspirinlike compound, salicylic acid, in organic vegetable soup compared with soup made from nonorganic vegetables.

Finally, a recent study by researchers at Rutgers University looked at the mineral content of organic versus conventional cabbage, lettuce, snap beans, spinach, and tomatoes, and found that the organic vegetables exhibited enormous increases in boron, calcium, cobalt, copper, iron, magnesium, manganese, phosphorus, and potassium. These findings were said to have shocked some of the researchers, who admitted they had begun the study as skeptics of the organic-is-better school of thought. Studies such as these are making believers out of huge numbers of people, who are now buying more organic produce than ever.

PRIORITIZING ORGANIC FOODS

Learning about current agricultural methods is like opening the proverbial can of worms; the more you learn, the less likely it is you will want to purchase nonorganics. Given herbicide and pesticide residues, antibiotic and hormone contaminants, and lowered nutritional value overall, conventionally grown produce becomes less and less appealing. And on top of the nutritional questions for individuals, there remains the fact that chemical-based agriculture is profoundly unhealthy for the entire environment. It depletes topsoil, which contributes to erosion; it dumps massive amounts of toxic chemicals into the land and waterways; it introduces genetically modified crops and their pollen into the environment; and it indiscriminately kills beneficial insects along with pests.

So what choices can you make, especially if you are on a limited budget, or faced with dining out or eating at a friend's house? These are hard questions, and obviously the answers may change with the circumstances. As your knowledge and commitment to eating healthier grows and deepens, so too will your own personal answers to these questions. *The Nutrient-Dense Eating Plan* certainly doesn't expect (or necessarily want) you to be perfect—that can be too stressful. Instead, begin with the understanding that you do, after all, live in an imperfect world, make the best choices possible, and learn to compromise when necessary.

I do not eat 100 percent organically. Social conventions and the willingness not to offend are important to me, as are the realities of living in America today. Whenever possible, however, I will choose the organic option. When I buy organic, I vote with my dollars. And when I can support an organic farmer, store, or restaurant, I buy organic. More Americans than ever are similarly supporting organic agriculture and farming, and in so doing, are changing the way food is produced. This is important for the welfare of future generations, too, because organic agriculture is much gentler on the environment. To me, these are all important considerations.

For those transitioning to a healthier diet, who are not yet entirely convinced of the importance and superiority of an organic-based diet, or who have important financial considerations, several studies have targeted the most important foods to buy organically. Such lists are a good place to start prioritizing the foods you wish to purchase as organics.

Do I know with absolute certainty which foods are most heavily contaminated with pesticides and other chemicals and therefore, presumably, the most dangerous? No, I do not. Chemicals are often individually chosen by farmers, although the corporations running these farms increasingly call the shots. Factors such as post-harvest handling also affect the final residue levels. Nevertheless, here is an alphabetical list of some foods thought to have the heaviest chemical exposure: Apples, grapes, green beans, mushrooms (button), peaches, peanuts, pears, potatoes, raisins, raspberries, spinach, strawberries, and winter squash. (One USDA study showed that the *least* contaminated crops were bananas and broccoli.) In addition to produce, I am especially leery of commercial chicken and eggs, all pork products, and all commercial dairy products.

THE ORGANIC SHOPPER

First, I want to say that because I strongly dislike the word *consumer,* I have chosen to use the word *shopper* instead. I find the connotation of consumer distasteful and demeaning, even if unintentionally so. To label people consumers puts them in a box and makes them little more than money generators, objects to be marketed to and exploited. It also implies a one-dimensionality, the notion that a person's primary role is to be complicit in a world where economics takes precedence over other, more human, values.

I think it is important for those contemplating a move to a more organic-based style of food shopping to realize the power and momentum behind this movement. Organic food purchases have consistently risen at an average of 20 to 25 percent a year over the past decade, and are increasing at more than *ten times* the rate of conventional foods, easily making organic shopping the fastest growing segment of the food industry. Surveys now indicate that a majority of American shoppers have consciously chosen at least some organic products, and that at least one-third of all households occasionally purchase organics on a regular basis. And the numbers keep mushrooming as awareness grows. Every year, millions of Americans are learning about the relationships between food, personal health, and the health of the environment.

The Organic Consumers Association lists the following ten reasons why people are choosing healthier organic foods.

1. People worry about untested and unlabeled genetically engineered food ingredients. To date, the government and industry refuse to label foods containing genetically modified organisms (GMO) although polls indicate 90 percent of Americans want labeling.
2. People worry about pesticide and drug (hormones, etc.) residues in their food.
3. People are concerned about irradiated foods. Again there are labeling and disclosure concerns.
4. People are concerned about *E. coli,* salmonella, and other diseases associated with food poisoning from conventional agricultural practices.
5. People are concerned about the use of toxic sludge as commercial fertilizer.
6. People are concerned about the inhumane treatment of animals by commercial interests.
7. People are worried about the use of rendered (recycled) animal parts in animal feed, particularly with mad cow disease (Creutzfeldt-Jakob disease) showing up in several cows in this country.
8. People are concerned about the effects of chemical fertilizer, pesticide, and feedlot run-off polluting drinking and groundwater.
9. People want food with a higher nutrient-density value than commercial produce provides.
10. People wish to see the preservation of family farms and smaller scale, appropriate farming.

SHOPPING FOR THE EARTH

The group, Mothers and Others for a Livable Planet, Inc., puts out a publication called *The Green Guide.* One issue published a list of guidelines for those who wish to "choose food in a way that is environmentally and socially responsible." I find this list a useful reminder for those who are beginning to sort out ways to increase the nutritional denseness—and overall integrity—of their diets. As you are seeing, shopping and eating in ways that are good for you personally are frequently also in harmony with the greater good of ecosystems and the entire planet. The suggestions in this synopsis of their list are mostly in accord with the principles of nutrient density.

1. Eat a variety of food. People rely on only twenty varieties of plants for 90 percent of their food, but diversity is important for your personal nutrient base, as well as for the broader environment (some believe that allergies can develop if the same foods are eaten too often).
2. Buy locally produced food. One of the big hidden costs in food production is the energy it takes to transport it. The average food item travels between 1,000 and 1,500 miles to get to your kitchen.
3. Buy produce in season.
4. Buy organically produced food.
5. Eat fresh, whole foods.
6. Eat fewer and smaller portions of animal products and seafood.
7. Choose minimally processed and packaged foods.
8. Prepare more meals at home.

The question of organics is no longer a mere philosophical question. Rather, it goes to the heart of nutrient density and eating healthily, and it goes beyond just cutting down on levels of pesticide residues. Eating organically has a twofold purpose: to *increase* your intake of dense nutrients, and to *decrease* the amount of toxins you ingest. Cutting down on toxins but keeping your nutrient intake at a subpar level is not good enough. Similarly, increasing your nutrient intake yet continuing your exposure to harmful chemicals is not good enough either.

If this seems a little extreme, that's because it is. But extreme problems call for extreme solutions. Instead of finger-pointing, nutrient-dense principles focus on solutions, and the happy solution is that nutrient-dense foods are available in abundance. Incorporating them into your life may involve rejecting some low-quality foods you like, but more important, it is about affirming the positive high-quality choices you can make.

Many people still resist the organic alternative. Some may feel threatened by the extent of change called for, while others strongly identify with the prevailing cultural norms of eating and so feel personally threatened by an indictment of conventional agriculture. I think it is important to address these feelings because such an approach can make people more aware of the contours of their personal, cultural, and culinary landscapes.

There may be flaws and kinks to be worked out concerning the organic alternative, but on the whole it is a reasonable way to begin the desired journey back to wholeness, healing, and health. Organic agriculture makes deep sense, because it is the basis of health, and healing must take place from the ground up. This is not a political statement or a philosophical position; it is common sense. It is also the heart of nutrient-dense eating.

CHAPTER 9

A Brief History of the American Diet

Patterns of food consumption for humans have changed enormously since prehistoric times. Shifts in technology and the environment, plus cultural factors have radically changed what and how people eat. Since the American diet has shown a similarly dramatic change in just the past several generations, it might be a good idea to look at some of the ways our cultural eating patterns have changed as well, so that we may find an answer to the question of whether the present American diet is more nutrient dense than that of our ancestors.

Since the dawn of the human race, there have been several key turning points in how people have gone about nourishing themselves. Our ancestors foraged, scavenged, and gathered whatever foods could be found. They relied on a broad and diverse range of foods for their nutrient needs, eating a mixture of protein, fats, and carbohydrates from a wide variety of sources, including eggs, fish and other animals, fruits, insects, nuts, seeds, and a wide range of edible vegetation. As hunting skills improved, some anthropologists theorize that the increasing amounts of proteins and animal fats in the diet helped fuel the development of the brain and central nervous system.

The next significant change in human development occurred when populations settled into communities and developed relatively stable regional ties. This was made possible by the domestication of certain animals for more reliable sources of food, milk, eggs, fur, and leather. The domestication of promising wild grasses and other grains, along with other crops, gave rise to the first agriculturally based civilizations, which ultimately led to the evolution of cities, and with them, national identities. Settling into one particular place, however, limited the breadth and choices of foods.

The next big shift in food consumption did not occur until the post-Renaissance period, at which point the European-based industrial revolution allowed for the widespread availability of milled flour. Throughout the next few centuries, white flour, white rice, and white sugar (all refined carbohydrates) suddenly became staples for large segments of the world's population.

In the twentieth century, further drastic changes occurred in the way people ate. Driven by advances in technology and chemical knowledge, coupled with an increasing need to find ways to profitably sustain food transportation and storage, corporations and food technologists brought various innovations into use, including synthetic agricultural chemicals, such as fertilizers and herbicides. Other technological changes included the discovery of how to cheaply hydrogenate (thicken and preserve) oils, the homogenization and pasteurization of milk, the creation of artificial sweeteners (aspartame, cyclamate, and saccharin), and the increasing development of synthetic dyes, monosodium glutamate, flavors, and other compounds to alter the appearance, color, taste, texture, and preservability of foods. The widespread introduction of hormones and antibiotics in raising livestock for meat, milk products, and eggs generated further shifts away from ancestral eating habits. Microwave cooking, along with the ubiquitous use of plastic wrapping and the ascendancy of fast-food restaurants have also shaped food output in both subtle and profound ways.

Today, continued alterations with uncertain results include experimenting with aquaculture (fish and seafood farming), cloning technologies, factory farming, genetic engineering, and other changes. While few claim that every one of these changes is bad, it is unalterably true that the end result is a large number of cumulative shifts amounting to a radical departure from ancestral eating patterns. These changes might not be consequential by themselves, but taken together, they constitute a complete revolution of food production and consumption. And, unfortunately, many of these revolutionary changes result in greatly diminished nutrient density. (*See* Chapter 10, The Current Standard American Diet [SAD].)

In many areas of the world today, food production still remains a largely local affair where foods are produced and eaten seasonably. Many of these societies—agrarian communities, some underdeveloped nations, and the dwindling populations of indigenous peoples—are closely synchronized to the land and to the food they grow. However, this type of lifestyle is rapidly becoming part of the past. Worldwide, globalization and corporate control over food production and distribution is radically changing the ways in which food is grown, who grows it, and who gets it. It is an unfortunate fact that, while enough food is available to feed every person on earth, there are still far too many who go hungry and develop malnutrition, with its dire consequences. It may seem difficult to grasp that what people eat at home affects others, but the interdependencies of food, global politics, and corporate business policies is an undeniable fact of life. Unfortunately, the loss of nutrient density has far-reaching implications, both at home and abroad.

Today, fewer people than ever before are involved in food production. In a world where specialization and narrowing fields of expertise are increasingly dominant forces, raising food is now mostly left to others. And while this leaves people free to pursue other interests, it also pulls them farther away from a basic human activity, and from nature herself. This trend, the distancing from the very sources of nourishment, may be the principal cause of the modern disconnect from nutritious, nutrient-dense eating.

TRENDS IN THE AMERICAN DIET

Significant changes have taken place in the growing and production of the food people eat. But what other trends can we trace in the American diet? And how have these trends affected the overall nutrient density of today's diets?

Some changes in diet have occurred suddenly, such as those that have arisen from the introduction of a new processing technology, a food additive, or a newly discovered artificial color. Other trends develop more slowly, as the public comes to adopt new cuisines or products. Many of our current food choices and patterns of consumption reflect these gradual (subtle) changes.

One trend that has been well documented in recent years is the tendency to eat more meals outside of the home. Eating on the run, grabbing foods based solely on convenience, and finding the cheapest snacks available is obviously not the best way to get nutrient-dense foods. Ironically, it is often young people, the very ones who tend to have among the highest nutrient requirements, who eat out and snack the most. According to one survey, teenage males are the most likely to eat out, but more than 70 percent of all the people surveyed eat one or more meals outside the home every day. This trend has increased steadily in all age groups since the mid-1960s, with the greatest rises reported among young children, teenagers, the poor, and women age twenty and over.

While eating out is not necessarily a bad thing (*see* Chapter 44 on dining out and nutrient density), the food choices people select often reflect poor nutritional awareness, with the foods eaten most frequently usually being the least nutrient dense. For example, the most popular products consumed away from home are empty-calorie carbonated soft drinks, followed by coffee. As for vegetables, the chief foods eaten outside the home are French fries, iceberg lettuce, and mashed potatoes, hardly the most nutrient-dense options. The most popular snack choice in America, by far, is potato chips. Although potatoes are relatively nutrient dense when baked or boiled in their skins, fries and chips are largely empty of any nutrient value.

Food technology is a mixed blessing. While less than 4 percent of the population now live on farms, Americans seemingly have an overwhelming abundance of food available to them. But the real question today is not about food, but about nutrients. And, due to today's food-processing methods, many nutrients are frequently destroyed or lost before the food even reaches the table.

Technology's marriage with food production has yielded some great successes, but much of the diet has suffered tremendously. Let us take a look at how differently people eat today compared with a century ago.

According to the United States Department of Agriculture (USDA) surveys, processing procedures have led to the following increases in consumer goods from 1909 to 1976.

- Processed fats and oils: up 139 percent;
- Processed fruits: up 913 percent;
- Processed vegetables: up 300 percent.

At the same time, the annual per-person consumption of *fresh* fruits dropped 611 percent, with per-capita consumption of *fresh* vegetables dropping 411 percent. The processed versions of these foodstuffs are far more nutrient deficient than their fresh counterparts.

These trends show a dramatic decline in four important constituents of the traditional, denser diet: fresh produce, foods rich in fiber, natural fats and oils, and whole-grain products. Additionally, processing usually results in a loss of both minerals and vitamins.

Statistics such as these reveal that contemporary diets are less nutrient dense. Processing may increase the availability of certain foods, especially those ordinarily available only seasonally, but it does little to ensure that needed nutritional components are retained.

At the same time that many basic nutritional constituents have been on the decline, other elements have been dramatically increasing. The consumption of nutrient-poor soft drinks rose more than 180 percent from 1960 to 1981, while corn-syrup consumption rose almost 300 percent during the same period. From 1940 to 1981, the volume of added food colors jumped an astronomical 1,000 percent.

Fresh produce (vegetables and fruits) is a key to a nutrient-dense diet. Fruits and vegetables supply needed fiber, minerals, vitamins, and a class of health-promoting compounds known as phytonutrients (plant nutrients). But the consumption of fresh produce has plummeted as the intake of processed fruits and vegetables has risen. Does ketchup compare favorably with real, whole tomatoes? Do potato chips, or boxed flaked potato buds have the same nutritional value as a fresh baked potato? Does filtered, pasteurized apple juice have the same value as an organic apple picked from a tree, or freshly pressed into cider?

To put this into perspective, here are further statistics from USDA surveys on the consumption of selected produce from 1910 to 1976:

- Fresh apples: down 75 percent;

- Fresh cabbage: down 65 percent;
- Fresh melons: down 50 percent;
- Fresh potatoes: down 74 percent.

These statistics reflect an alarming trend in the overall nutrient density of the American diet. Consumption of fresh produce, whole grains, and other crops has declined, only to be replaced by enormous increases in consumption of salt, sugar, refined oils, artificial colors, and other additives.

One of the most alarming trends is the huge role that sugar and other refined carbohydrates have assumed. According to one study, sugars now average at least one-quarter of the average American's caloric intake. Not only does sugar contain empty calories devoid of minerals and other nutrients, it actually *depletes* the body of nutrients because so many are required for its metabolism.

Other alarming trends in the nation's eating habits include:

- Approximately 35 percent of the red meat sold in the United States is highly processed (bologna, frankfurters, salami), and approximately 85 percent of the calories in these foods are from fat;
- From 1919 to 1976, the intake of fat rose by 27 percent, primarily in the form of processed and hydrogenated vegetable oils, with margarine consumption alone jumping 650 percent between 1910 and 1976;
- Ninety-five percent of all flour used today is refined white;
- Soft-drink consumption jumped from 192 servings per person in 1960 to 493 servings per person in 1976.

This unprecedented shift toward diets laden with so many empty calories simply means that Americans are eating more and more of less and less. Sugar, soft drinks, processed foods, alcohol, and convenience and snack foods have replaced the wholesome, nutrient-rich foods that our bodies require.

Food surveys and nutrient-intake data confirm that, because of this, many Americans are not getting even the already low, minimum RDA levels for many vitamins and minerals. Nor are they getting sufficient quantities of phytonutrients, or other substances whose beneficial role in health is still poorly understood.

Americans are a diverse group whose eating patterns vary widely. Yet fast-food chains and national brands are increasingly responsible for establishing a homogenized food culture. Since much of what is readily available is highly processed and nutritionally suspect, it is important to adopt healthful habits and make an earnest effort to obtain the most nutritious foods available.

Some of the at-risk categories that many fall into include:

- People who have an aversion to certain healthy foods, for example, fish, vegetables, and salads;
- Older people who have poor appetites and low incomes;
- Single people who feel it's no fun to cook for themselves;
- People who skip breakfast and settle for coffee and a high sugar-content food;
- People who take medications that interfere with nutrient absorption or metabolism;
- Teenagers who live on snacks, fast foods, and sodas;
- Weight watchers and calorie counters who too drastically limit their intake of nutritionally beneficial, nonfattening foods.

These and other trends add up to an alarming case for malnutrition. Despite the rosy pictures painted by advertisers, corporate lobbyists, and political apologists, the writing is clearly on the wall. In the face of statistics showing unprecedented levels of depression, diabetes, heart disease, obesity, and numerous other problems, it is simply astounding that so many people continue to have their heads in the sand when it comes to the relationship between health and diet.

In the late 1960s, the Health, Education, and Welfare Department (HEW) launched a comprehensive survey that revealed the following data:

- Deficiencies of B_1 and B_2 (riboflavin) were commonplace;
- Iron deficiency was a public health problem, especially among adolescents, infants, older people, and pregnant and lactating women;
- Low levels of vitamin A in young people was a serious concern.

Prior to this information, which shocked many in government and the scientific community, it was easy to believe—as the food-processing industry repeatedly said—that the United States was the best-nourished country in the world. Yet studies such as this illuminated the fact that malnutrition could occur in this country, and actually *was* occurring, and to people of all backgrounds and social strata. The myth that all of the required nutrients could be easily obtained just from eating a balanced diet was shattered.

Additional surveys indicated that infants and children generally had substandard levels of a wide range of nutrients, especially iron and vitamins A and C. Furthermore, pregnant women and people over sixty showed "major nutritional and dietary inadequacies." In 1977 and 1978, the Nationwide Food Consumption Survey uncovered other serious nutritional deficiencies, along with signs that certain negative trends were only marginally improving. In 1980, the government concluded the National Health and Nutrition Examination Survey II, or NHANES II. This data revealed that serious nutritional inadequacies continued to persist among Americans. The findings indicated that:

- 90 percent of all low-income girls, 25 percent of all men, and 75 percent of all girls between the ages of twelve and eighteen did not get the recommended calcium requirements;
- 90 percent of all women over the age of thirty-five were deficient in iron;
- 25 percent of all American women fail to get the RDA for protein;
- 25 percent of all Americans had substandard intakes of vitamin C.

What these alarming studies indicate is that the nation is nutritionally lacking in many areas. In the subsequent chapters, I will show that there is a solution to this national dilemma. Attaining, maintaining, and sustaining a nutrient-dense diet can be easily accomplished. It is not difficult, austere, or punitive, and it is delicious.

CHAPTER 10

The Current Standard American Diet (SAD)

If one word could represent the Standard American Diet (SAD), it would be *processed,* which is the manipulation of food for various reasons. Generally, the motivation behind processing food is, of course, good. No one would argue with the desire to extend the shelf life of food, or the goal of creating a safer, potentially less contaminated product. And some foods simply have to be processed in order to liberate their nutrients or to make them more absorbable. Food processing covers an enormous range of steps and technologies, from plucking feathers, separating chaff from grain, to boiling, salting, or smoking food. Ancient Mesoamericans learned centuries ago that mixing lime (calcium) with their corn rendered it more nutritious and helped prevent vitamin deficiencies. Despite the usefulness of many ancient processes, however, food is now frequently *overprocessed.*

Processing has two principal downsides. The first is that processing can result in a loss of the quality and quantity of nutrients. And second, processing can alter food, allowing harmful new compounds or changes in the food's chemistry to occur.

Today, the scope of food processing is unprecedented. Not only are highly processed foods available in unparalleled amounts, but they are aggressively marketed. Perhaps what is most disturbing is the lack of reliable research on the long-term effects of ingesting many of these highly processed foods.

Processing refers to alteration, change, and manipulation of foods, from the starting point of agriculture all the way to food preservation techniques, packaging, and storage. As a result of these technologies, a large percentage of food today no longer comes in its natural form, but in various recombined ways that yield novel, unusual, and even frightening combinations.

Processing encompasses a huge list of methods: Canning and freeze-drying foods, chemicalized agricultural practices, genetic manipulation of crops, homogenization and pasteurization of milk products, hydrogenization of oils to make shortenings and margarines, milling whole grains to refine flour by removing the bran and germ (and unintentionally, most of the fiber, trace minerals, and vitamins), puffing grains to yield breakfast cereals, the unprecedented use of high-fructose corn syrup, saccharin, aspartame (NutraSweet) and other artificial sweeteners, MSG and other flavor enhancers. These practices almost always result in far less nutrient density than is found in the unadulterated whole foods produced by nature.

It is important to understand what processing does to nutrients in order to select foods that are less *tweaked,* and therefore more nutrient dense. Though processing is vigorously defended by the powerful and influential agribusiness and food-processing companies, a large, impartial body of scientific evidence points to the loss of nutrients in processed foods and the introduction of synthetic and untested substances as causes for concern, if not alarm. People genuinely concerned about the quality of their diets and the overall status of their health are questioning many of these practices of food production, and are looking instead for wholesome, minimally processed foods. They are, in fact, looking for nutrient density.

The Nutrient-Dense Eating Plan can give these people what they are looking for. In direct contrast to the SAD diet, this plan is based on whole, minimally processed, nutrient-packed foods that have much in common with more traditional Paleolithic and macrobiotic diets. In recent decades, people who value healthy eating have sometimes been jokingly referred to as *health nuts* or *granola heads,* yet this type of eating is simply a return to common sense, to the nutrient-dense foods that our ancestors ate for tens of thousands of years. In contrast, many of the processing techniques have only been around for a handful of decades.

Fast Food and MSG

It is impossible to overstate the significance of monosodium glutamate (MSG) in today's fast-food world—it has forever changed how people eat and taste. MSG is not part of the ancestral diet, but is a chemical added by the food industry to restore *brightness* (the industry's word) to processed foods that have had much of the original flavor cooked out or degraded. MSG works by overstimulating, or tricking, the taste-bud receptors, and is everywhere today—from secret sauces to ketchup to salad dressing to canned and packaged soups. This excitotoxin directly affects your brain's chemistry through stimulation (excitation) of specific receptor sites, and is considered by numerous reputable scientists to pose a threat to many susceptible individuals, including infants, small children, and pregnant and nursing mothers. A sensitivity to MSG can result in depression, excessive thirst, headaches, an inability to think clearly, nausea, and numerous other symptoms. I strongly recommend an excellent book on this topic, *Excitotoxins: The Taste That Kills,* by Russell Blaylock, M.D., a highly respected neurosurgeon.

Unfortunately, these new processing techniques and chemical additives have often been poorly tested, and their long-term effects on health are seldom if even properly investigated. Eating the results of these technological breakthroughs is akin to being an unwitting participant in an unprecedented experiment in human nutrition and health. Perhaps it is time to rethink who the *real* nuts are.

THE EMERGENCE OF THE SAD DIET

What *has* happened to America's eating habits? At the beginning of the twentieth century, Americans primarily ate their three meals a day at home. Most food was locally produced, fresh, and grown without chemicals. It was simple, straightforward, and uncomplicated. Today, the majority of meals are eaten outside the home, often in fast-food restaurants or as snacks on the run (foods not equated with nutrient density).

Many of these changes have been steady, persistent, and cumulative. Fast-food establishments simply did not exist prior to the 1950s. Today, such chains as McDonald's, Wendy's, Burger King, Pizza Hut, Taco Bell, Arby's, and Dairy Queen practically define the American landscape. Similarly, the omnipresence of 7-Eleven and similar convenience stores has made low-quality junk food an overwhelming reality in the lives of most people. These franchises are certainly convenient, but nutritious and healthful?

Cheap food is abundant and more available to the vast majority of Americans than ever, thanks to efficient transportation, refrigeration, and related technologies. However, a serious look at the *quality* of what is available shows another story.

The bottom line is that very few people on the low-quality SAD diet feel really healthy. The unprecedented prevalence of cancer, diabetes, heart disease, obesity, and other chronic conditions would strongly suggest that the real issues surrounding food should focus on *quality*, not *quantity*.

Convenience is undeniably wonderful, but if people realized the price they paid for these so-called *benefits* in poor health, they would rise up and demand better for themselves and their families. Feel-good foods that taste good and are filling are not enough. Foods that are depleted of nutrient value and full of empty calories must be replaced by more nutrient-dense foods that give people what they really need, want, and deserve, a return to the principles of nutritional common sense.

From production to finished product, food consumption surveys and dietary data show how food processing touches virtually every aspect of the SAD diet, and just how extensively processed foods have insinuated themselves into daily life. The near-universal acceptance of processing technologies reveals how far removed people have become from the eating habits of their ancestors.

For some, questioning the health and safety of the American way of eating is almost treasonous, shaking to the core much that is held sacred in American culture. Pride in America's ability to feed herself is deeply ingrained. A rich heritage of technological and agricultural accomplishments exists today, with food production drastically different from how it was traditionally practiced.

The family farm, producing food for the local community, is largely a relic of the past. The gradual blurring of the boundaries between agriculture and the giant chemical companies is at the heart of food production today, with the ultimate consequence that, except for the relatively small (but growing) organic movement, all food grown today is chemical-reliant.

FOOD DISPARAGEMENT

One primary example of the power of the food-producing industries lies in the so-called food-disparagement laws. These laws, lobbied for and won by vested interests in the food-production world, hold that it is *illegal* to disparage or criticize certain foods, contending that to do so could create economic problems for the companies that produce it. The fact that these laws put corporate food interests ahead of free speech, informed public opinion, and the right to share information shows just how extensively those who control the food supply are able to influence matters. The famous 1998 court case, in which television talk show host Oprah Winfrey was sued by the Texas Cattleman's Association for allegedly slandering beef in the wake of scares over mad cow disease, illustrates how far industry will go to protect its self-interest. Winfrey won the case in the end, but the court proceedings tipped the hand of the beef industry, whose message was, Do not bite the hand that feeds you, and do not question the quality of the food on your table or at your grocery store. The fact that food lobbies are willing to use legal intimidation to protect their interests is a frightening reflection of the extent to which agricultural interests push their agenda on American society.

Food disparagement laws struck many legal experts, social commentators, and writers as highly questionable, even unconstitutional. A real fear exists that such laws could lead to a repressive atmosphere where serious questioning of industry practices would not exist. The fact that such fears could exist in the United States is chillingly evocative of George Orwell's writings. The reality that an entire industry could take such measures at the expense of open public discourse, concerning something as essential to life as our food supply, is deeply shocking, but it is an unfortunate truth that food has become both an economic and a political issue, instead of the agricultural, humanistic one it should be. Being perhaps the most intimate and immediate link with the larger world, food is ultimately about people. Yet now it is related more to global politics, and to how power moves around the world. Ultimately, controlling food allows for the control of people.

Because food should not be about power, politics, or economics, but about feeding people and keeping them healthy, it is fortunate that more and more people are establishing fundamental, healthy relationships with their food, their environment, and their communities. For those people, the SAD diet is no longer a viable option. This book and similar ones are increasingly pointing the way to a healthier relationship with food, and with the world.

CHAPTER 11

The New Nutrition

Today's new nutrition is based on a rapidly expanding understanding of how the human body functions. New understandings about cellular and tissue physiology as well as genetics have revolutionized an appreciation for the role nutrients play in critical biochemical reactions. This has become the meeting ground for a new mutual appreciation of the relationship between the formerly disparate fields of nutrition and biochemistry.

Antioxidant biochemistry, cellular genomics, endocrine physiology, immunology, and orthomolecular medicine, plus other fields, have much to offer such traditionally separate medical disciplines as cardiovascular medicine, gastroenterology, gerontology, oncology, psychiatry, and rheumatology. Leading these emerging new interdisciplinary connections are medical innovators, original thinkers, and researchers from many fields, including biochemists, clinicians, nutritionists, medical anthropologists, statisticians, and others. Plus, entirely new fields, such as environmental medicine and psychoneuroimmunology, are rapidly evolving in response to this fertile and exciting intellectual environment. Even whole new industries are forming. Producers are working to develop new designer foods and nutraceuticals (compounds that supply concentrated or specific nutrients), phytonutrients, and other increasingly important biochemicals. Even clinical laboratory technology, led by innovators such as North Carolina's Great Smokies Diagnostic Laboratory in Asheville, are actively involved in exploring and documenting the interface between nutrition and its role in creating health and preventing the manifestations of disease.

That clinically established diseases, along with various states of subclinical unwellness, are frequently associated with a nutrition-based cause has been most eloquently championed by such renowned health educators as Jeffrey Bland, Ph.D., who has single-handedly articulated this marriage of research-based, biochemically grounded nutritional science with the clinical acumen of many health professionals and physicians.

The outcome of this nexus has been a dialogue that has spurred on the disciplines of researcher and clinician alike. The results have led to a newly emerging understanding of both the causes and the processes of disease, as well as to a more sophisticated appreciation of how the human body sustains and builds health. In particular, the role of diet, accompanied by a growing appreciation for the functions of food and other nutritive substances, is advancing rapidly.

What this means is a greater understanding of how foods and their nutrients interact with the human body. The new nutrition is saying that food is capable of much more than merely supplying essential nutrients and the basic elements of energy production. Beyond these traditional and still-valid functions, food-sourced nutrients can reinforce and optimize health in numerous ways. Whereas traditional nutrition assigned a value to food only according to its ability to supply specific nutrients (vitamins, minerals, EFAs, and so on), today's nutrition now encompasses interesting and important new functions—antioxidant, steroidal (plant phytosterols), structural (EFAs), and substances as diverse as prostaglandins and neurotransmitters—that alter physiology and optimize function.

The new nutrition has a lot to offer because it can make the most of the various factors in a person's specific biochemical makeup, while offering protection against certain lifestyle or genetic risk factors. Based on this new nutritional knowledge people can self-select diets that are truly in their best interests.

This opportunity to use nutrition to consciously balance physiology and lessen the risk for specific diseases, while increasing creative energy, and quite possibly longevity, should not be minimized. This is powerful information that is truly capable of helping individuals make positive nutritional choices in their lives.

Rampant consumerism, the onslaught of media-backed advertising, the weakening of federal watchdog activism and protection, and the unprecedented emergence of enormously powerful multidimensional corporations that have virtually total control over food production from field to table, has had the net effect of limiting both quality and choices of foods offered in America. This emphasis on corporately controlled foods in mainstream American fare has not presented a pretty picture for several decades.

On the other hand, over the years a small, enduring subculture of American eating has quietly but steadily gained adherents and popularity. The health food movement gained a permanent niche in the natural green movements of the 1960s and 70s, and is now a vibrant and robustly growing subculture in its own right. Statistics reveal that the health food sector of agriculture is the fastest and most reliably consistent growth area in farming and food production. Over the past decade, sales of organics have maintained an annual 20 percent growth rate—unheard of, unprecedented, and in sharp distinction to the flat-sales picture of other, more conventional sectors of the food industry.

Paralleling Americans' surging interests in alternative medicine, the rising sales of organics and health foods seem to be reflecting an enormous change in the consciousness of ever-increasing numbers of people. Self-responsibility, personal empowerment, and freedom of choice over how to nurture, heal, and nourish define this new realm of healing. The new nutrition that underlies it provides an opportunity to move forward in ways that reflect the need for healing on a human scale.

CHAPTER 12

Phytonutrients and Nutrient Density

The story of nutritional progress and the breakthroughs in nutritional understanding over the past few decades have largely been centered on phytonutrients, plant compounds that have biological activity. Phytonutrients are responsible for taste, color, and other unique characteristics of plants. The pungent, unmistakable smell of garlic is due to sulfur-containing phytonutrients. So is the spicy-sweet taste of cinnamon. Capsaicin, the compound in chilies and jalapeño peppers responsible for their hot taste, is a phytonutrient. There are literally thousands of these plant-derived substances, which interact with normal biological processes at the cellular level.

Understanding phytonutrients helps to sort out the often complex relationship between diet and health in a whole new way. Garlic's phytonutrients can favorably influence cholesterol levels. Cinnamon has been investigated for its ability to help the body regulate and metabolize sugar. Cayenne and other hot peppers can improve blood flow and circulation, and they have been studied for their ability to block pain receptors.

These phytonutrient compounds are sometimes referred to as accessory nutrients. Unlike vitamins and minerals, which are considered essential for health, phytonutrients are not absolutely necessary for *preventing* specific diseases. However, many of them definitely play important roles in *optimizing* health by enhancing normal biological functioning, improving resistance to stress, toxins, or disease organisms, serving as antioxidants (buffering against radiation and other environmental assaults), and acting as donors of biologically important precursor molecules, to name a few.

Utilizing their genetic uniqueness, plants can synthesize an astonishing array of molecules of varying complexity primarily out of the basic elements of carbon, hydrogen, nitrogen, oxygen, phosphorus, and sulfur. Vitamins were the first, and best-studied, examples of this plant-created chemistry, and were relatively easy to isolate and study due to their essential roles in health. Now, with advances in analytical techniques aiding scientists, researchers are turning their attention to the thousands of compounds in foods that range from blueberries and garlic to broccoli and pomegranates.

PHYTONUTRIENTS AND THE IMPORTANCE OF DIVERSITY

This new appreciation for phytonutrients demonstrates the importance of a diverse diet. The presence in food of hundreds of thousands of these accessory nutrients means that eating a diverse diet will ensure a similarly complex chemical environment in the body. This may be important for several reasons. In nature, complex, diverse ecosystems are the most stable because they are the most highly resistant to adverse conditions, such as disease, environmental changes, population pressures, or predators. By contrast, monoculture (one-crop variety) agriculture farms and plantations are highly vulnerable to disease and other environmental stressors. In order to keep them relatively healthy, in an attempt to maximize yields and stave off problems, large quantities of agricultural chemicals are applied. Left alone, a monoculture farm or field would soon be overrun by invading species from adjacent ecosystems, as nature moves in to recreate a more diverse and natural environment.

Similarly, eating a restricted diet where most of the nutrients repeatedly come from the same foods, could limit the body's chemical diversity because exposure to a rich mix of molecular species is curtailed. This is not a far-fetched idea; many people (children especially) limit themselves to a narrow range of foods. In my experience, such behavior is all too common, and food surveys reflect this lack of diversity in the American diet. For many Americans, the most frequently eaten vegetables are iceberg lettuce, potatoes (usually as chips or fries), and tomatoes (most frequently consumed as ketchup, which one former administration, in a school-lunch cost-cutting frenzy, even tried listing as a vegetable instead of a condiment). The most frequently eaten fruits are apples (as juice concentrate), bananas, and oranges (also as juice), hardly the most nutrient-dense choices available. And, thanks to genetic tinkering and the corporate patenting of varieties, there are fewer variations of produce and consequently less phytonutrient diversity available than ever before.

What does all this have to do with nutrient density? The answer is simple. The density level of accessory nutrients in the typical SAD diet is lower than at any time in history. If people eat a markedly monoculture-based diet, and therefore limit the rich abundance and diversity of biologically active molecules, they run the risk of creating an ever more susceptible and fragile internal environment. Further, limiting the diversity of your diet increases the likelihood of inviting nutritional deficiencies.

And this is exactly what is happening. Although the food industry and its corporations are consistently touting the contemporary diet as the best in human history, the health of the American population stands in stark contrast to these rosy claims. If the SAD diet was truly nourishing and health-building, then Americans would not be the most heavily medicated population of any country—but we are.

Due to an emerging awareness of these beneficial phytonutrients, people are being encouraged to eat at least five to seven servings of produce—fruits and vegetables—a day. This means eating as much *fresh* produce as possible from a variety of sources, including different strains and varieties (there is even further benefit in eating organic, local-grown produce). By following this general guideline, you are much more likely to serve your body's needs by supplying a dense assortment of these biologically important molecules.

CLASSES OF PHYTONUTRIENTS—ALLIES IN HEALTH

Phytonutrients, chemical compounds manufactured by different plants, are the molecules responsible for the color, smell, and taste of different foods. But phytonutrients do far more than just give spices their aroma or fruits and vegetables their deep, luscious colors. Certain volatile oils in cinnamon, for example, have been shown to improve glucose tolerance, making them a potentially useful ally in dealing with blood-sugar disorders, such as diabetes or hypoglycemia. And anthocyanins and other strong pigments in fruits are now well known for their antioxidant capabilities.

Due to the increasing recognition of their importance as nutritive-supporting compounds, this book uses the phytonutrient contributions of certain foods as one of the criteria for evaluating their overall nutrient density. Various phytonutrient-dense foods are described throughout this book, even if they are not particularly high in specific vitamins or minerals. Pomegranates are a prime example. Although a good source for potassium and a fair source of vitamin C, they are not outstandingly nutrient dense in the classic sense. However, the potent level of antioxidant activity in pomegranate juice qualifies this fruit as nutrient dense for purple-pigmented flavonoids.

SPECIFIC PHYTONUTRIENTS

There are literally tens of thousands of known phytonutrients, and the actual amounts of specific phytomolecules probably runs into the hundreds of thousands or even millions. This complexity shows the astounding depth and breadth of variety of plant life on earth. The opium in poppies, the spiciness of black pepper, the unique smell of cinnamon, the sulfur in garlic, the brilliant reds, yellows, purples, and other colors of flowers, fruits, and vegetables—all this diversity in the plant kingdom comes from phytonutrients.

I could never begin to list the astounding number of phytocompounds here, and in any case, the vast majority of these molecules have incomprehensible chemical names recognizable only to the trained chemist. Nonetheless, scientists have categorized phytonutrients into several basic categories. Some of the more general classifications are listed below to help pinpoint the specific contributions of some favorite foods.

Chlorophyll

People may not think of chlorophyll as a phytonutrient, but it is probably the most basic and important of all plant molecules. Chlorophyll is the compound responsible for harnessing the solar radiation of the sun, enabling a green plant to convert sunlight (along with CO_2) into sugars and other carbohydrates. Thus, chlorophyll represents the most basic level of synthesis for plants to produce more complex compounds. While some compounds are synthesized in the absence of chlorophyll, as in plant roots or mushrooms, chlorophyll is still considered the most fundamental substance for creating and sustaining life. Even the atmosphere's oxygen is a byproduct of chlorophyll's conversion of sun and carbon dioxide into more complex molecules.

Carotenoids

Chlorophyll is also important because it is associated with other pigments that may absorb different wavelengths of light and thereby act as antioxidants. These pigments, called carotenoids, are responsible for the yellows and oranges seen in different fruits and vegetables, as well as in the colors of autumn leaves. Beta-carotene, found abundantly in carrots, pumpkin, and squash, and lycopene, a red pigment found in tomatoes, pink grapefruit, watermelon, and guava fruits are two better-known examples of carotenoids.

Nature seems to value carotenoids. To date, scientists have identified the molecular signatures of more than 600 different carotenoids, and many appear to have tissue-specific properties (they offer more protection to particular tissues). Breast, colon, lung, and retinal tissues are all known to respond to different carotenoids, and research continues to clarify these important relationships. Cryptoxanthin, lutein, xanthophylls, and zeaxanthin are some of the carotenoids known to exhibit biologically active and protective properties for the eyes and other tissues.

Flavonoids

Flavonoids are important as the largest single class of phytonutrients, with several thousand having been identified so far. These compounds have been heavily researched for their roles in health maintenance, as they provide a wide array of biologically supportive functions, including as antioxidants, chelators of heavy metals, and modulators of allergic responses. Known for their ability to inhibit cancer, many are important immune stimulants and have antibacterial and antiviral properties as well.

The flavonoids are usually subdivided into five major categories. The active components of green and black teas are the catechins and epicatechin, compounds that are responsible for the well-documented antioxidant properties of beverages made from the tea plant, *Camellia sinensis.* Another well-known category of flavonoids includes the anthocyanins, which are the pigments found commonly in many berries and other fruits. Responsible for blues, deep purples, and red colors, these pigments are increasingly being recognized as potent antioxidants.

Other important, but less well-known categories of flavonoids include the flavanones, such as naringenin found in grapefruit and tangerines, the flavones found in numerous herbs and grains, including chamomile, and the flavonols, a group of related molecules also found in a wide range of plants, including apples, buckwheat, onions, and others.

Additional well-known flavonoids include the important bioflavonoids hesperidin, quercetin, and rutin. These and other bioflavonoids have traditionally been used by the alternative medical community to treat allergies, inflammation, and venous problems. Silybin and its related compounds, the active constituents of the milk thistle plant, are flavonoids that have been extensively studied for their specific ability to detoxify certain chemicals and poisons, while supporting liver function.

Limonoids

Limonoids are yet another class of fruit-derived phytonutrients and one commonly found in the peels of citrus fruits. Limonoids appear to have antitumor effects as well as being immune-system stimulants. They also have mucolytic properties (they break down mucus from the lungs).

Sulfur

Sulfur-containing compounds in plants form a unique category of phytocompounds. Foods as diverse as broccoli, cabbage, garlic, leeks, mustard, and onions all contain important sulfur phytochemicals. Some of these compounds, allyl sulfides, isothiocyanates, sulforaphanes, and sulfur indoles, are being actively studied for their potential as anticarcinogenic agents, and may further help scientists understand how cancer formation occurs.

Additional Beneficial Phytonutrients

Many plants have their own unique contributions to make to the complex world where plant chemistry and human biochemistry interface. Hot peppers, such as jalapeños, are renowned for their production of capsaicin, a potent blood-vessel dilator and analgesic. Ginger root, long used for various medicinal purposes, including the treatment of motion sickness, nausea, and the queasiness of early pregnancy, contains a complex array of compounds called gingerols. Licorice root, also traditionally used for medicinal purposes, and now known to have important influences on the adrenal glands, produces a beneficial compound called glycyrrhizin. Curcumin, from the spice turmeric, is another phytonutrient, and is being looked at for its promise as an anti-inflammatory agent and for its ability to suppress the formation of blood clots.

Similarly, aromatic oils from diverse sources, such as cinnamon, oregano, peppermint, and rosemary, are all derived from phytonutrient molecules, each with unique ways of interacting and influencing human physiology and functioning. Other actively studied biomolecules from plants include saponins from whole grains and legumes, isoflavones from soybeans, and phytosterols, which are plant hormones that may have mild effects on the human body.

Other important phytonutrients include ellagic acid, a polyphenol found in blackberries, raspberries, and other berries and lignins, a type of plant fiber found in flaxseeds and whole grains. And there are a broad range of interesting mushroom-derived compounds, which appear to be highly supportive of the immune system.

LIVE BETTER WITH PHYTONUTRIENTS

Research and surveys have shown there is less disease in places where people eat more vegetables and fruits. This is one of the rare, unequivocal findings in contemporary nutrition, and it speaks volumes about the importance of ingesting a diet rich in diverse sources of phytonutrients. The diversity and nutrient density of the diet simply must be increased to adequately nourish and protect people from the stresses and toxicities of today's world.

Nutrients are classically defined as nourishing substances. Traditionally, that role was relegated to vitamins, a few minerals, and essential fatty acids, along with proteins. Today, phytonutrients are joining that group and are assuming an ever-larger place in nutritional understanding, as science increasingly documents how these accessory nutrients safeguard health and enhance the quality of life. By incorporating as many of these phytonutrient-dense foods, spices, and condiments into the diet as possible, your body will have a more diverse micro-environment of antioxidants and other biologically significant biomolecules with which to build resiliency and health at the cellular level.

CHAPTER 13

The Denseness of Color

Nature has always provided clues as to the whereabouts, abundance, and readiness (ripeness) of food. Appearance, smell, and color have all been ways in which animal and human foragers have been alerted to the presence of possible food sources.

Colors are important in several ways. As discussed in Chapter 12, science now understands that the presence of color is an indication of certain unique properties in pigmented plants. The chemistry of color, which is about the interrelationship of special chemical bonds, electrons, and sunlight, is important to the science of nutritional antioxidants and phytochemicals, and plant pigments are turning out to be one of the newest, most exciting areas of nutrition.

One of my earliest mentors in the field of nutrition was the legendary nutrition expert, chiropractor, and naturopathic physician, Dr. Bernard Jensen. I heard Dr. Jensen speak several times when he was in his eighties, after the many decades he had spent traveling and treating patients. In every lecture, Dr. Jensen would emphasize the importance of color in a healthy diet. One of his favorite recommendations was for people to eat what he called rainbow salads. In Dr. Jensen's view, by eating fresh produce rich in greens, oranges, purples, reds, and yellows, people would be sure to get a full spectrum of color nutrients.

Although Dr. Jensen studied and taught before the full benefits of today's chemical and analytical techniques were available, he was right. Bright-red bell peppers, deep-red tomatoes, emerald-green broccoli, sunny-yellow crookneck squash, vibrant-orange carrots, violet-purple cabbage, and the deep purples and blues of berries and cherries are all clues to some of the beneficial nutritional secrets locked inside the cells of fruits and vegetables.

For many years, researchers, scientists, and nutrition experts have told the public that eating a lot of fresh fruits and vegetables is one of the best things they can do for their health. Although studies have consistently showed a strong correlation between health (reduced rates of cardiovascular disease and cancer, and overall lowered mortality) and fresh produce consumption, the exact reasons were unclear. For years, basic assumptions centered on high fiber, low fat, and the presence of beta-carotene in these foods, but recently scientists have been zeroing in on other constituents of these foods.

The big clue for many of these researchers was the beta-carotene connection. Beta-carotene is a precursor to vitamin A, a fat-soluble vitamin found mainly in animal fats, such as dairy and egg yolks. Beta-carotene is, however, found primarily in plant foods. It is a strongly pigmented compound responsible for the orange in carrots and in many other vegetables. And, it is a powerful antioxidant.

Beta-carotene is in the carotenoid family discussed in Chapter 12. In nature, and in foods, there are hundreds of these related compounds, all with varying degrees of antioxidant activity. Most do not exhibit vitamin-A activity, but many can scavenge free radicals to varying degrees.

Investigating the carotenoids has turned out to be exciting work, yielding a lot of useful information about plant chemistry and helping to expand the knowledge of nutrition. Yet the carotenoids are only part of the pigment picture. It turns out that the chemistry of color in the world of plants is much broader and more interesting than anyone might have suspected when carotenoids were first discovered.

Carotenoids, in turn, belong to a still larger group of phytonutrients known as flavonoids, which contain other phytonutrients such as anthocyanins. These flavonoids contain many of the compounds responsible for the reds, blues, and purples found in fruits, such as berries, grapes, or pomegranates. Like the carotenoids, anthocyanins also exhibit strong antioxidant, and therefore anti-inflammatory, properties.

Although scientists have been interested in flavonoids for quite some time, analytical techniques in the past few decades have allowed research to take off, and it is now well understood that flavonoids have a variety of useful functions in biological systems. They are not considered *essential* in the same way as vitamins, but, as outlined in Chapter 12, they have been shown to be strong promoters of health, acting as strong antioxidants, stimulants of the immune system, chelators of heavy metals, modulators of immune responses, cancer-cell inhibitors, and carcinogen reducers, and at times, exhibit bacteria-inhibiting properties.

With all their beneficial effects, it is no wonder that research has begun to zero in on flavonoids and pigment-inducing compounds. In one study, the most nutrient-dense sources of food antioxidants were found to be beets, blueberries, broccoli, Brussels sprouts, kale, oranges, plums, red grapes, spinach, and strawberries. What is striking about this list is the colorfulness of most of these vegetables and fruits. Foraging ancestors would definitely have noticed these and other similarly colorful plants and investigated them for their edible potential.

Today, since colorful produce can indicate the presence of healthful foods, it is not necessary to be enticed by artificially colored beverages, baked goods, candies, meats, and seafood (most farmed salmon today has red dyes added for consumer appeal). The nutrient-dense shopper is instead attracted to the vibrant, *natural* colors that beckon from farmer's markets, the produce section of the local store, or home gardens.

Natural color is often a sound indicator of the healthiness of food. Farmers and nutritionists know, for instance, that during the spring when the grass is higher in chlorophyll and various carotenoids, butter and cream have a strong yellow color, and are also richer in vitamin A. Similarly, eggs from chickens that roam free and forage on grubs, insects, and plant material have a brighter, more intense orange yolk than the pale yellow ones that come from factory-raised chickens.

One of the first connections between color and health was made as a result of the relationship between red wine and cardiovascular health. The pigments responsible for the reds and purples of grape skins were soon discovered to be strong antioxidants. Researchers theorized that these antioxidant molecules offer protection from hardening of the arteries by slowing down the oxidation of cholesterol and other fats that can lead to atherosclerosis. Interestingly, white wines made from grapes lacking these pigments do not seem to confer the same degree of protection from cardiovascular disease. This difference led researchers to understand that the protection red wine provides comes from the grapeskin pigments, not the alcohol, as originally thought. Nonalcoholic grape juice is, therefore, thought to be just as protective as red wine.

Blackberries, black cherries, blueberries, pomegranates, purple grapes, and raspberries may all be delicious, but they have something else in common—anthocyanins. These unique pigments, called polyphenols or phenolic acids by scientists, are renowned for their powerful antioxidant free-radical scavenging abilities. Similar to other flavonoid compounds discussed, anthocyanins hold a promise for being able to slow down, or possibly prevent, the onset of some cancers, heart and vascular diseases, and other inflammatory processes. Researchers are also investigating the ability of anthocyanins to improve functioning, and possibly reverse some of the signs of aging in the nervous system.

Another important color for health is yellow. Many of the yellows in the plant world come from carotenoids and are often found in conjunction with chlorophyll. Yellows are also present in many nonyellow vegetables, but the color may be masked by the green chlorophyll pigment. Some of these yellow carotenoids, such as lutein, cryptoxanthin, and zeaxanthin, are abundant in such foods as corn, spinach, and squash. These particular carotenoids are being actively investigated for their ability to retard and prevent the formation of cataracts, which (as with hardening of the arteries) are thought to result from oxidation of the lens tissue. Oxidative reactions involving the interaction of sugar and proteins in the lens of the eye are thought to be a major factor in cataract development.

An important yellow compound is found in the spice turmeric, which is used both alone and as part of curry blends. Turmeric is becoming renowned for its powerful anti-inflammatory and antioxidant properties, and it is also being investigated for its ability to reduce fibrinogen, an important marker for certain forms of cardiovascular disease, clotting, and strokes.

Another interesting yellow food is bee pollen, collected from flowers by bees. In addition to its beautiful spectrum of yellow and orange colors, bee pollen is a concentrated source of amino acids, minerals, and unique phytonutrients. For years considered a true *health food,* bee pollen still enjoys a remarkable reputation as a powerful source of energy and nutrients.

Two other important nutrient-dense foods that are yellow are nutritional yeast and unrefined oils from flaxseeds and wheat germ. Nutritional yeast is one of the best sources of B vitamins, and its striking yellow color is due to the presence of large quantities of vitamin B_2, or riboflavin, a yellow-pigmented B vitamin (*see* Chapter 30, Nutritional Yeast). Unrefined wheat germ oil and flaxseed oil are sometimes referred to as liquid gold—these rich, unprocessed oils are important nutrient-dense sources of essential fatty acids, and their vibrant yellow-gold color is due to the presence of carotenoids.

Lycopene, another pigment found in certain foods, is a unique, recently discovered, red carotenoid, and is the principal pigment found in tomatoes. Lycopene is also found in guavas, pink grapefruits, and watermelons. In the past several years, lycopene has had a lot of media attention as research has demonstrated that men who consume tomato products more frequently have a reduced risk of prostate cancer. Other studies are linking lycopene with a reduction in sunburn, yet another indication of its protective, antioxidant capabilities.

Finally, there is the color green, so commonplace it could be taken for granted. As discussed in Chapter 12, chlorophyll is the original color pigment and highlights the ingenuity of plants. The conversion of the primeval, toxic atmosphere on this planet to one with the proper oxygen content for life is due to photosynthesis, the reaction of the chlorophyll molecule with sunlight. This true miracle of alchemy, the conversion of solar light energy to matter (molecules of carbohydrate), is the basis for all life on earth, and serves as a great reminder of the importance of color, and of the special chemical structures that make color—and life—possible.

Today, thousands of synthetic molecules are added to food in attempts to manipulate its appearance, perishability, smell, taste, and texture. Dozens, perhaps hundreds, of chemicals are used to change its color as well. Unfortunately, synthetic dyes do not have a good safety record. Over the years, several dyes have been pulled off the market due to their carcinogenic risks. Many of the dyes currently favored by the food industry are known or suspected carcinogens. Other dyes have not been adequately tested, either alone or in combination with other dyes, a common feature in foods of the SAD diet.

Nutrient-dense foods supply a vast array of nutrients, and color can now be considered a vital component, along with amino acids, essential fatty acids, vitamins, minerals, and accessory phytonutrients, such as fiber. Ingesting colors is taking in the energy, vitality, and brilliance of the world and letting it make you shine. Nutrient-dense eating means participating in, and celebrating, the color and beauty of the world.

CHAPTER 14

Anti-aging and the Nutrient-Dense Eating Plan

Is there anyone who would not like to forestall aging and the seemingly inevitable degenerations of form and function that accompany it? Probably not. Research in gerontology (the science of aging) has consistently demonstrated that the best, and only consistent, way to extend the life span of animals is through feeding them a nutrient-dense diet, without overfeeding them (animals and people who eat nutritiously, yet sparingly, consistently live longer).

Aging is a complex subject that has traditionally resisted scientific analysis and understanding. What *is* well known is that the cumulative interchange between an organism and its environment triggers changes on a cellular level, and those, in turn, lead to changes associated with an overall decline in the functioning, responsiveness, and efficiency of the organism. Typical changes associated with aging may include a decline in the immune system's responsiveness, a decreased ability to regulate blood sugar, a loss of muscle strength, neurological changes, and more. Throughout the world, researchers are actively searching for the common themes and mechanisms that underlie these changes.

In recent years, two principal themes underlying aging have consistently emerged at the forefront of gerontological studies. The first concerns the role of antioxidants in preventing or limiting free-radical damage to cells and tissues. The second centers around a newly emerging field known most simply as caloric restriction. Nutrient density is central to both themes.

ANTIOXIDANTS AND NUTRIENT DENSITY

The concept of free radicals as a mechanism for cellular injury and disease was first advanced by the chemist Denham Harman, M.D., Ph.D., in 1957. Free radicals are unstable and highly reactive molecules that attack, or borrow, needed electrons from adjacent and neighboring molecules in an attempt to stabilize themselves. Unfortunately, in so doing, they unbalance their neighbors and tend to generate chain reactions by breaking chemical bonds, ultimately altering the chemical structure of large numbers of molecules in the process. This runaway chain reaction of molecular events can lead to cellular damage, tissue inflammation, and changes in the function of tissues and organs, sometimes leading to pathology and disease.

For years after Harman's theory was first published, the significance of this concept was obscured. The importance of free radicals seemed too subtle, and other more obvious causes of disease were being actively investigated. New generations of drugs were being developed, and free radicals remained of minor interest.

In time, however, improvements in chemical analytical techniques led to an increased appreciation for the role of free radicals. The significance of such molecules as DNA became better understood, and with this understanding came the realization that such molecules are prone to degradation and damage. Scientists began to accumulate information verifying that free-radical-induced oxidation of biologically important molecules was profoundly significant. Research began to confirm that free-radical-mediated changes could affect the membranes, nucleus, and mitochondria of cells in virtually all body tissues.

Accompanying this explosion of research and information on free radicals was a simultaneous increase in understanding of the role and function of antioxidants. Free radicals act to initiate and propagate oxidative chain reactions and molecular damage, and the role of antioxidants is to terminate such reactions, often by sacrificing themselves. Scientists began to understand that naturally occurring antioxidants are designed exactly for this protective role, and that many essential minerals and vitamins perform these functions in the body. Selenium and zinc are two such well-known minerals, while the best-known and best-understood antioxidant vitamins are C and E.

In recent years, many scientists have shifted their focus to accessory nutrients, as they have realized that antioxidant activity goes far beyond vitamins and minerals, and that antioxidant activity is an indispensable part of the survival strategy of all plants and animals. This is the direct result of evolutionary processes occurring in an oxygen-rich atmosphere, and is also a consequence of living in a solar system where life is based around a star that generates ultraviolet radiation. Antioxidants in plants and animals are what allow life to thrive under what would otherwise be impossibly adverse circumstances.

As a result of this expanded awareness, many recent studies have begun to focus on plant-based antioxidant molecules. These food-sourced molecules are the same phytonutrients (phytochemicals) formed by the fruits and vegetables that make up the human diet, and are highly relevant to *The Nutrient-Dense Eating Plan,* which emphasizes consciously selecting as many of these foods as possible. The denser these phytonutrients are in your diet, the more they can help you resist the free-radical changes associated with poor health, lowered resistance to disease, and aging.

CALORIC RESTRICTION AND NUTRIENT DENSITY

In addition to the science behind free radicals and antioxidants, research has also unequivocally shown that maintaining a high level of nutrients while limiting or restricting calories allows every species examined to reach their maximum life span. Lowering calories while maintaining optimal levels of nutrients is, in fact, how nutrient density increases. The concentration of nutrients, relative to total caloric intake, is how the denseness of nutrients in food is actually defined.

Interestingly, the only common thread among all the animals studied (from flies and other invertebrates to many species of mammals, and even primates) is that, when the diet has one-third fewer calories than usual, but approximately the same level of nutrients, the test animals consistently outlive their peers, often to a highly significant degree. Why is this phenomenon so widespread, consistent, and reproducible? The answer seems to lie in the reduced metabolic processes occurring with caloric restriction. By slowing the overall metabolic rate, cells tend to generate fewer metabolic waste products, many of which are capable of creating oxidant stress and cellular damage, and overwhelming the antioxidant system. Over time, as oxidant damage accumulates, the changes associated with aging occur.

Research is bearing out this hypothesis. Studies of animals on calorically restricted but nutritionally dense diets show a reduction in the stress response normally associated with accelerated aging. One scientific theory proposes that aging occurs as a response to the stress of oxidatively damaged proteins and other molecules. Since an excess of calories generates an extra metabolic load on the system, the best diet would be the most efficient one. Perhaps nutrient density could be referred to as the less-is-more school of nutrition.

INCREASING YOUR HEALTH SPAN

What has most intrigued researchers is that this phenomenon—undereating without malnutrition—also supports healthiness, in addition to longevity. Not only do animals live *longer* on calorically restricted but nutrient-adequate diets, they live *better,* with less disease. It can be said that these diets increase the quantity *and* the quality of animals' lives.

The idea that a nutrient-dense diet induces increased biochemical efficiency is what links caloric restriction, nutrient density, and antioxidant capability as unifying principles in understanding aging, longevity, and disease reduction. The connection seems to work because the caloric reduction associated with nutrient-dense foods in the diet lowers the metabolism, while simultaneously supplying high levels of antioxidants. This means fewer free radicals are produced, and this reduces the potential for damage to the body's cells.

These findings apply to various aspects of aging. One well-known sign of aging is a decline in the cell's ability to regulate glucose, the body's principal fuel. Scientists have found that primates on calorically restricted diets maintain their glucose and insulin levels far better than animals allowed to eat all they want. Since glycation—the attaching of glucose to protein molecules—is another well-known biochemical mark of aging, it is interesting to note that animals on reduced-calorie diets show less glycation damage. These glucose-damaged proteins are known as advanced glycation end products, or AGEs.

The clear message of *The Nutrient-Dense Eating Plan* is that incorporating nutrient-dense foods is the most straightforward way to ensure a high quality of life throughout life, and especially into old age. I call this combination of increasing your life span while reducing your risk of disease, your *health span.* The equation is, health span = longevity + reduced disease risk. Science has repeatedly shown that only a nutrient-dense diet consistently satisfies this equation.

CHAPTER 15

The Wholeness of Whole Foods

One of the guiding principles of nutrient density is that whole foods are, generally speaking, more desirable than heavily processed or synthetic foods. Yet, what is it about whole foods that seems to give them their edge?

Whole foods are foods as nature intended them, complete in and of themselves. Part of the problem with processing foods is that processing alters food, sometimes for the better but more often for the worse, by either removing important constituents or adding harmful ones. Whole foods are typically simpler, humbler foods. They are also closer to the foods consumed by humans for the vast majority of time.

In fairness, I must say that processing is not universally bad. Some processing techniques are necessary, even beneficial. A problem only arises when a society becomes dependent upon heavily processed foods and excludes naturally occurring whole foods.

Sugar is a prime example of how a whole food can be altered to its disadvantage. In its natural state, as sugar cane, it is a whole, complete food, full of healthy minerals and vitamins. Yet, when refined, it is nothing but empty calories that are ultimately damaging to health. (*See* Chapter 34, Sweets.)

Whole foods in nature are incredibly complex in their chemistry. Science is just starting to understand how to identify all the compounds and molecules in foods. Since this is an expensive and daunting task, the supplement industry often finds it easiest to identify and isolate a single compound within an herb or plant. For marketing purposes, they then attempt to equate the efficacy of the whole plant with this one compound. This is similar to the pharmaceutical industry isolating and synthesizing single molecules to be patented and sold as drugs. It may be the easiest and most profitable way to ensure consistency and purity, but it doesn't reflect the synergy of the plant's chemistry. Foods are not drugs, although the mentality of the drug industry has definitely invaded the arena of agriculture, nutrition, and food production.

When foods get refined or processed, they often lose the complexities, subtle balances, and benefits found in the original, whole foods. Oranges are not just a natural source of vitamin C, they offer much more. Equating oranges and vitamin C does a disservice to the myriad of other biologically active constituents present in fresh citrus fruit, such as bioflavonoids, enzymes, and pigments.

Eating whole foods allows you to appreciate the complexity and the beauty inherent in nature. Whole foods provide you with small but often important amounts of a wide variety of nutrients that are not reproduced in isolated supplements. When I teach, I often make the point that nutrition is still a very young science, still in the early phase of the learning curve, and scientists therefore need to be much humbler about what they know and do not know. Much of what is of value in whole, natural, and wild foods is still not known, understood, or appreciated.

This idea of humility is important. To put too much faith in man-made synthetic or highly processed foods is as unwise as it is arrogant. Nature seems to be pretty smart. The more you learn, the clearer it becomes that, in nature, little, if anything, is wasted. There is some redundancy, but even that seems to have an important function, similar to backing up important information on a hard drive to a disc or CD.

At this point, scientists have isolated and identified the functions of some fifty or so of the essential inorganic minerals and organic molecules known as vitamins. At the same time, they are also slowly discovering a huge array of other, less easily classified compounds with their own biological activity. Many of these compounds are just now being studied, while others have hardly been looked at, but at least science is beginning to appreciate the magnificent symphony of substances that make a whole food the unique, intricate miracle it is.

One of the most difficult tasks facing science is understanding the way that various substances interact with one another. Called synergy, these interactions seem to imply that many compounds help strengthen each other. Sorting out these complex interactions can pose problems for scientists who tend to prefer relatively simple questions with fewer variables. Unfortunately for science, complexity and subtlety is much more in keeping with how the real world works.

Two good examples of synergy at work are vitamins C and E. The overwhelming majority of vitamin C on the market today is sold in pill, capsule, or powder form. Virtually all vitamin C is manufactured by a small handful of companies and sold as purified, crystalline ascorbic acid. Mixed into multivitamin preparations, or sold alone, consumers almost always get this same product—the only variables being colors, fillers, flavors, and occasionally, a small amount of added bioflavonoids or a bit of acerola cherry. Because this ascorbic acid is not directly derived from food, it is not identical to the vitamin C found in nature. In a strawberry or a kiwi fruit, for example, ascorbic acid is found in an intimate partnership with numerous other compounds, including enzymes and pigments, such as carotenoids and other related molecules, such as bioflavonoids.

Is the activity of vitamin C substantially different if it is obtained from a grapefruit as opposed to a multivitamin? Unfortunately, this is not an easy question to answer. Certainly the companies that market supplements want you to believe there is no difference between the two. My belief lies on the side of nature. Although the differences may be subtle, I feel strongly that nature has a lot more experience and know-how than any laboratory technician or corporate strategist.

Similar to vitamin C, vitamin E also illustrates the importance of properly understanding the interrelationships and complexities of nutrients found in nature. Vitamin E is a fat-soluble antioxidant that protects lipid-rich tissues, such as cell membranes and other sensitive structures, from certain classes of free radicals.

Vitamin E is commonly identified with alpha tocopherol, the chemical name given to the molecule that is easiest to isolate and measure from foods such as soybeans, spinach, and many nuts and seeds. However, it has been known for many years that this molecule always coexists in nature with several other closely related tocopherol molecules that have similar chemical shapes. For years, the purpose for these molecular cousins was not known, and scientists concluded that they must be unimportant. Typical vitamin-E preparations, therefore, contained only alpha tocopherol, and not its underappreciated relatives. Recent research, however, has revealed that some of these related molecules *do* have specific functions, and may fulfill some roles that alpha tocopherol alone cannot.

This example demonstrates just how young the science of nutrition really is. Knowledge on the subject is still evolving, and that is why it is crucial to take many nutritional conclusions with a grain of salt. Nature undoubtedly provides many more subtle nutrients than are presently known—only a minuscule fraction of the tens of thousands of food molecules ingested daily have been studied, no more than a couple of handfuls of vitamins and minerals—a compelling argument for choosing whole foods and a diverse diet whenever possible.

Does this mean I am antivitamin/mineral or against all supplements and believe in getting these from elements only from foods? Certainly not. I feel that the better-quality supplements have a definite role to play in rounding out diets, especially in the earlier stages of transitioning to a denser diet. For a variety of reasons, supplements make sense, particularly when they are taken as adjuncts to real food, but I believe that, *when possible,* your primary source of nutrition should come from whole foods. Supplements are *not* beneficial if people justify their poor eating habits by rationalizing that their multivitamin will allow them to compromise in their food choices. And, for those on tight budgets, I feel that the money some people spend on supplements could be better put to use by purchasing higher quality foods.

FOOD AS A TEACHER

In ways not yet understood, the entire tapestry of a food can nourish people. There may be large numbers of substances in foods that, *even in small amounts,* may be extraordinarily important to health. Currently, nutrition is viewed as a means for the body to obtain specific substances, called nutrients (minerals, vitamins, essential fatty acids, and so forth). But what if nutrition involves more than just these separate, material substances? The *wholeness* of whole foods could prove to be one of the leading edges of nutrition's journey into the twenty-first century.

I am referring here to the *net* effect of food in people. Instead of viewing food merely as a collection of isolated, specific substances, perhaps food might convey something less tangible as well. It might provide *information* on a larger scale. In addition to nourishing with nutrients, food might have something to *teach.* This is a novel concept, I realize, yet one that has its own logic and intuitive reasonableness, and comprises the beginning of a truly holistic view of food.

FOOD AS INFORMATION

Food as information implies a holistic view that does not separate or isolate individual constituents of food. Instead, the messages carried by food are ingested and interpreted by your body in individual ways, which take into account your time of life, state of health, unique biochemical and genetic individuality, and the quality, consistency, and appropriateness of the food itself. In this way, food uniquely intersects with your life in ways that reflect your individual circumstances.

What messages can food convey? The answer is that food carries its own history with it. How and where it was grown, the environment it came from, even the intentions of the people who produced it are all part of the overall message that comes with food. In the deep message of holism, everything is connected. Information is never lost from the system, it simply moves around. The totality of the experience, or the history of the food, remains.

In this way, food carries a sort of integrity that speaks of ingesting values, ethics, principles, and consistency. If food is raised in ways that do not correspond with deep-seated wishes for a healthy planet, clean local ecosystems, fair and equitable distribution of food, happiness for food producers and consumers, as well as the animals used and eaten, then anyone eating that food ingests these inconsistencies and mixed messages along with their meal.

Clearly this is a much deeper view of food than is conventionally held. Yet, perhaps it is not too far-fetched. Once again, one of the most important principles of the perennial philosophy of food is that *you are what you eat.* Who says you have to limit this notion to the ingesting of material substances? People certainly swallow beliefs, views, and propaganda, without giving these matters much thought. And food is, after all, a nexus or hub that represents a meeting place of many realities.

This implies a deeper and broader sense of responsibility. Seen in this way, *what* you eat becomes a more conscious act and indicates the importance of cultivating a deeper sense of mindfulness over what has too often become a culturally reflexive habit. Instead of abdicating food choices to corporate business decisions and a chemical-based agricultural system, through the simple act of eating, you can begin the process of reclaiming the world, starting with the immediate and intimate local access of your own body. This is an application of the principle that charity begins at home and points to where you can begin the healing process in your own life. For those who eat *and* have a social conscience, the mindful message of the wholeness of whole foods can point out a direction that helps to complete themselves and the world.

NUTRITION AS INFORMATION

Scientific literature on cellular functioning and physiology is revealing the many ways that food speaks to the body's cells. For example, receptor sites in cell membranes have emerged as a new field of study that is revolutionizing people's understanding of the food-health relationship.

Membranes are the brains of cells, the means by which they communicate with each other and with their environment. Messages from the rest of the body must be received, routed, and ultimately, interpreted by the membranes surrounding each cell in the body. Sensitive membranes also encircle the genetic codes in the nuclei of cells and act as conduits for information arriving in the form of food-derived molecules. This information speaks to your genes, which in turn, allow your cells, and hence your body, to respond in appropriate, or inappropriate, ways.

Nutrition as information implies that people's bodies are intelligent enough to sort out the messages being sent to them. If your cells receive consistent messages of health via a rich supply of nutrients, they will respond accordingly. If you send your cells the message that you do not care about what you are eating, and you repeatedly bathe your cells in an unwholesome environment with fewer nutrients and more toxins, then it would be unrealistic to expect superior health in return. This is yet another application of the age-old principle, you are what you eat.

THE INTELLIGENT BODY

Another theme that runs through this book is respect. The concept of nutrition as information also means understanding that your body is *intelligent*. Even though intelligence is usually thought of as something that resides in the brain and nervous system, this is a broader, deeper view of intelligence. Your cells and your body also have the wisdom to sort out or discriminate between the kinds of messages they are being sent. If you are smoking cigarettes, are you respecting your lung or heart cells? If you smoke and think it somehow does not matter to your body, then aren't you guilty of seeing your body as little more than an unfeeling servant? In this respect, is eating junk food any different from smoking cigarettes or abusing your body in other ways?

Realizing that your body *does* understand and respond to the messages it receives is the beginning of understanding what it means to inhabit your body with respect, mindfulness, and compassion. This is precisely the kind of relationship that *The Nutrient-Dense Eating Plan* seeks to foster.

RESPECTING THE WHOLENESS OF NATURE

When you begin to respect yourself in this way, you also begin to grasp the meaning of interconnectedness. The more you open up to the possibilities of relating to your food, your body, and your world with compassion and awareness, the more you will begin to think and act holistically. Eating whole foods that are nutrient dense and unadulterated then becomes, not an obligation, but a natural extension of your deepening view of the web of life.

When food is broken down and its constituents isolated, purified, and separated, it almost seems as if something precious is being violated. Although breaking the complex, subtle interconnections of food constituents is sometimes unavoidable, I believe it is done far too frequently, and often with no other motivation than to create a profitable new market.

A recent experience I had with eggs illustrates this point perfectly. At a friend's house, I was offered eggs for breakfast. Looking at my plate, it took me a moment to figure out what was not quite right, until I realized that the lack of yellow in the omelet before me indicated it was made solely with the whites. My friend, it turned out, had used a box of preseparated egg whites, thinking that these high-protein, no-cholesterol abominations were a healthy improvement over regular eggs. I viewed this fragmented food quite differently, of course. (*See also* Chapter 27, Eggs, for a full discussion of cholesterol.)

As they say, it's not nice to fool Mother Nature. Or manipulate her. Doing so may invite trouble, or at least, unforeseen consequences. Breaking foods down unnecessarily, as in separating or powdering eggs, is often a subtle form of manipulating—fooling around with—nature. Whole foods, on the other hand, are an acknowledgment of nature's wisdom, and they also provide the opportunity to affirm respect for her and the food she so generously provides.

The wholeness of whole foods is clearly a central topic in this discussion of nutrient density, as whole foods are really the heart of *The Nutrient-Dense Eating Plan,* communicating vitally important messages to your body, and cells. The message that whole foods carry is integrity, and this wholeness provides an important opportunity for you to experience that integrity in the very essence of who you are. If you believe you are what you eat, then the principles of nutrient density hold the promise of profound healing because they give you the opportunity to reclaim your own wholeness of being.

PART 2

Nutrient-Dense Foods

CHAPTER 16

Vitamins

The first two chapters of Part 2 discuss vitamins and minerals. Vitamins are organic, carbon-based, compounds required, in small amounts, for the biochemical reactions of life to occur. By definition, vitamins cannot be made in the body from other compounds, but must be obtained from outside sources, usually, food. For this reason, they were deemed *vital amines* by the chemist, Casmir Funk, in 1912. Since the discovery of B_1, the first vitamin, some thirteen additional vitamins have been isolated, chemically analyzed, and studied.

Vitamins are broadly categorized into two main groups, depending on their solubility in water or lipids. There are the water-soluble vitamins, comprised of vitamin C and the B-vitamin group, and the fat-soluble vitamins—A, D, E, and K. Foods vary widely in their specific contributions of vitamins. Some foods are dense for one or more vitamins and weak in the others (no single food offers high levels of the entire vitamin spectrum). In this chapter, I will focus on the most nutrient-dense sources for each vitamin.

NATURAL VERSUS SYNTHETIC VITAMINS

In nature, vitamins are not found isolated and alone, separate from their surroundings. Instead, they usually form complexes in association with related, synergistic molecules. This is what sets vitamins found in nature apart from the isolated, synthetic versions sold in bottles. Vitamin C in foods, for example, is always found in conjunction with various bioflavonoids—phytochemical molecules that exhibit related antioxidant properties. Commercially sold vitamin C, by contrast, is virtually always chemically pure ascorbic acid, isolated from its naturally occurring neighbors. In the fat-soluble category, vitamin E is commonly sold commercially as isolated alpha tocopherol, but in vitamin-E food sources, alpha tocopherol is never found by itself. Instead, it is part of a mixture of tocopherol molecules—beta tocopherol, delta tocopherol, and gamma tocopherol. Today, the vitamin industry is based almost solely on synthetic, isolated vitamins, which are cheaper to produce, measure, and standardize than their natural counterparts. There are, of course, a few exceptions to this rule, but more than 99 percent of all vitamins are, in fact, synthetic versions of what normally is found in food.

Nonetheless, science is beginning to unravel how these different molecules interact and synergistically support one another in nature. Honoring this naturally occurring complexity of food is, of course, a guiding principle of nutrient density. Nutrition should not come out of a bottle. Good nutrition is about real food for real people.

THE WATER-SOLUBLE VITAMINS

The body must take in water-soluble vitamins on a daily basis, as it cannot store them for any length of time.

Vitamin C

Vitamin C, probably the best known of all the vitamins, was first discovered when the British surgeon James Lind uncovered the link between scurvy and a diet deficient in fresh produce, particularly fruit. Due to this connection, first seen in the eighteenth century, vitamin C has been known as the *antiscorbutic* (ascorbic) factor. Although largely unknown today, scurvy is characterized by bleeding gums, bruising, diminished immunity, lassitude, and a weakening of collagen-based tissues. Since blood vessels, including capillaries, owe their strength and integrity to collagen, severe vitamin-C deficiency, or scurvy, can lead to hemorrhaging, and possibly death.

Although science now equates vitamin C with the single ascorbic-acid molecule, in fresh fruits and vegetables it is part of a complex admixture of bioflavonoids, polyphenols, and (often) proanthocyanins, a type of plant pigment. It is interesting to note that Indian tribes of the upper regions of North America treated scorbutic English sailors with extracts of pine tree bark, which contains virtually no ascorbic acid, but does have abundant quantities of proanthocyanins.

From an evolutionary point of view, ascorbic acid is an interesting molecule. Most animals, from insects to reptiles to birds to mammals, are able to manufacture abundant amounts of this molecule in their own bodies, yet humans and other primates cannot. In most mammals, for example, ascorbic acid is made in the liver from glucose. Evidently, some evolutionary mutation or defect rendered our distant common primate ancestors, including the higher primates (chimps, gorillas, and humans), incapable of making this important conversion. Evolving in a tropical climate, such as equatorial Africa, however, allowed early humans to be dietarily supplied with acorbate through fruits and other easily foraged plant foods rich in vitamin C. This hypothesis, that our early ancestors lost the gene for manufacturing ascorbic acid from glucose, was first put forth by the renowned chemist, Linus Pauling, and is now widely accepted as both plausible and probable. It also accounts for the fact that many people may not get enough vitamin C to optimally meet their needs, and is grounds for the contention that the current recommended levels of vitamin C are far lower than those needed for optimal health.

As Pauling and others have pointed out, most mammals can manufacture far larger quantities of ascorbate from blood glucose than humans usually obtain in their diets. More important, animals tend to produce massive amounts of it in response to stress. Due to this, many researchers believe that the RDAs for vitamin C are merely adequate to ward off obvious signs of deficiency, but are far too low to help people deal with the acute or chronic stress many face today. Because of this, many scientists and nutritionists believe that vitamin C should be supplemented at a much higher level than the amount typically ingested in a normal diet.

As an extremely important biomolecule, ascorbic acid is involved in numerous biologically crucial reactions. Ascorbic acid is therefore responsible for the synthesis of a large number of vitally important molecules including bile acids, certain proteins, collagen, corticosteroids, histamine, and norepinephrine, among others. Vitamin C is also crucial for wound healing, helps with many allergic reactions, and positively affects the functioning of white blood cells. Through its role in supporting adrenal function, vitamin C is also known to help people respond to stressful situations and challenges.

Fortunately many excellent food sources of vitamin C are available. Some of the most nutrient dense are bell peppers, broccoli, citrus fruits, kiwi fruit, papaya, parsley, strawberries, and green leafy vegetables, including collards, chard, kale, mustard, and spinach. Dairy, eggs, meats, and seafood are considered poor sources. Vitamin C is also important because its presence improves the absorption of iron from vegetable sources.

The B Vitamins

The other major group of water-soluble vitamins are known as the vitamin B family. Though often referred to as the B family, these molecules are not directly related to one another in a chemical sense. Instead they are related through their common functions of helping to metabolize (liberate) energy from carbohydrates, fats, and proteins. The numbers designating the various B vitamins—B_1, B_2, B_3, and so forth—do not signify any particular chemical or functional purpose, but were simply the numbers assigned to the corresponding molecule based on the order in which it was discovered. Thiamine was the first B vitamin to be chemically isolated and mapped out, and so is called vitamin B_1, while the second B vitamin discovered, riboflavin, is referred to as B_2, and so on.

Metabolically active foods, such as nuts, seeds, and whole grains, tend to be the best sources of B vitamins, as are liver and other organ meats. The most consistently reliable source of B vitamins is nutritional (Brewer's) yeast (*see* Chapter 30, Nutritional Yeast).

Vitamin B_1—Thiamine

Vitamin B_1, or thiamine, is a crucial element in carbohydrate metabolism as it facilitates the pathways that obtain glucose and energy from more complex sugars. Since glucose is a vital fuel for many tissues, a thiamine deficiency often results in symptoms in the cardiovascular and nervous systems, which are heavily dependent on glucose.

The classic result of a thiamine deficiency is beriberi, which can manifest as anorexia, edema, an enlarged heart, mental confusion, mental weakness, and peripheral paralysis when the deficiency is severe. While these symptoms will not typically all appear together, a chronically inadequate intake of thiamine may result in at least some of these symptoms. These symptoms may reflect an increased need for B_1 in older people, either because of a poor diet, poor absorption, or a decrease in metabolic efficiency.

It is also well known that long-term abuse of alcohol can lead to a thiamine deficiency. Altered mental functioning in alcoholics, including certain forms of dementia and short-term memory loss, is thought to be caused by alcohol's interference with the absorption and availability of thiamine in the diet. Diets high in refined carbohydrates, such as white flour, white rice, and white sugar, can also put you at risk for a B_1 deficiency.

The most nutrient-dense food source for B_1 is nutritional (Brewer's) yeast. Other nutritious sources include liver and other organ meats, nuts and seeds, and whole grains. Of all the nuts and seeds, sunflower seeds are the most nutrient dense for thiamine, but Brazil nuts, hazelnuts (filberts), macadamia nuts, pine nuts, pistachios, and sesame seeds are also considered excellent sources.

Vitamin B_2—Riboflavin

Vitamin B_2, or riboflavin, is a necessary component of various important coenzymes involved in biochemical reactions, and its presence helps to activate these reactions. Vitamins B_6 (pyridoxine) and B_3 (niacin) require riboflavin in order to become fully active. Several forms of dermatitis, including sores and cracking around the mouth, are often associated with an inadequate intake of riboflavin.

The most nutrient-dense source of riboflavin is nutritional yeast. One serving can supply up to 90 percent of your daily riboflavin needs. Some green vegetables, including asparagus and broccoli, are also good sources. Eggs and raw (unpasteurized and unhomogenized) dairy are also good sources, as is liver.

Vitamin B_3—Niacin

Vitamin B_3, known as niacin or nicotinic acid, is one of the more interesting B vitamins. This supplement is responsible for the well-known niacin flush, a reaction that often brings on redness, warmth, and a flushed, itchy feeling, caused by its ability to dilate peripheral blood vessels. People take niacin for a variety of reasons, including its much-documented ability to lower cholesterol levels.

Niacin's principal biochemical function is its role as the central component in two important energy-producing enzymes, nicotinamide adenine dinucleotide, NAD, and a slightly different version, NADP. These are present in every cell of your body and are responsible for numerous important metabolic reactions, including the breakdown of sugars (glycolysis), cellular respiration, and fatty-acid metabolism.

Deficiencies of vitamin B_3 can result in dementia, depression, dermatitis, inflammation of mucous membranes, and intestinal problems, such as diarrhea. Fortunately, a nutrient-dense diet can supply adequate levels of this important vitamin. Brewer's yeast and many high-protein foods, such as fish, legumes, meats, and nuts and seeds are all nutrient dense for niacin. Peanuts are the most nutrient-dense nonmeat source of niacin. Because it is so important, the body requires higher levels of niacin than any other B vitamin.

Vitamin B_6—Pyridoxine

Vitamin B_6, or pyridoxine, is another very important B vitamin. Besides its primary role in energy production, B_6 is linked to protein metabolism, and is directly involved in numerous chemical reactions involving amino acids. The more protein you eat, the more B_6 you need. B_6 is also used for fat metabolism as well as in various detoxification pathways.

The most nutrient-dense foods for B_6 are chicken, eggs, fish, meats, and organ meats, including liver. For vegetarians, the best sources, besides nutritional yeast, are asparagus, bananas, hazelnuts (filberts), legumes, pistachio nuts, sesame seeds, sunflower seeds, and whole grains, including brown rice and oats. Dairy is a poor source of B_6.

Vitamin B_{12}—Cobalamin

Vitamin B_{12}, cobalamin, is an important B vitamin that is necessary for the synthesis of nucleic acid (DNA, RNA). The classic sign of a B_{12} deficiency is a unique form of anemia known as pernicious anemia. While the better known, classic iron-deficiency anemia results in small red blood cells, pernicious anemia is characterized by enlarged, pale blood cells. B_{12} deficiency particularly targets the nervous system, and can lead to demyelination of the spinal and peripheral nerves, dementia, and other neuropsychiatric symptoms.

In nature, B_{12} is only found in animal products, and vegetarians are more at risk of developing B_{12} deficiencies than people who include meat in their diets. Fortunately, your body has the ability to store B_{12} and can usually go for three to seven years on a low B_{12} diet before symptoms begin to appear. However, people do vary, and the symptoms could manifest sooner than later. It should also be pointed out that, while some vegetarians claim that blue-green algaes and some root-crop vegetables can contribute B_{12} to the diet, most scientists dispute this. These researchers point out that, although algae and some bacteria (those clinging to the roots) can synthesize some close cousins of B_{12}, these molecules are not identical to real B_{12}, and probably have little if any effect on preventing pernicious anemia or the other symptoms of B_{12} deficiency. For this reason, most nutritionists believe that long-term vegetarians, and especially vegans, would do well to consider using B_{12} supplements.

Another at-risk group are older people, both as a result of a lifetime of suboptimal intake catching up with them, and because B_{12} is relatively difficult to absorb. A common sign of aging is a reduction in stomach-acid secretion, which makes it even more difficult to absorb B_{12} from food. Many of the neuropsychiatric symptoms associated with aging, including disorientation, fatigue, mild depression, and short-term memory loss, could be attributable to poor B_{12} status. Unfortunately, relatively few doctors have been adequately trained to look at B_{12} levels, and so this deficiency frequently has gone undiagnosed and untreated in the past.

The most nutrient-dense sources of B_{12} include red meats (beef, buffalo, elk, and lamb), and especially liver, which is the single most nutrient-dense source of B_{12} known. Eggs also have respectable amounts of B_{12}, as do raw dairy products, fish, and other forms of seafood.

Biotin

Biotin is another vitamin in the B family. Like most of the other Bs, biotin is an essential co-factor in several enzymatic reactions, including the synthesis of fatty acids and gluconeogenesis (the synthesis of glucose from fats and proteins). Classic signs of biotin deficiency include depression, dry scaly skin, hair loss, hypoglycemia, increased cholesterol, and seborrheic dermatitis, found in infants under six months of age. Biotin is available from such nutrient-dense sources as egg yolk, liver, soy, and yeast.

Folic Acid

Folacin, folate, or folic acid are often interchangeable terms for molecules of pteroylglutamic acid, an important biological molecule that acts as a coenzyme for the transfer of small, but important one-carbon fragments from one compound to another, for such diverse functions as amino-acid metabolism, detoxification, and nucleic synthesis. One important consequence of inadequate folic acid is impaired cell division and changes in protein synthesis, which is most noticeable in rapidly dividing cells and tissues, and can lead to anemia and other problems. Neural tube defects, a developmental problem involving the spine that occurs early in pregnancy and results in spina bifida, is known to be directly related to inadequate intake of folate by pregnant mothers.

The words folate and foliage have the same origins, which underscores the connection between folate and green vegetables, considered nutrient dense for folate. Liver, peanuts, sunflower seeds, and yeast are exceptionally rich sources, and beans, hazelnuts (filberts), legumes, sesame seeds, and walnuts are also considered nutrient dense for folate.

Pantothenic Acid

Pantothenic acid is a component of the very important biomolecule, coenzyme A, which serves a variety of critically important functions in the body. It is involved in gluconeogenesis (synthesizing glucose from fats and proteins), the metabolism of fatty acids, the release of energy from carbohydrates, and the synthesis of several important molecules, including steroidal hormones and other vital proteins. Deficiencies of pantothenic acid can cause a variety of symptoms, including abnormal pigmentation, adrenal stress, a loss of fertility, neuromuscular difficulties, and problems with growth and development. Pantothenic acid is widely distributed in nature, and a good, well-rounded nutrient-dense diet should supply adequate amounts. The densest sources of pantothenic acid are eggs, legumes, meats, nuts and seeds (especially sunflower seeds), and whole grains.

THE FAT-SOLUBLE VITAMINS

The fat-soluble group of vitamins have lipidlike characteristics and can be stored longer than the water-soluble vitamins in the body's fatty tissues and liver. They are most commonly in the fat found in foods, including avocados, dairy, eggs, meats, and nuts.

Vitamin A

Vitamin A, retinol, is a fat-soluble vitamin that is essential for the proper functioning of the immune system, lungs, membranes, skin (epithelial tissue), vision, and the ability of cells to differentiate and grow properly.

Vitamin A is obtained either in a preformed state from animal products, including calves liver, dairy products, eggs, and fish liver oils (cod-liver oil), or in the form of plant-based carotenoids, such as beta-carotene. With vegetarian-source carotenes, the body must convert these pigments to retinol, a process that is considered relatively easy for some and more difficult for others. The scientific community has concluded that six units of beta-carotene are needed to yield one unit of retinol.

Vitamin-A deficiency is a problem recognized throughout the world, and symptoms include corneal and other visual problems, keratinization (scaly hardening of the skin), night blindness, a reduction in immunity, and lowered resistance to viral and other infections. The densest sources of vitamin A include animal fats, such as butter, calves liver, cod-liver oil, cream, and egg yolk. Provitamin A (beta-carotene) is found principally in green leafy vegetables, such as beet greens, collards, kale, parsley, and spinach, as well as the yellow/orange vegetables, such as carrots, pumpkin, and squash.

Vitamin D

Vitamin D is an interesting and unusual fat-soluble vitamin, which many scientists consider more hormonelike than a vitamin. Unlike all other vitamins, vitamin D is generally not obtained from food at all. Except for such fatty fish as cod, halibut, salmon, and sushi, and the fortifying of dairy products with an artificial form of D, this vitamin does not naturally exist as a food-sourced substance. Surprisingly, the principal source of vitamin D is the sun. Commonly referred to as the sunshine vitamin, vitamin D is produced by the effect of ultraviolet sunlight radiation acting on the cholesterol present in skin tissue. This light/chemical conversion alters cholesterol into another form that is then carried to the liver and kidneys, where it is converted to its active form as vitamin D.

According to Reinhold Veith, Ph.D., a leading authority on vitamin D, insufficiencies of this vitamin rank at the top of vitamin deficiencies for people living in the temperate (northern) latitudes. Today, as people tend to spend more time indoors, and use sunscreens when outside, vitamin-D adequacy is probably at an all-time low, with the probable result that vitamin-D deficiencies are widespread and routinely misdiagnosed.

Many nutrition experts feel that the two most at-risk groups for a vitamin-D deficiency are the very young and the elderly. Thanks to the fortification of dairy products, rickets, the principal vitamin-D deficiency in the young, is quite rare, but there is still a concern because young bones are actively growing and developing, and need vitamin D. In recent decades there has been a well-documented decline in time spent outdoors due to the influences of computers, shopping malls, and television, and people are therefore deprived of needed sunshine. Older people are at risk because they also spend much of their time indoors. In addition, older skin produces less cholesterol and is therefore less efficient at generating vitamin D.

Vitamin D facilitates the absorption of calcium by providing the kidneys with a key hormone needed for calcium metabolism. In addition, several researchers have pointed out that the average vitamin-D intake (through sun exposure) declines the farther north you go, while certain cancers—breast, ovarian, and prostate—become more prevalent. This same correlation holds for hypertension, multiple sclerosis, and other diseases. Although no definitive evidence linking vitamin D with these diseases has yet been confirmed, research into a possible link is being investigated.

Vitamin E

Vitamin E, alpha tocopherol, as its most common form is known, is actually composed of a group of related tocopherol molecules known for their antioxidant activity. As fat-soluble vitamins, the tocopherols help to protect lipid-rich tissues, such as cellular and mitochondrial membranes, from oxidation. Vitamin E also helps reduce the stickiness of platelets and other elements in the blood, thereby reducing the risk of clots, infarctions (a loss of blood supply to the heart, causing a heart attack), and strokes. Vitamin E is helpful in reducing inflammation (phlebitis or vasculitis) in blood vessels. Vitamin E also plays an important role in muscular functioning, protection of the nerves, and reproduction.

The best sources for vitamin E include egg yolk, green leafy vegetables such as spinach, many raw nuts, in particular, almonds, Brazil nuts, hazelnuts, peanuts, and sunflower seeds, and unprocessed vegetable oils—the most nutrient dense being unrefined wheat germ oil. (*See also* Chapter 15 for additional information on vitamin E.)

Vitamin K

Vitamin K is probably the least understood fat-soluble vitamin. Its principal role involves the formation of blood-clotting factors, and it may be involved in the proper formation of bone calcium. Vitamin K comes mainly from green leafy vegetables, and it is thought that small amounts are synthesized by intestinal bacteria.

CHAPTER 17

Minerals

Literally every biochemical reaction and process in your body requires the presence of vitamins and minerals, which function as catalysts, facilitating the reactions that allow life to occur. Vitamins are organic, carbon-based molecules, and are complex chemical structures. By contrast, minerals are single elements. Though simple in makeup, minerals are equally important and necessary for life and health.

Traditionally, vitamins have gotten a lot more attention than minerals. From their earliest discovery, vitamins have always had an aura of mystery and promise. Discovered for their roles in preventing (or curing) specific diseases and problems, vitamins have always seemed to be a magic key that could unlock the closed doors of health and bring in its light. Even the very name, which comes from the concept of a *vital amine,* connotes the idea of a key to life itself. Minerals, on the other hand, have generally seemed more prosaic and down to earth, as simple elements commonly found in soil and other ordinary places.

Yet, if minerals suffer from this basic, subtle lack of respect and appreciation, it is not because they are unimportant to health. I often think of minerals as the spark plugs of the body, providing cells with the charge needed to get them running.

Similar to vitamins, minerals are often present in insufficient amounts for optimal functioning of the cells in your body. But minerals don't just need to be present in adequate amounts, they also need to be in the proper ratios with each other in order to be most effective, so it is necessary to look at the relative, as well as absolute, quantities of these important elements.

By definition, vitamins are *organic* (carbon-based) molecular compounds that plug into specific biochemical pathways in order to facilitate reactions in the body. Minerals, by contrast, are *inorganic* elements that also need to plug in at highly specific points along these pathways in order to serve as catalysts helping to speed up or slow down the body's processes.

Although there are more than a hundred known minerals, only about twenty-two are considered essential for human health. Of these, there are two basic categories: the major minerals, and the trace elements. Land-based minerals are widely dispersed throughout the crust of the earth, with soils varying dramatically in specific mineral composition, due to geological and other factors. Oceans, on the other hand, represent a more consistent picture of mineral composition, having come into equilibrium eons ago. Seawater is a mixture of virtually every mineral element found on earth. Although ultratrace elements exist in the oceans in extremely minute amounts, they may prove biologically important, because deficiencies of trace minerals are becoming more common throughout the world. In the future, ocean water, seafood, and sea vegetables may become increasingly important options for obtaining these vital elements.

MINERAL DEFICIENCIES

How can elements so commonly found in the earth be missing or deficient in the diet? Why should you be concerned about mineral density anyway? The answers can be found by looking at current agricultural practices, food production, processing, and lifestyle factors.

Many studies have documented that the mineral content of foods today is lower than in the past. The principal explanations for this decline have to do with the deteriorating quality and condition of contemporary soils due to current agricultural practices, and the genetic selection and breeding of plant varieties for appearance, ease of storage, and shelf life at the expense of nutrient content.

A plant's ability to absorb minerals is contingent on several factors, including the health of the soil and the types of fertilizers and other agricultural chemicals used. The uptake of trace minerals requires living, healthy soil, with microbes to secrete organic acids into the soil and create the proper conditions for plant roots to absorb minerals. In chemically treated soils, microbial activity is often close to zero, and in this semisterile soil climate, there is a dramatic reduction in the uptake of trace elements.

The mineral composition of plants is measurable; numerous studies have examined the relationship between soil health and plant-mineral denseness. Consistent findings of superior mineral content in organic produce underscore the importance of healthy, living soil for the absorption of minerals by plants.

Synthetic fertilizers have also done much to change the mineral profile of edible plants. In order to grow large, *apparently* healthy plants, you need little more than the basic macronutrients, and commercial fertilizers focus on these: nitrogen, phosphorus, and potassium, or N, P, and K for short. Using this sort of simplistic fertilizer may foster abundant plant growth, but these plants are nutritionally hollow. While they look good on the outside, the diversity and density of other minerals present in their tissues is greatly diminished.

Then there is the fact that many of the varieties of produce planted today by large agribusiness-dominated farming operations are heavily standardized, hybridized forms. Losing many of the older, more nutritious varieties as a trade-off for more marketability is yet another sacrifice that is ultimately paid by the consumer, and future generations.

Lastly, the heavy processing of many foods further lessens what nutrition is ultimately available to the purchaser. Milling whole wheat into white flour, for example, can lead to an 80 percent loss, or more, of the minerals originally in the grain. Chromium, copper, manganese, magnesium, and zinc are just some of the minerals that are drastically reduced by processing technologies.

However, not all the blame for poor mineral status can be blamed on agribusiness and the corporate interests that dominate the food markets today. Individual lifestyle patterns can also undermine the mineral density of your diet. Heavy sugar consumption, for example, depletes the body of certain minerals. Similarly, heavy alcohol consumption will also strip minerals from the body, potentially aggravating an already dangerous situation. For all these reasons, in *The Nutrient-Dense Eating Plan*, optimal mineral intake is one of the highest priorities.

THE MAJOR MINERALS

Calcium, magnesium, and phosphorus, and the electrolytes chloride, potassium, and sodium are the minerals found in the largest amounts in the body. All are required in relatively substantial amounts for optimal health and functioning.

Calcium

Of all the minerals, calcium is probably the best known, probably because it is the most abundant mineral in the body. The bulk of it, the part you hear most about, resides in the matrix of skeletal bone. But nonskeletal calcium, found in cells, in cell membranes, and in extracellular fluids, where it is vitally involved in such diverse functions as blood clotting, muscle contraction, and nerve transmission, is also crucial for your health.

Many foods provide abundant quantities of calcium. The dairy industry would have you believe it is impossible to get sufficient calcium in the diet without milk, but this simply is not true. Many nutritionists believe the big emphasis on getting enough calcium is exaggerated, and that the most important thing is not the sheer amount of calcium in your diet, but your ability to *retain* the calcium you ingest.

Studies of other cultures bear this out. In other parts of the world where dairy is not a major part of the diet, and where people consume far less calcium than in America, osteoporosis is not a common problem. There are many factors in the SAD diet, such as alcohol, caffeine, and sugar, that deplete the calcium in your body.

Soda, with its large contribution of phosphorus (phosphoric acid), upsets the body's calcium balance. The body interprets this sudden excess of phosphorus as a deficiency of calcium, and to compensate, calcium is pulled from its storage place in the bones to make more of it available in the bloodstream. When this is repeated over time, a chronic soda drinker develops a calcium deficiency and a much higher risk of developing osteoporosis. Some prescription medications can also interfere with the absorption, metabolism, or retention of calcium. The solution to osteoporosis in these cases, is not to consume more calcium, but to consume less of what creates such imbalances.

The most nutrient-dense sources of calcium are green vegetables, such as broccoli, collards, kale, and spinach, many beans and legumes, nonhomogenized raw milk and cheeses, sardines and other seafood with the bones cooked in, and tofu, when prepared with calcium sulfate. Almonds and sesame seeds are particularly rich in calcium, and many other nuts and seeds are nutrient-dense sources of calcium as well, including hazelnuts (filberts), peanuts, pistachios, sunflower seeds, and walnuts. Still other excellent sources include blackeyed peas, blackstrap molasses, figs, and tempeh.

Chloride

Chloride is typically found with sodium in salt. Chloride is abundantly supplied in most diets and is rarely a nutritional problem.

Magnesium

All minerals work by acting as catalysts to facilitate enzymatic reactions in your cells. For these reactions to occur, it is crucial for the right mineral to be in the right place at the right time, so it could be said that optimal health is dependent on the presence of these minerals.

The importance of magnesium can be easily understood by the fact that magnesium is required for more of these biochemical reactions than any other mineral. Researchers have documented more than 300 enzymatic reactions that are dependent on magnesium, and they cover the full spectrum of physiological activities. The ability to transport molecules across cell membranes, DNA transcription (the transfer of DNA information to RNA), glycolysis (the breakdown of sugar to release energy), muscle contraction and relaxation, nerve transmission, and protein synthesis are all magnesium-dependent processes. Clinically, such conditions as asthma, high blood pressure, menstrual cramps, and migraine headaches have responded well to magnesium supplements or to the addition of magnesium-rich foods to the diet. Inadequate magnesium intake can lead to cardiovascular problems, including cardiac arrhythmias, and high blood pressure. Alcoholism, the consumption of a diet dominated by highly processed foods (SAD), and generally poor nutrition are the primary reasons for inadequate magnesium. Processing whole-grain wheat and turning it into refined white flour, for example, makes the finished product lose more than 80 percent of the original magnesium content.

Many unprocessed plant-based foods are nutrient dense for magnesium, including nuts and seeds, particularly almonds, Brazil nuts, sesame seeds, and sunflower seeds. Chocolate, too, is rich in magnesium, especially unprocessed cocoa powder and dark chocolate, which is made with a higher percentage of magnesium-containing cocoa solids than milk chocolates. Hazelnuts, peanuts, and pistachios are also good sources. Other foods that are relatively nutrient dense for magnesium include leafy, dark green vegetables, tofu made with magnesium salts, and whole grains (especially quinoa and amaranth). Most fruits are relatively low in magnesium, with the exception of bananas and apricots. Mineral, or hard, water can also contribute magnesium to the diet. Several studies have even demonstrated a reduction in risk for hypertension (high blood pressure) and strokes in populations consuming magnesium-containing water. Meat and dairy are considered poor sources of magnesium.

Phosphorus

Phosphorus is closely involved with bone metabolism and is an important mineral linked to the metabolism of calcium and magnesium. As with many other minerals, the ratio of phosphorous to other minerals, particularly calcium, is highly significant. A phosphorus deficiency is unusual, however, since this mineral is present in nearly all foods, so the major concern with phosphorus stems from people getting too much, often due to its use as an additive in many processed foods. Fast foods may contribute 30 percent or more of its daily intake, and when consumed in excess relative to calcium, phosphorus may cause problems with the parathyroid glands, thereby upsetting calcium metabolism. Some researchers suspect this imbalance could be a possible contributor to the development of osteoporosis and related problems. Sodas are a major source of excess phosphorus because they contain phosphoric acid. A diet that is excessively high in protein but low in calcium-containing foods may also lead to an imbalance in the phosphorus/calcium ratio (*see also* Calcium section above).

Potassium and Sodium

The importance of the electrolyte potassium lies not so much in the absolute amounts of this mineral from the diet, but in its presence relative to another electrolyte, sodium. Most people get adequate amounts of potassium, but because of the high amounts of sodium added to processed food, the SAD diet has led to a reversal of the normal, healthy potassium/sodium ratio.

Potassium is widely present in unprocessed foods, particularly fruits, meats, nuts, seeds, vegetables, and whole grains. Blackstrap molasses is a very nutrient-dense source of potassium, as are many fruits, including figs and oranges. Since most of these foods have very low sodium levels, the normal diet of our ancestors consisted of much more potassium than sodium. For example, 100 grams of raw peanuts contain more than 700 milligrams of potassium, yet have less than 20 milligrams of sodium. Salted peanuts, however, may have as much sodium as potassium, and often more. This is true of many processed foods (*see* Table 17.1). Salt (sodium) is frequently added to food at an astronomical rate, and many researchers and nutritionists believe this imbalance is responsible for many of the health problems affecting consumers of the SAD diet.

TABLE 17.1. POTASSIUM AND SODIUM LEVELS OF PROCESSED AND UNPROCESSED FOODS

Food	Potassium	Sodium
Peanuts (raw)	705 mg	18 mg
Peanuts (roasted, salted)	612 mg	772 mg
Potatoes (boiled, no salt)	379 mg	4 mg
Potatoes (boiled, salted)	287 mg	256 mg
Potato chips	381 mg	755 mg
Whole-wheat flour	405 mg	5 mg
White flour	107 mg	2 mg
Wheat crackers	183 mg	795 mg

When examining the role of electrolytes, we can see how upsetting this ratio could lead to so many health problems. Electrolytes (chloride, sodium, and potassium) play key roles in the dynamics of blood pressure, cell membranes, the electrical charges between cells, and regulating water balance. Electrolytes are therefore of critical importance in helping to regulate the subtle interplay between the intracellular and extracellular environment. They are also crucial for the electrical activity of the heart and the proper functioning of muscles and nerves, and a chronic imbalance of electrolytes can lead to edema, high blood pressure, a lowered metabolic efficiency, and muscle weakness. Different types of salt seem to have different effects on electrolyte balance. Refined salt appears to be more detrimental to sodium-sensitive individuals, while unrefined sea salts (*see* Chapter 33) may be better tolerated, possibly due to the presence of trace elements not found in refined salt.

TRACE ELEMENTS

In addition to the major minerals (required in relatively large amounts), there are the essential trace elements, including chromium, copper, iodine, iron, manganese, selenium, sulfur, zinc, and sometimes fluoride and molybdenum, which, though not required in the same quantities, are nonetheless essential for optimal functioning and health. (In addition, there are a number of ultra-trace elements that are typically present in very small amounts, provided a diverse, mainly organic, diet is eaten. To ensure an adequate amount of ultra-trace elements in your diet, try to eat generous amounts of sea vegetables and use high-quality, unprocessed sea salt.)

Chromium

The trace mineral chromium plays an essential role in the metabolism of sugar and other carbohydrates because it is intimately involved with the functioning of insulin and glucose tolerance. The most nutrient-dense source of chromium is nutritional yeast, but other dense sources include black pepper, calves liver, some microbrew beers, wheat germ, and whole grains.

Copper

Copper is an important, but often overlooked, mineral in human nutrition. As with many minerals, copper is often paired with another element, zinc, which has traditionally grabbed most of the spotlight. Overshadowed by its more popular relative, copper is nonetheless essential and is frequently undersupplied by the SAD diet.

Similar to other trace minerals, an adequate copper supply is often contingent on healthy, balanced soils and on crops that can incorporate it into their tissues, not always a guarantee given today's agricultural practices. Copper is essential for numerous enzymatic reactions and for antioxidant systems involving protection of the heart and the vascular tissues. Copper is also necessary for bone metabolism, brain and nerve-cell development, heart rhythm, immune responsiveness, nerve transmission and function, and the synthesis of hemoglobin.

Copper deficiency is known to affect the strength and integrity of connective tissue, such as collagen. Therefore, insufficient copper can lead to an increase in aneurysms and strokes, and other problems including anemia, demyelination of the nerves, immune dysfunction, loss of pigmentation in hair or skin, and skeletal defects.

An excess of fructose, fruit sugar, is known to interfere with copper absorption, and can lead to a deficiency. This has now become a bigger concern due to the food industry's shift to high-fructose corn syrup as the commercial sweetener of choice in many prepared and packaged foods.

The most nutrient-dense sources of copper include cocoa and dark chocolate, liver, nutritional yeast, oysters and shellfish, some microbrew beers and, depending on the soil in which they grow, whole grains. Other relatively dense sources of copper include black pepper, and several types of nuts and seeds, particularly Brazil nuts and sesame seeds.

Iodine

Iodine's importance comes from its role as a key part of the thyroid hormone, which is crucial for the overall regulation of the body's metabolic rate of functioning. This trace element is well known for its role in preventing goiter (enlarged thyroid tissue), which can develop when the body tries to trap as much of this essential micromineral as it can. Severe iodine deficiency can even lead to cretinism and mental retardation.

Iodine is found primarily in seafood and sea vegetables (the most nutrient-dense source of this element). It is also to be found in land plants grown in soil containing adequate levels of iodine. Since many inland and mountainous regions contain very low levels of available iodine, the United States began the iodization of salt in 1924, resulting in a drastic reduction in goiter and other problems associated with iodine deficiency.

Additional sources of iodine include an excess from the dairy industry's use of it as a disinfectant to cleanse storage tanks and milking equipment, and its use as a dough conditioner in many commercial breads. Although neither commercial dairy products nor commercial breads are considered appropriate foods in a nutrient-dense diet, the excess of dietary iodine in the SAD diet has been a cause of concern for some nutritional researchers. Both too much and too little iodine have been equally linked to thyroid problems, including a hyperactive thyroid (thyrotoxicosis), and some goiters.

Iron

If calcium is the best known of the major minerals, iron is probably the most widely studied and appreciated of the *trace* elements. As the central component of hemoglobin, the principal pigment and oxygen carrier of blood, iron is intimately associated with life itself. Yet iron deficiency and its result, anemia, is the most prevalent mineral deficiency worldwide—ironic since iron is widely distributed throughout nature.

In addition to its importance for hemoglobin and the formation of healthy blood cells, iron is an essential element in numerous other biological functions. Myoglobin, an important protein in muscle metabolism, is iron-dependent. Apathy, fatigue, and lowered immune functioning are frequent symptoms of iron deficiency, as are learning disabilities. Some researchers feel attention deficit disorder (ADD) may also be related to iron insufficiency.

In the diet, iron is found in two principal forms: heme and nonheme iron. Heme (short for hemoglobin) iron comes from animal sources, such as fish, meat, and poultry. Nonheme iron is obtained from vegetable sources. The most nutrient-dense sources of heme iron include organ meats, red meats, and the dark meat of poultry. Nutrient-dense foods for nonheme iron include blackstrap molasses; cocoa solids (found in the highest percentage in dark chocolates); dark green leafy vegetables, such as beet greens, chard, collards, and kale; and raisins. Ascorbic acid (vitamin C) is thought to enhance the absorption of nonheme iron, which, relative to the heme form, is poorly absorbed.

Manganese

Manganese (not to be confused with the major mineral, magnesium) is an essential trace element involved in collagen and bone formation, energy production, glucose tolerance (sugar metabolism), overall skeletal growth, and reproductive integrity. In addition, manganese is an essential component of several antioxidant enzymes.

Manganese is present in a wide variety of plant foods, but again, soil composition has to be considered when looking at the ability of plants to supply this trace mineral in the diet. Black tea is considered one of the most nutrient-dense sources of manganese, along with cocoa, legumes, nuts (almonds, sesame seeds, sunflower seeds, walnuts, and especially hazelnuts) and whole grains. Dairy, poultry, and meat are considered poor sources of manganese.

Molybdenum

Molybdenum may seem like an obscure trace element, but it is as essential as any of its mineral relatives. Molybdenum's importance stems from its biochemical role in several key enzymes as a promoter of antioxidant function. Its other principal role involves the metabolism of certain amino acids. Molybdenum is adequately supplied by most healthy diets, as it is present in beans, lentils, nuts, peas, and whole grains. However, as with the other trace elements, adequate molybdenum is dependent on healthy, mineral-rich soils.

Selenium

Selenium is an important, well-studied trace element with impressively documented effects for maintaining and promoting health, including cancer prevention, cardiovascular health, and immune functioning. Selenium's main benefits are attributable to its crucial role in several antioxidant enzymes, including glutathione peroxidase, the principal enzyme involved in neutralizing harmful hydroperoxide free radicals. Numerous studies have documented the relationship between selenium intake and a reduced risk for several cancers, including those of the colon, lung, prostate, and rectum. Other studies have shown that people with skin cancer have lower levels of selenium in their blood than those without skin cancer.

Selenium deficiencies have also been associated with cardiomyopathy, a disease of the heart muscle. Other research has found positive associations between selenium intake and mood. Further, selenium is known to be vitally important for proper thyroid functioning, as it is essential for the biochemical conversion of the inactive form of thyroid hormone (T-4) to the active form (T-3) in the body.

The most nutrient-dense source of selenium is the Brazil nut. Most organ meats, such as kidney and liver, are dense sources, as are garlic, nutritional yeast (which is also a dense source of chromium and copper), and seafood. Although many grains are potentially good contributors of selenium, the amount of selenium in soil is known to vary widely, with some soils being very high in this mineral, while others are extremely depleted. This is another good argument for eating a diet containing foods grown from a variety of regions.

Sulfur

Sulfur is an important trace element that is incorporated into connective tissue and numerous proteins. In particular, sulfur is needed by the hair and skin, where it is found in abundance. It also activates numerous cellular enzymes.

The most nutrient-dense sources of sulfur include broccoli, Brussels sprouts, cabbage, cauliflower, chives, eggs, garlic, leeks, mustard greens, onions, and shallots.

Zinc

Zinc is a versatile metallic mineral that is necessary for most of the body's metabolic pathways. It is involved in the activation of more than 200 separate enzymes and is indispensable for cellular replication, growth and maturation, immune functioning, the metabolism of nucleic acids and protein, reproductive development, and wound healing. Zinc deficiencies are most likely in alcoholics, older people, and some vegetarians. A generally poor diet, liver disease, pregnancy, and surgery can also lead to a deficiency. Symptoms of insufficient zinc intake include altered taste and smell, changes in the quality of hair or skin, an increased susceptibility to colds, and poor wound healing. More than half the world's population is believed to get inadequate zinc from their diets.

The most nutrient-dense sources of zinc include eggs, liver, organic meats, oysters and other shellfish, and many nuts and seeds. Brazil nuts, sesame seeds, and sunflower seeds are especially dense sources for vegetarians, who tend to be more at risk for low-zinc intakes than meat eaters. Cocoa is also a good vegetarian source. Though controversial, many researchers believe that compounds called phytates, found in wheat and other cereal grains, can interfere with the uptake of zinc by binding to it and preventing its absorption. For this reason, vegetarians should pay even more attention to the densest sources of zinc.

ULTRA-TRACE MINERALS

In addition to the better-known major minerals and the less-known trace minerals, there is a class of elements called ultra-trace minerals. As the name implies, the ultra-trace minerals are found in extremely small amounts in foods and in the body. However, the fact they are not needed in substantial amounts does not mean they are unimportant. The ultra-trace minerals may buffer you from stressors or disease states in ways that are still not fully understood.

Human blood roughly parallels the salinity of the oceans, from which our distant ancestors (and all life) presumably evolved. Due to the forces of erosion and the movement of water and soil toward the seas, the oceans contain at least some of every element found on land. This includes such ultra-trace elements as antimony, boron, gold, rubidium, tin, titanium, and literally dozens of others. Although trace elements are present only in minuscule amounts there, the oceans constitute an important reservoir of these rare elements—in even small quantities of seawater, chemical analysis can detect their atoms.

The principle of diversity has been extensively mentioned in the pages of this book. An environmentally diverse farm, forest, or ocean is far healthier, more disease-resistant, and more resilient to sudden changes or stressors than any less diverse, monocropped system. People eating narrow, culturally or agriculturally limited food selections, especially food grown on depleted soils, may develop questionable levels of some of these ultra-trace minerals. In lieu of drinking seawater, and especially for those who do not live in a coastal region, eating more seafood and sea vegetables, and sprinkling your food with high-quality sea salts, might be effective ways of ingesting these diverse, and still underappreciated, elements.

CHAPTER 18

Protein from the Land

Protein, in an adequate quantity and quality, is a basic requirement of a healthy diet. A good understanding of how protein works for your specific lifestyle, metabolic needs, and unique genetic requirements is important, and nutrient-dense principles can help.

In nature, protein rarely occurs alone. In animal sources, it is usually accompanied by various fats. When supplied by plants, it is found in the company of carbohydrates and phytonutrients. Soy protein, for example, is present in soybeans, along with isoflavones, phytoestrogens, and other biologically active molecules. Protein is also typically found in conjunction with certain B vitamins, such as B_6, which is needed to help metabolize the protein.

Proteins are usually very large, complex molecules that act as key structural components of cells and tissues, including skin, collagen, and even bone. They also may be directly incorporated into biological molecules such as hemoglobin, hormones, nucleic acids (DNA), and neurotransmitters. Protein is the principal dietary source of nitrogen, an important component of amino acids, the most basic units of protein molecules.

Proteins are generally broken down during the digestive process, either into individual amino acids or very simple clumps of two to three amino acids called peptides. Once absorbed, many of these amino acids are recycled and reassembled as parts of a new protein. The body's ability to assemble needed proteins on demand requires a reservoir of available amino acids, as well as the presence of specific vitamins and trace minerals. Usually, this pool is adequate to meet most of your body's needs, but in times of extreme stress and metabolic demand, there may not be enough of these required amino acids to go around. Such protein malnutrition can result in a wide variety of negative consequences.

What are the most common food sources for protein, and what are the best and worst choices? Regardless of your lifestyle, *The Nutrient-Dense Eating Plan* can show you the best options for meeting your protein requirements. Broadly speaking, protein originates from several key areas of highest density—eggs, legumes, meats, nuts and seeds, seafood, whole grains, and for some, dairy products.

Protein quality is determined by the availability and proportion of the amino acids it supplies. For adults, eight essential amino acids are required to make complete proteins, and the diet should be dense for all of these. If your diet is consistently lacking in one or more of these essential amino acids, problems could arise. However, the well-known principle of protein combining or complementing amino acids for complete amino-acid availability means that most diverse diets should have no problem supplying all of your essential amino-acid needs.

MEATS

Meat is definitely one of the more controversial subjects in contemporary nutrition discussions. In this book, I intend to put aside the often difficult and intensely personal feelings people have about the farming, killing, and eating of animals. While such personal ethical and moral questions do have their place in any serious discussion of nutrition, *The Nutrient-Dense Eating Plan* does not tell people what to do or how to make such individual choices. Its purpose, instead, is to focus on the nutritional facts. If a person chooses to eat animal products, then that person should know what the safest, most nutrient-dense options are, and why. (Similarly, if someone chooses to avoid animal-based foods, then that person, too, should know exactly which foods are the most nutrient dense within the limits of that diet, in order to eat as healthily as possible.)

All meats are nutrient dense. They are high in easily absorbable iron, essential and nonessential fats, many of the B vitamins, selenium, zinc, and of course, protein. However, the quality and healthiness among the types of meat that are offered today varies considerably. The diets of many ancestral people show that animal protein was often a central part of their food supply. Traditional cultures and presumably our distant paleoancestors, got their meat from hunting—wild game was often the predominant source of their protein and many other nutrients. Today, most people get their store-bought meat prebutchered and packaged. Many studies point out the need to look carefully at the quality of such meat; more and more people have become aware that the majority of today's meat is produced with agricultural chemicals, including antibiotics and hormones, such as synthetic estrogens. There is also a growing awareness that the feed used to fatten farmed animals is questionable because it is grown with herbicides, pesticides, synthetic fertilizers, and related agricultural chemicals. Unnatural practices, such as feeding vegetarian animals (cattle and chickens) animal byproducts may also have the unforeseen, tragic consequences of mad cow disease and a similar sheep disease, scrapie. Being at the end of the food chain, humans should be properly cautious about what they are consuming.

Fortunately, some good alternatives are available. For meat eaters, I recommend using only the cleanest, safest, most natural meats possible. Increasing numbers of ranchers are raising grass-fed, free-range, antibiotic- and hormone-free meats, including beef, buffalo, chicken, elk, lamb, and venison, so consumers actually have more choices than ever before. Although meat raised this way is more expensive, I feel it is well worth the price. In terms of poor health and its associated costs, cheaply subsidized meats could make you end up paying a much higher price in the long run.

Studies of the wild game and foods our paleoancestors ate have revealed that such meat is consistently higher in minerals, lower in overall fat, and higher in essential fatty acids than commercially raised meats. Buffalo, for example, is lower than beef in cholesterol and total fat, and higher than beef in calcium, iron, magnesium, and protein. In addition, it has a better balance of the omega-6 and omega-3 essential fatty acids.

There is no question that these meats are nutrient-dense. In terms of daily requirements, a single serving of buffalo can contribute up to one-third of the requirement for protein, one-third of iron, 20 percent of phosphorus, 10 percent of vitamin B_3 (niacin), 15 percent of vitamin B_6, 30 percent of zinc, and 50 percent of the recommended daily serving of selenium.

Similarly, lamb can be a great, nutrient-dense alternative to beef or chicken. Lamb is particularly dense in niacin, pantothenic acid, protein, selenium, and zinc. Elk and venison are also excellent sources of protein, and are, overall, much leaner and lower in calories than commercial meats. Furthermore, these animals are raised with far fewer chemicals, drugs, and hormones.

My personal choices for meat-based proteins lean toward buffalo, elk, and lamb. I generally avoid chicken as it can be so chemically intensive. If I were served certified organic chicken, however, I would eat it, but I would never order it from a restaurant, unless I was certain it was organically raised. I feel the same about all pork products. I really consider pork unfit as a food, a feeling based partly on the way it is produced and partly on the way the animals are treated; I also consider pigs to be highly developed, intelligent animals. I fully admit this is not a scientifically based attitude, but nutrient-dense eating also involves a good bit of trusting your own instincts. To me, the wild, or less-domesticated animals, such as buffalo and elk, are more suitable food choices. As I have emphasized, many of the nutrient-dense principles about eating more naturally are attuned to ancestral patterns of eating.

LEGUMES AND WHOLE GRAINS

Whole grains, such as amaranth, barley, brown rice, kamut, millet, quinoa, teff, and wheat, are good sources of plant-based proteins. Grain-based proteins are incomplete in their amino acids, but even so, it is relatively easy to achieve a healthy balance of amino acids simply by eating a dense and diverse diet. Legumes, such as lentils, split peas, and the many dried beans, also are good sources of plant-based protein, and combined with brown rice or another whole grain, can supply all eight essential amino acids.

NUTS AND SEEDS

For our foraging ancestors, nuts and seeds meant a ready, nutrient-dense source of energy and protein. Almonds, Brazil nuts, hazelnuts, peanuts, pine nuts, pistachio nuts, pumpkin seeds, sesame seeds, and sunflower seeds are all useful, protein-rich, and nutrient-dense foods. However, as with most plant-source proteins, including legumes and whole grains, it is helpful to have a diet of diverse types of proteins, in order to balance out their incomplete amino acids.

EGGS

Of all protein sources, eggs are considered by scientists of nutrition to have an almost ideal proportion of amino acids for human health. Eggs are a consummate nutrient-dense food, as they are rich in many nutrients in addition to protein, including lecithin, vitamin A, cholesterol, and the mineral sulfur. Sulfur is actually supplied in the form of certain egg-containing amino acids, which have sulfur as their main constituent. In contrast, most amino acids are characterized by nitrogen, not sulfur. Sulfur amino acids are specialized and have numerous functions in the body; they are often used to make structurally important proteins, such as keratin, which is found in hair. A typical hen's egg contains approximately 8 to 9 grams of protein, all of which is highly bioavailable for use by the body.

DAIRY

Dairy is definitely a good source of protein. However, in general, *The Nutrien-Dense Eating Plan* does not endorse commercially produced dairy because of the numerous issues associated with its production, such as the heavy reliance on agricultural chemicals, including antibiotics and hormones. And because of potential problems associated with homogenization and pasteurization, I do not endorse even the organic brands of dairy products *unless* you are in the early stages of transitioning to a more nutrient-dense diet. The nutrient-dense solution to quality dairy lies in finding certifiably safe raw milk products in your area. Such dairy definitely exists in many parts of the country and is well worth seeking out.

CHAPTER 19

Protein from the Sea

Traditionally, seafood has always been considered one of the ideal protein sources. Now, some seafood is also being recognized as supplying copious amounts of the omega-3 essential fatty acids, which makes it doubly nutrient dense.

OCEANS AT THE CROSSROADS

As the single largest ecosystem, the world's oceans may well govern the health of the planet as a whole. They are the true lungs of the world. They act as a buffer for temperature control, a reservoir for oxygen and water, and they have been the home to much of the world's protein supply. The oceans are also mankind's true womb, the original birthplace of our evolutionary journey. The salty blood that runs through your veins is said to reflect your oceanic origins.

These days, however, much of the news concerning the oceans of the world is troubling. Reports of serious threats to the health of coral reefs, fish populations, sea mammals, sea turtles, shores, and the waters themselves, are everywhere. Agricultural and industrial runoff (including mercury) from every continent, overfishing, the use of the oceans and seas as toxic dumping grounds, and the closing of some public beaches as unsafe, all seem to indicate that the great and vast oceans of the planet represent both a battleground and a crossroads.

If so, then the foods obtained from the oceans will ultimately reflect the consequences of these destructive acts. There is still much that is safe and healthy in the world's waters, but for the first time in human history, it is vital we become better informed in order to minimize the risks, optimize the benefits, and act to help safeguard a healthy and adequate supply of seafood for future generations.

Research has linked fish consumption with many health benefits, including a lowered risk for arthritis, heart attacks, high blood pressure, prostate cancer in men, and strokes. Because of its nutrient denseness, seafood can help you meet your dietary needs for calcium, essential fats, iodine, and protein. And, as discussed in Chapter 24, Sea Vegetables (Seaweed), plants from the oceans can be uniquely nutrient-dense sources of phytonutrients and, most particularly, of hard-to-obtain trace minerals. So what is there to worry about?

CAUTIONS FROM THE SEAS

For the first time in human history, there are very real concerns regarding the sustainability of current harvests. Around the world, many formerly abundant populations of fish have crashed or been dramatically reduced, and many previously robust fish industries have all but ceased to exist, due to a lack of fish. Cod, orange roughy, sea bass, shrimp (now primarily farm raised), swordfish, tuna, whiting, and even shark, are just some of the fish in grave danger of being fished to near-extinction.

Toxic contamination of certain varieties of fish seems to pose a definite problem to human health as well. Recently, mercury contamination has received a lot of publicity, and will probably continue to do so. As a neurological poison and biological toxin, mercury runoff into the oceans from land-based industries is a major, long-term problem because this heavy metal tends to bio-accumulate up the food chain. As larger fish consume smaller fish, the mercury in the predators' bodies builds up. Therefore, certain species of fish (the larger, longer-lived species in particular) tend to have higher levels of mercury stored in their bodies. Most of these species have traditionally been, in fact, the most desirable for humans as food sources. But because of concerns over mercury contamination, increasing numbers of specialists are cautioning against eating these larger species of free-ranging ocean fish, such as king mackerel, sea bass, shark, swordfish, tilefish, and some tuna species, including ahi.

Other concerns with contaminants are centered on farmed seafood, or aquaculture, a rapidly expanding enterprise that includes salmon, shrimp, tilapia, and several other commercially important species. As a result of the types of feed used, some studies have found that levels of polychlorinated biphenyls (PCBs) are much higher in farm-raised salmon than in the wild varieties. Other concerns with farmed fish include the use of antibiotics and chemicals, genetic modification of the fish, the presence of parasites and disease, and the lowered nutritional quality, including lowered levels of omega-3 fats.

However, if you choose carefully, and with an awareness of where the food comes from, I believe you can still eat healthy, high-quality, nutrient-dense seafood as a way of getting good protein.

THE NUTRIENT-DENSE CHOICES

So, what choices do you have if you want healthy, nutrient-dense seafood? While several species of formerly popular fish are no longer widely available, others are still relatively abundant and safe. *The Nutrient-Dense Eating Plan* recommends eating fish and seafood from the cleanest coldwater sources possible—the Arctic and northern waters of the Pacific and Atlantic oceans; these fish include halibut, mackerel, sardines, and (wild) salmon. In addition to their high quality, a relatively large quantity of these fish still exist, although their numbers are lower than in the past.

Salmon and sardines, in particular, are good sources of omega-3 essential fatty acids, while halibut is a great source of protein. The caliber of protein in most seafood is, in fact, excellent. A four-ounce serving of salmon contains 25 grams of protein, which is close to half a day's protein requirement for most adults. Similarly, a single serving of canned sardines can supply 30 to 50 percent of your daily need for protein, while contributing anywhere from 20 to 40 percent of your calcium requirements, in addition to omega-3 essential fatty acids.

Sardines are probably one of the most underutilized and underappreciated foods today. They deserve a much wider audience. Although many canned foods have a less-than-fresh connotation (bringing to mind overcooked canned vegetables or ultrapasteurized condensed milk), canned sardines are a convenient way to buy and store a ready-made, nutrient-dense source of protein, fats, and (especially) calcium. They also supply approximately 10 percent of the RDA for iron, as well as a modest amount of healthy (nonoxidized) cholesterol. Roy Walford, M.D., a much-respected gerontologist and author, highly recommended sardines as a nutrient-dense source of nucleic acids in *The 120-Year Diet,* a book he wrote on anti-aging and caloric restriction.

In the years ahead, the conditions of the oceans will continue to get attention and scrutiny from scientists and the media. In order to preserve the legacy of abundance from the seas, a lot of hard work will have to be done. As you can see, nutrient-dense eating gives you a lot of opportunities to take responsibility—for your own health, and for the health of the planet, your home.

CHAPTER 20

Fats and Oils

Of all the components in people's diets, the most controversial and least understood seem to be fats. Though they play an essential role in human health, our culture's ongoing fat phobia has created an atmosphere in which it is difficult to find an objective appreciation for this important class of nutrients. Instead of being celebrated for their numerous biological functions, fats and oils seem to receive a disproportionate load of the blame for people's nutrient-weak diets and overall poor health. This includes obesity, now considered epidemic, which probably has more to do with the *types* of fats being eaten today because, according to nutrient-dense wisdom, there is nothing intrinsically unhealthy in fats themselves.

The Nutrient-Dense Eating Plan differs from much of today's prevailing wisdom by strongly distinguishing good fats from bad fats. Like every other category of foods, fats and oils can be looked at from the perspective of their quality, or denseness. When not taken in excess, the right fats and oils have vitally important contributions to make to the human diet. Therefore, in order to be able to evaluate them properly, it is important to understand their functions in your body and what benefits individual fats and oils can offer nutritionally. This is especially true of the lipids, since they have the capacity to help or harm, depending on their freshness, quality, and source, and on how they are altered by processing or refining.

Much of the hysteria surrounding fats in the diet is due to the numerous correlations drawn between fat intake, cancer, heart disease, and obesity. This is understandable in light of the fact that most of the edible oils are actually highly processed, refined products of questionable nutritional value. From an historical/evolutionary standpoint, these oils are unnatural and unprecedented. Looking at fat intake from a nutrient-dense perspective, you can begin to see what constitutes good, natural fats, and how they can build, rather than destroy, your health, when used discerningly.

DIFFERENCES BETWEEN FATS AND OILS

Fats and oils are collectively known as lipids, a miscellaneous class of organic substances not ordinarily soluble in water, that are composed principally of chains of carbon atoms, along with atoms of hydrogen and oxygen. Lipids include the animal fats, cholesterol, molecules known as phospholipids, and vegetable oils. Fats are lipids that are solid at room temperatures. Oils are lipids that are liquid at room temperature. These distinctions are of great importance biologically and nutritionally, and are due to differences in the chemical bonds that hold these molecules together.

THE FUNCTIONS OF LIPIDS

Though commonly misunderstood, fats and oils play a crucial part in the big picture of human health, and their multiple roles affect how the body functions on many levels.

Lipids in Cell Membranes

As noted, what sets lipids apart from other biologically important substances is their insolubility in water. Since most of your body is composed of water or water-soluble compounds, this distinction is of great consequence. By keeping water out, lipids are primarily responsible for compartmentalizing key structures, and keeping the boundaries of your tissues intact. Lipids are essential components of all cellular membranes; without them you would, for example, quickly become waterlogged when you went for a swim or took a shower. Cellular and intracellular membranes are among the most important structures in the body, playing a key role in maintaining the shape and integrity of cells and tissues.

Membranes are also the means through which cells become aware of their surrounding environment, including cell-to-cell communication. Membranes are essentially the *skin* of the cells, and their lipid components help facilitate communication and responsiveness between the cells and their environment. The vigilance of white blood cells, for example, results in the healthy functioning of the immune system, and these cells are, in turn, dependent on the normal functioning of their cellular membranes as they seek and destroy foreign invaders, pathogens, and other potentially harmful substances.

This notion of boundaries is central to many of the functions of lipids. Cell membranes are highly selective in actively distinguishing between what should enter the cell and what should be kept out. Keeping potentially toxic substances out, while allowing in such necessary compounds as nutrients and other important building blocks, is therefore largely dependent on the integrity and health of the membranes. *And the health of these membranes is, in turn, largely determined by what types of fats and other lipid materials they consist of.* Much of the current understanding of how the immune system functions is, in fact, based on this knowledge of how cell membranes operate, and their vital importance and subtle complexities are increasingly being appreciated by biologists and physiologists.

Lipids as Energy Sources

Lipids play numerous other roles as well. Fats and oils are unparalleled as energy sources. Proteins and carbohydrates each supply approximately four kilocalories of energy (a unit of heat) per gram, but fats and oils provide approximately nine kilocalories per gram, more than twice that amount. This gives fats more than *twice* the energy density of protein and carbohydrates. Burning fats for fuel provides you with an abundant source of energy, and spares such substances as amino acids from being utilized for energy production, preserving them for their important roles in building proteins. And, in addition to supplying you with a concentrated source of fuel, fats provide you with warmth and protection. Fats cushion, insulate, nourish, and protect vital organs.

Lipids as Transporters of Fat-Soluble Vitamins

Fats also act as the vehicle for carrying the fat-soluble vitamins A, D, E, and K, all of which need a lipid-rich medium in order to be effectively absorbed. In fact, a diet that is too low in fats could end up creating a deficiency of these important fat-soluble vitamins, which have astonishingly diverse functions, including antioxidant activity, the metabolism of calcium, the proper clotting of blood, and the regulation of immune functioning.

Lipids as Creators of Compounds

Lipids are also important because they can combine with other substances to make additional classes of biologically important compounds. Phospholipids, such as lecithin, and lipoproteins are being increasingly recognized for their roles in maintaining normal functioning and health. Another famous lipid, cholesterol, is so vital that it is produced in the body. Cholesterol will be fully discussed later (*see* Chapter 28, Dairy), but suffice it to say here that cholesterol and its related kinfolk, steroidal and adrenal hormones, constitute an extremely important class of biological molecules. Without these lipid-based molecules, life as we know it could not exist.

Lipids as the Source of Essential Fatty Acids

Lipids are also the source of essential fatty acids (EFAs). As the name implies, EFAs are *necessary* for the proper functioning of the human body. In the same way that you rely on food to supply you with the essential compounds called vitamins, your diet must also give you a certain amount of essential lipids, or fatty acids.

Most fatty acids (the functional units of lipids) are not indispensable, or essential, but do, however, serve as useful sources of energy and as building blocks for more complex molecules. On the other hand, the essential fatty acids, EFAs, *must* be present, or people will begin to experience deficiencies, which can include behavioral disturbances, a decline in fertility, growth retardation, hair and scalp problems, heart and circulatory problems, inflammatory changes, miscarriages, poor wound healing, problems with immune functioning, skin disorders, and other problems.

A nutrient-dense diet rich in healthy sources of fats and oils will provide adequate amounts of these essential, useful lipids. In contrast, the SAD diet often provides marginal quantities, and worse, contributes substantial amounts of unhealthy fats, such as highly processed, oxidized, and trans fatty acids. Fat phobia toward these commercial oils is certainly justified, but on the other hand, you should *not* avoid high-quality, minimally processed, and naturally occurring fats and oils. In the nutrient-dense diet, these foods are actually valued and sought out.

OILS TO USE, OILS TO AVOID

Good oils are extremely healthy and important, and your body can find many ways to utilize them. Their presence signals messages of abundance and health. Poor-quality oxidized or rancid oils, on the other hand, can be quite detrimental, acting as potent generators of harmful free radicals that can attack and damage cell membranes and other sensitive tissues. What's more, evidence is emerging from scientific studies that the wrong types of lipids can signal the cell's nucleus to alter its gene expression (how the cell's genetic code manifests itself), altering its metabolism, and resulting in the possibility of cancer and other diseases.

Refined and Hydrogenated Oils

The Nutrient-Dense Eating Plan strongly discourages consuming hydrogenated oils, partially hydrogenated vegetable shortening, any margarine or shortening containing hydrogenated fats, and trans fatty acids. Additionally, the crops that yield cottonseed and peanut oils receive some of the highest levels of pesticides, so these oils should also be curtailed or eliminated, as should butter-margarine combination spreads, nonorganic butter, and refined vegetable oils. I also recommend eliminating, or at least drastically cutting back on, all fried foods, including deep-fried tacos, egg rolls, French fries, fried fish and chicken, potato and corn chips, and tempura. When the oils used to cook these foods get exposed to the high temperatures needed for deep frying, they begin to rapidly degrade, a process that leads to free-radical formation. While *all* free radicals are considered potentially harmful, free radicals from oils are considered particularly damaging. I would also limit the amount of oil-based salad dressings you use because these oils are almost always highly refined. And for the same reason, I would avoid the oil and vinegar offered at salad bars or restaurants.

In *The Nutrient-Dense Eating Plan,* I particularly emphasize avoiding hydrogenated oils if you desire to build and maintain good health. It is becoming common knowledge that hydrogenated and partially hydrogenated vegetable oils are completely unnatural, man-made, altered fats used solely to extend the shelf life of processed foods and confer a desired texture (crispiness, for example) in these products. Other than these commercial uses, hydrogenated oils have no beneficial use in the human body whatsoever.

The negative effects of these fats are due to the presence of trans fatty acids, the chemical byproducts of the hydrogenation process. These trans fats are seldom encountered in natural diets, and current research is studying their effects. You should be very careful about introducing these easily incorporated, but unrecognizable (in terms of evolutionary exposure) and unprecedented, molecules into your body.

Unfortunately, until a scientific consensus is reached on the risks from hydrogenated trans fats, food processors and their corporations will continue to use these mutant fats because, as of now, it is far too profitable to stop. This trend may slowly be changing, but why wait for them to change the makeup of their products? You can reach your own personal conclusions, based on scientific research and common sense, and you can follow the principles of nutrient density, which state strongly that hydrogenated oils have no place in a health-oriented diet.

The leading source of hydrogenated oils and trans fatty acids in the typical American diet is margarine. It is virtually always made from the hydrogenation of vegetable oils and has long been (erroneously) promoted as a healthier alternative to butter. Some margarines use corn oil as a base, while others use soybean or safflower oil. Many health food stores carry margarines made from soybean oil, and people often buy these products in the mistaken notion they are somehow safe, healthy products, due to soy's reputation as a healthy food. Clever labeling that employs pastoral or country scenes is, of course, designed to reinforce that concept.

Margarine is far from the only source of trans fats in the American food supply, however. Hydrogenated vegetable shortening is widely found in a broad range of packaged and canned products, which routinely use this processed vegetable fat to increase the shelf life and create a crisp texture in their products. Virtually everyone on the SAD diet ingests hydrogenated oils and its trans fats every day.

Since it was never nature's intent to have these fats as part of your food supply, the human body simply does not have the means to metabolize or utilize them. Therefore, they tend to build up in body tissues, increasing as time goes on. Breast cancer, cellulite fat deposits, and obesity are all linked to trans fat ingestion.

Many of us who have lectured and written on the implications of ingesting hydrogenated oils for more than twenty-five years are amazed at the number of people who continue to buy margarine and other offending products, and do not bother to read the labels prior to buying them. This tells me people have been inadequately informed about the seriousness of the threat these hydrogenated oils pose to their health. The broad presence and acceptance of these substances in the food supply seems to provide them with some kind of legitimacy in the minds of the public. It is easy to dismiss hydrogenated substances as a not-too-serious problem—a classic example of a threat that affects people gradually, cumulatively, and imperceptibly. In terms of *The Nutrient-Dense Eating Plan,* however, the elimination of hydrogenated oils is essential in learning how to dramatically improve your diet and your health.

What *is* known about hydrogenated fats? For one thing, these fats were not in the American diet until the 1930s, but their usage has greatly increased from that time until the present. Today just about every mainstream food company uses them extensively. Hydrogenated oils are now so commonplace that virtually all packaged products contain them. Hydrogenated vegetable shortening is the basis of all commercial margarines, and is equally ubiquitous in all baked goods and pastry-type products. Breads, breakfast pastries, cakes, candies, cookies, corn and potato chips, crackers, desserts, muffins, premade pizza crusts, tortillas, snack foods, and many other foods are almost always guaranteed to contain partially hydrogenated oils. My personal policy regarding shopping is simple: I always read the label on any product I might buy, and as soon as I see the words *hydrogenated vegetable oil* or *partially hydrogenated vegetable oil* (or *shortening*), back on the shelf it goes.

Am I making too much out of something that may only be present in certain foods, and then only in small amounts? The fact is, since they are foreign to your system, there are no enzymes or biochemical processes available to the body to get rid of them efficiently. Trans fats get metabolized out of your body very slowly, and if you have been eating the typical SAD diet that is loaded with them, you have, as I said, been steadily accumulating these trans fats in your tissues.

Currently, research is investigating links between levels of trans fats in the body and risks for certain cancers, heart and vascular diseases, and other problems. The well-known Harvard-based nutrition researcher, Walter Willett, has stated that hydrogenated oils constitute ". . . the most significant culprit in generating heart disease, cancer, and diabetes." And, in July 2002, the National Academy of Sciences declared that trans fatty acids were, quite simply, unsafe for consumption.

The Good Oils

Fats often accompany many of the most delicious, fun foods, so if you have to avoid all the negative lipids, then what does that leave you with? Can you still enjoy food if you have to eliminate so many foods you have grown up with and genuinely enjoy?

Fortunately, the answer is yes because there are still many excellent, nutrient-dense sources of healthy fats and oils available to you. As you have seen, *The Nutrient-Dense Eating Plan* strongly recommends seeking out *the highest quality* carbohydrates, proteins, and fats, so there is no contradiction between eating healthily and eating deliciously.

Take a look at some of the most delicious, highest-quality sources of good fats and oils. They make up a very long list, which includes avocados, butter (organic only), eggs (boiled), flaxseed oil, nuts and seeds (almonds, Brazil nuts, pine nuts, pumpkin seeds, sesame seeds, sunflower seeds, walnuts), olives, sardines and other oily fish (cod, halibut, haddock, mackerel, salmon), moderate and fatty cuts of meats (buffalo, elk, lamb, organic beef, venison), and nut butters (almond butter, pumpkin seed butter, sunflower seed butter, tahini).

Fatty acids play numerous vital roles in multitudes of biochemical reactions involving the production of energy within cells. Because they are critically important for transporting electrons and interacting with oxygen, fatty acids are central to life itself. It is no wonder, then, that nature has provided so many nutrient-dense foods to ensure an abundant supply of these important molecules. EFAs are frequently present in metabolically active foods. Nuts and seeds, for example, are among the richest sources of EFAs, because they must contain all the nutrients necessary to support a new generation of organisms and ensure that sprouting plants get a robust, healthy start in life.

Furthermore, plants growing in colder climates tend to have higher amounts of essential fatty acids than their southern counterparts. Walnuts, a northern nut tree, have higher levels of essential fatty acids than pecans, which grow in southern climates. The northern-adapted flax plant is perhaps the richest single plant source of the important EFA known as linolenic acid. Flaxseed oil, available in health food stores (where it should always be refrigerated), is a truly superb supplemental food; it is an important addition to a nutrient-dense diet. Other good, plant-based sources of healthy oils include raw almonds and sunflower seeds. Freshly pureed nut butters, such as almond butter and sunflower seed butter, are particularly convenient ways to get healthy oils into your system. As with all oily foods, always store them in your refrigerator to maintain their freshness.

Similar to plants, fish from the coldest waters tend to have the highest levels of EFAs in their body tissue because a greater percentage of unsaturated body oils help keep them from freezing in Arctic waters. Cod, halibut, mackerel, and salmon are especially good sources of these polyunsaturated essential fatty acids. Many studies are backing up claims that coldwater fish are extremely important nutritional aids in treating a wide range of disorders and problems. Besides being useful sources of essential oils, sardines and anchovies are dense sources of protein and calcium. Cod-liver oil has been used as a potent health tonic for generations, and more recently, sushi and other forms of seafood have also been highlighted for their importance in maintaining, treating, and building health.

Eggs and Essential Oils

The egg is one of the most versatile and nutrient dense of all foods. Eggs contain a wide spectrum of crucially important nutrients, including protein and several important vitamins. Though less appreciated for their healthy lipids (cholesterol included), they can be a wonderful source of good fats as well. Egg yolks, which contain the fats in whole eggs, are approximately 30 percent lipids, and in free-range eggs, one-third of these fats are essential fatty acids. Unfortunately, the feed used for commercially raised eggs seldom contains EFAs, so the fats from those eggs have lower EFA levels.

Eggs are also nature's finest source of phospholipids. Made from a combination of fat molecules and the mineral phosphorus, phospholipids are complex, biologically important compounds with a variety of crucial functions, particularly in cell membranes and neurons, and are considered vitally important to brain and nervous-system functioning. The best known of the phospholipids is lecithin, and egg yolks are nature's most nutrient-dense source of this important phospholipid.

Dairy products can be a good source of fats as well, but a high percentage of them are saturated fats. These can be used for energy, but in general dairy contains few essential fatty acids.

Cooking Oils

Cooking oils need to be quite stable in order to resist breaking down during exposure to high temperatures—heat, light, and oxygen are the three biggest enemies of unsaturated oils. Unsaturated oils contain chemically vulnerable multiple double bonds, the weak links in lipid molecules and the places most susceptible to oxidation upon exposure to heat and light. When double bonds become oxidized, free radicals are generated, and the result is rancid oil molecules.

Highly unsaturated (polyunsaturated) oils, are therefore more prone to oxidative breakdown compared to saturated fats. Not too long ago, everyone was saying that polyunsaturated oils were, by far, the healthiest way to go. Today, however, many nutritionists are revising their thinking. Saturated fats are less vulnerable to oxidative damage than unsaturated fats, more stable, and therefore safer to use for sautéing and frying at the higher temperatures these methods require.

In line with this, I recommend butter, coconut oil, ghee (clarified butter), or olive oil for frying or sautéing. Although *The Nutrient-Dense Eating Plan* prefers boiling, poaching, or steaming to frying, when frying or sautéing is unavoidable, these saturated oils tend to stand up to the heat better and don't break down as easily when exposed to the high temperatures in a skillet or wok. While none of these fats supply the essential fatty acids that nuts, seeds, or coldwater fish do, they will at least not be as prone to creating harmful free radicals as their more unsaturated relatives are.

Coconut Oil

Coconut oil, also known as coconut fat or coconut butter (due to its high percentage of saturated fatty acids, it is solid at normal room temperatures), is a unique and underappreciated lipid with some surprising qualities. As a saturated vegetable oil, coconut oil is heat-stable for high-temperature sautéing and frying. It keeps very well, as it resists rancidity better than most fats. When unrefined, it has a delicious, mild coconutlike taste and aroma that enhances many dishes, and often evokes Southeast Asian cuisine.

Several studies have shown that coconut fat in the diet can improve indicators of cardiovascular health by lowering cholesterol overall, and raising the good form of cholesterol (HDL), while lowering the bad form (LDL). It has been noted that Polynesian and Indonesian cultures traditionally relied on coconut butter as their principal cooking oil yet did not suffer from heart disease, but it is also important to note that they use it very sparingly. It is ironic that cultures such as ours, which principally use unsaturated oils and hydrogenated oils (margarines and shortenings) have enormously high levels of cardiovascular disease.

Coconut oil is also unique in that it is made up of a high proportion of short- and medium-chain triglycerides, known to be more readily available for energy production. Several researchers have shown that coconut oil can reliably stimulate overall metabolism and, when used in moderation, can help cause gentle, natural, consistent weight loss without dieting.

Finally, coconut oil contains a substantial percentage of a specific fatty acid known as lauric acid, which has strong antiviral and antifungal properties, and is known to support the immune system. Some doctors even recommend coconut oil to help restore a better balance of intestinal flora, because lauric acid may help suppress growth of the yeast, candida.

Due to their origins, coconut and palm oils are often referred to as tropical oils. In the 1980s, there was a lot of negative publicity about the dangers of these oils. As a result, many people now believe that saturated tropical oils, such as coconut oil, are unequivocally bad for the arteries and the heart. However, much of this bad press was created by competing interests in the vegetable-oil industry, which may make it suspect. There is at least some evidence that saturated vegetable oils, such as coconut and palm oils, behave differently in the body compared to saturated fats from animal sources. Since a high proportion of the saturated fatty acids in these tropical oils are in the form of medium-length chains, they get used more readily for energy production, and do not get deposited in atherosclerotic plaques.

I believe the many qualities of coconut oil—its stability to heat, the presence of compounds such as medium-chain fatty acids, and its taste—all qualify it for a prominent place in nutrient-dense cooking.

Butter

Being more saturated than most vegetable oils, butter is similar to coconut oil, and is therefore desirable for baking, cooking, or light sautéing. Composed of a broad spectrum of fatty acids, butter can also be a dense contributor of fat-soluble vitamins, particularly vitamin A.

Since butter is a dairy food, my focus centers on whether or not it is organic. Most agricultural chemicals, including antibiotics, fungicides, pesticides, and synthetic hormones, are fat soluble, so they will accumulate in fatty tissues and foods, butter included. Therefore, if you choose to eat and cook with butter (as I do), then it is doubly important to buy certifiably organic brands—the right thing for you and the environment.

Many people who are lactose and dairy sensitive avoid butter. However, since butter is virtually 100 percent fat and contains only trace amounts of the proteins and carbohydrates found in whole milk, many of these dairy-sensitive people find they can use butter with no problem. Over the years, I have rarely encountered a lactose-intolerant patient in my practice who could not tolerate butter.

Finally, it should be noted that all the commercial butter on the market, including the organic brands, is derived from pasteurized milk. Though I am unaware of any studies on how such butter compares nutritionally to butter from raw, unprocessed whole-milk cream, I can say there *is* a clear difference in texture and taste. I do, however, regularly purchase commercial, organic brands of butter because fresh cream butter is seldom available. On the occasions I do find it (in rural areas or at farmer's markets), I consider it a treat, and gratefully appreciate every mouthful.

Olive Oil

Along with butter and coconut oil, olive oil completes the big three cooking oils. Whole books have been written about olive oil, stacks of research articles attest to its health benefits, and olive oil has gained media attention due to its seemingly protective relationship in heart disease. Along with garlic, olive oil is one of the principal components of the well-studied Mediterranean diet, which is, in fact, associated with lower-than-usual levels of cardiovascular disease, although this effect is probably related more to the overall nutrient density of this eating lifestyle than to olive oil alone.

Depending upon the extraction techniques used, olive oil is classified as pure, virgin, or extra virgin. The most natural oils are graded extra virgin, which means that only mechanical means (presses) are used to squeeze out the oil. This grade of olive oil has the most color and flavor, and the highest levels of organic acids, pigments, and other compounds. Virgin olive oils come from the second pressing, and additional means, such as heat, are used, if necessary, to improve the efficiency of

Benefits of the Mediterranean Diet

There are five main nutrient-dense aspects to the Mediterranean diet. First, besides the high consumption of garlic and olive oil, there is the use of many antioxidant-rich plant foods, such as the herbs basil, oregano, and rosemary. Then, there are the antioxidant phenolic pigments associated with red wine, also considered important aspects of the diet's heart-healthy qualities. And the diet includes a high level of fish and other beneficial seafoods known to be nutrient dense for essential fats. Finally, the Mediterranean diet is traditionally low in excess sugar, fried and refined oils, hydrogenated oils, and pasteurized, homogenized dairy products. All of these taken together, olive oil included, make it a very healthy diet.

extraction. This oil has less flavor and fewer of the original pigments compared to the extra virgin grade, but is still relatively good-quality oil. Pure olive oil sounds good, but is actually the most highly processed of the three grades. In this case, chemical solvents (usually hexane or a related petrochemical) are applied to the leftover olive skins, pulp, and seeds, in order to pull out any remaining oil and ensure that nothing is wasted.

Similar to the process used to produce many other foods today, olive growers frequently use herbicides, insecticides, and synthetic fertilizers. But organic olive oils are widely available and are highly recommended to help reduce the overall burden of chemicals in your body and on the land that grows these wonderful trees.

Flaxseed Oil

There are two major families of essential fatty acids, named omega-3 and omega-6 after their chemical structure, and they are the sources of the two principal essential fatty acids, linolenic acid and linoleic acid. As with vitamins and the essential minerals, these two essential fatty acids are absolutely necessary for your health. Alpha-linolenic acid is classified as an essential omega-3 fatty acid, and is less common in the normal diet. Linoleic acid, far more common in the SAD diet, is the omega-6 essential fatty acid.

Many researchers in the health field today believe these two families of fatty acids are out of balance in people's diets. They point out that the diets of most indigenous people, as well as those of our distant ancestors, consisted of much greater quantities of omega-3 oils than the diets of today. In fact, today processing and the widespread availability of oils dominant in omega-6 fatty acids has led to a ratio that is far from the historical norm. Packaged and fast foods are typically very high in the omega-6s and almost devoid of the omega-3s. Since the metabolic pathways these two families take in the body are so different, many researchers believe there could be a strong link between this unprecedented imbalance and many of the inflammatory disease states so prevalent today.

Fortifying your diet with omega-3 fats is one solution to this imbalance. The two classic sources of oils rich in omega-3 fatty acids are coldwater (marine) fish and flaxseed oil. Although flaxseed is not the only oil that contains omega-3 fatty acids, it is unique in that more than half its fats are these rare alpha-linolenic fatty acids. Although flaxseed oil has only been readily available since the 1980s, it is now widely used, and I consider it an exceptionally important nutrient-dense food. It is certainly the densest vegetarian source of linolenic acid. Flaxseed oil should always be bought refrigerated and stored in your refrigerator. Try to avoid leaving it out after using it—oils are incredibly sensitive to heat, humidity, light, and oxygen. What I appreciate about the companies that make this product is the obvious care they put into the production and packaging of their oil. Virtually all flaxseed oil sold in this country is packaged in either brown glass or opaque black plastic bottles that are flushed with nitrogen or argon (an inert gas), which eliminates most of the oxygen from the bottle. Then, almost every brand is shipped and stored under constant refrigeration.

Flax and similar quality oils are sensitive to heat so it is best not to cook with them, but rather to incorporate them in salad dressings, or other cold foods, such as egg salad, guacamole, hummus, tofu spread, and tuna or potato salad. I also use flax oil as a condiment, drizzling it on brown rice (or other grains), steamed broccoli, or other vegetables, in place of olive oil or melted butter.

Cod-Liver Oil

Although many people groan at the thought of taking a spoonful of cod-liver oil, the fact is, grandma was right. This fresh oil, pressed from North Atlantic cod, is extraordinarily rich in the omega-3 fatty acids, EPA and DHA, and is also a superb source of the fat-soluble vitamins A and D. I find that cod-liver oil is especially useful in the fall and winter months when there is less daylight. It is probably no coincidence that this time of the year correlates with: (a) an increase in colds and flu; (b) seasonal affective disorder (SAD) and other forms of depression; and (c) a decrease in vitamin-D synthesis. Cod-liver oil is very important for pregnant and lactating mothers—research on DHA strongly associates this nutrient with the intelligence and immunologic health of infants. There is no doubt that cod-liver oil, an acquired taste for some, is an extremely unique and important nutrient-dense food. There are several reliable companies that take care to deliver safe, clean, well-tested, fresh oil, and their products are easily found in health food stores. Keep a refrigerated bottle on hand and take a spoonful of nutrient-dense health from time to time.

FATS AND OILS—A FINAL WORD

The subject of fats and oils has been embroiled in controversy, conflicting points of view, and confusion for a long time. In particular, the American public has been confused about the relative healthiness of saturated fats versus unsaturated ones. Instead of a serious inquiry into their relative merits, however, oversimplified answers have been widely disseminated. For example, people have been taught that all tropical oils, including healthful coconut oil, are bad for them. At the same time, until recently there has been little discussion of truly important topics such as trans fatty acids (hydrogenated oils), and the risks posed by processed, highly refined oils.

No wonder consumers are confused. While the fat content of many fast foods are at an all-time high, marketing and advertising budgets have often centered around claims of low fat, no fat, and no cholesterol. Yet, such fat phobia flies in the face of common sense, as well as basic nutritional understanding. When fats come from healthy sources, and are taken in moderation, they are actually very important foods that support health in fundamental ways.

Balancing the intake of essential fatty acids has led to well-documented favorable changes in a long list of conditions, including behavioral and learning problems; blood-lipid regulation; improved immune functioning; improvements in some forms of arthritis; lessening of depression, eczema and skin problems; reduction in blood pressure and risk of stroke; and restoration of fertility.

Anthropological evidence also supports the importance of a diet rich in essential fats. Aboriginal, indigenous, and prehistoric people (those who ate the so-called Paleolithic diet) traditionally consumed diets rich in eggs, nuts, and seeds, seafood, and wild game—all excellent sources of essential fatty acids. But indigenous and ancestral people never consumed synthetic hydrogenated oils or refined vegetable oils. Instead, their fats mostly came from animals, with additional oils coming from nuts, seeds, and whole grains, which were usually consumed as part of the whole food, and rarely extracted. In addition, these diets had a more balanced ratio of the omega-3 and omega-6 families than the diets of today.

When properly understood, healthy fats taken in moderation do not have to lead to heart disease, obesity, or any of the other ills that have been frequently attributed to them. Instead of fat phobia, the principles of nutrient density once again show how it is possible to use a combination of trust in the goodness of real foods and your own intuitive wisdom to understand how to nourish yourself in a healthy way. Since there *are* fats to be avoided, the trick is to know which they are, while at the same time knowing how many wonderful and healthy nutrient-dense options you have.

If at times it appears that the so-called experts want the American public to remain confused and a little off-balance, it could be because they want to create a vulnerability and suggestibility, which translates into marketing opportunities for them. It is not always easy living in the midst of a fast-food world, especially with all the advertised claims and confusing hype, but nutrient-dense principles can give you the confidence to make better decisions as you begin to trust in really good food.

CHAPTER 21

Grains—The Staff of Life

Sometime around ten thousand years ago, people started to turn away from the more nomadic lifestyle of hunting, gathering, and foraging, and began to practice animal husbandry, raising and breeding livestock, and the cultivation of various plants and wild grains, marking the beginnings of an agricultural-based lifestyle. This new and more intimate relationship with the land and regional plants is thought to have ushered in a more sedentary way of life that ultimately allowed villages to evolve into towns, nation-states, and ultimately, civilization as it is today. It also fostered unprecedented changes in the availability of grain-based foods, thus changing forever the way humanity would eat.

Today, the legacy of those early agricultural practices—the domestication of wild plant varieties through selective breeding and hybridization techniques—can be seen in mankind's dependence on a handful of cereal crops as staple sources of many nutrients. Although many other grains are grown and consumed around the world, corn, rice, and wheat are the big three in terms of human and animal consumption and, as they have for millennia, constitute the backbone of diets for countless people.

THE LAND OF WHEAT

America is a wheat-based culture. Bagels, breads, breakfast cereals, buns, cookies, crackers, English muffins, pastas, pastries, pizza crusts, pretzels, rolls, and many other products are made almost exclusively from wheat flour. Instead of diversity, the SAD diet offers a steady stream of flour-based foods that are consumed throughout the day.

Traditionally, grains such as wheat and the breads made from them are known as *the staff of life,* meaning that people could rely on them in times of scarcity as well as in times of plenty. Of course, a staff should aid and support, but cultural overreliance on wheat often makes it seem like more of a crutch than a staff.

Many cultures around the world tend to rely on one principal grain for their primary support: Asian cultures have rice-based diets; Central Americans principally use corn, or maize; and North African populations chiefly use millet, or sometimes a grain called teff. These nutrient-dense whole grains certainly play an important role in the diets of many people, and the consistent availability of such foods is reassuring, especially when other foods become scarce.

However, the wheat that is typically used in America often resembles a *hollow* staff, one that would have a hard time really supporting anyone, because milling and processing turns it into refined white flour that is anything but nutrient dense. What is left over after the whole-wheat berry has been stripped of its original bran (fiber), essential oils, minerals, trace phytonutrients, and vitamins, is white flour, basically a dead food with little more than empty carbohydrates (starch) and some wheat protein, mostly in the form of gluten. Since there is essentially no nutritional value left, even insects and other pests do not want it, making its one big advantage that it stores very well.

Wheat left whole, on the other hand, retains its vital germ, the nutritious bran layer, vitamin E, several of the B vitamins, and various minerals, including iron, magnesium, and selenium. In addition to these nutrients, whole wheat contributes phytocompounds, such as fiber and flavonoids, and other beneficial compounds, such as lignins and saponins.

Overall, whole wheat is a pretty good grain that is moderately nutrient dense if you keep two main guidelines in mind. First, always choose organically raised wheat. Second, pay attention to the freshness and quality of the flour. Naturally occurring oils in the germ layer of the wheat kernel, soon after being milled into flour, become exposed to light, warmth, and oxygen, which very quickly turns them rancid. Intact, unmilled whole-wheat berries can keep for a long time, however, due to the presence of tocopherol molecules. This naturally occurring vitamin E performs its antioxidant function of protecting the delicate oils so the sprouting wheat plants will be able to harness them. After the berries are ground into flour, however, this vitamin E gets quickly used up.

In addition, many flour products also contain inferior oils, shortening, and sugar, further diminishing the nutrient density and quality of the finished product. Then too, the majority of the 100 percent whole-wheat products on the market are probably made from flour that has sat around for an extended period of time, and most of them are not organically grown, in any case. Given all this, it is my belief that the vast majority of wheat products on the market are not particularly nutrient dense.

To be fair, I have found products, generally in small bakeries, local health food stores, farmer's markets, and co-ops, that are fresher and more nutrient dense than the usual offerings.

ALTERNATIVE BREADS

Although breads and other baked goods are extremely commonplace in the American diet, I do not consider most of them nutrient dense. True, there is a wide spectrum of quality available, and some products are moderately nutrient dense. But, as you progress through the tiers (*see* Chapters 41–43), you will find that many nutrient-dense practitioners drop most flour products from their diets. This may seem a bit radical to those who cannot conceive of a diet without bread. For some, a diet without wheat is almost unthinkable.

But there is a category of *alternative breads* that may be a bridge for those considering a transition to a flourless way of eating. Many of these alternative bread products are made with grains that have been sprouted and then baked at low temperatures. These are much more nutritious than normally milled flour because the sprouting process activates enzymes which, by initiating the growing process, awaken the life force of the plant. Sprouted baked goods are not milled, they are flourless, and their gluten content is dramatically reduced, making them more digestible and less irritating for people than conventional breads. These baked goods go by different names, depending on the brand. You might encounter Essene bread, Ezekiel or Manna bread, or, as the Sunnyvale Bakery in Britain calls it, simply Sprouted Bread.

THE BREAD SPECTRUM

There is an enormous range of quality available in the world of flour, grain, and baked goods. The typical commercial loaf of bread familiar to most Americans usually contains refined white flour, surrounded by dough conditioners, flavoring and color agents, leavening agents, preservatives, refined and hydrogenated oils, sugars, texture enhancers, and other artificial ingredients. The irony is that the bread of our ancestors, the staff of life, was a relatively nutrient-dense, simple food, consisting of a few quality ingredients, including freshly ground flour, water, perhaps a little oil, some yeast, and a little salt. Such breads are still available today, but conscientious shoppers may need to read a few labels before they find one that reflects that quality and simplicity.

What follows is a list of some superior breads and companies I have found. Although by no means a complete list, it does contain a few of the more widely available, high-quality brands found in health food stores throughout America. There are also many smaller, local or regional bakeries throughout the United States that are producing very high-quality breads. (*See also* Appendix A, Recommended Resources and Appendix C, Label-Reading Workshop, for specific breads.)

- Best nonorganic bread: *Great Harvest Bread Co.*—Freshly milled, whole-grain, simplicity of recipes
- Best sprouted breads: *Ezekiel, Sunnyvale, Nature's Path*—Fresh, organic, simple
- Best gluten- and wheat-free bread: *Food for Life*—Taste, texture, quality

- Best whole-grain bread: *Bavarian Organic, Whole Rye*—Simplicity, quality (non-wheat)
- Best non-whole-grain breads: *Local handcrafted breads*—Freshness, simplicity

ADDITIONAL GRAINS

So far, I've limited my discussion of grains to wheat, noting that American culture relies on wheat to an extreme degree. The rest of the world, however, has numerous other grains that fill the niche that wheat has in the West, and often with a superior degree of nutrient density.

Amaranth

Amaranth is an extremely nutritious grain that comes courtesy of the pre-Columbian Aztec and Mayan civilizations. Amaranth has one of the highest percentages of protein of any cereal grain. It is also a high-quality protein, since it contains more of the amino acid lysine, giving it a more balanced profile of amino acids. Amaranth is also very dense for calcium and iron. It can be enjoyed as a cereal, used as a flour, toasted, or popped like popcorn.

Barley

Sometimes considered the world's oldest grain, barley has been cultivated for at least 8,000 years. It is comparable to wheat in terms of its protein and vitamin content, but is much more nutrient dense with respect to its fiber content. Much of the fiber in barley is the form called beta-glucan soluble fiber, the type that has been shown to effectively lower serum cholesterol levels. Barley is also dense in calcium, folic acid, magnesium, niacin, and zinc.

Buckwheat

In spite of the name, buckwheat is unrelated to wheat. Buckwheat is a cereal with no gluten, yet is high in protein, B vitamins, calcium, and iron. Buckwheat is often ground into flour, and is also commonly roasted and cooked as kasha.

Corn

Corn is one of the world's staple foods, having been a staff of life for Native American people for thousands of years. Today, corn is found in a wide array of forms and foods, and is even a source of nonnutrient-dense products, such as cornstarch and (high fructose) corn syrup. Even corn oil is extracted and used from this versatile cereal grain.

For many people, corn is still used as an important source of nutrients, including protein. Although not a complete protein, it is still easily complemented with other protein sources, and so makes useful nutritional contributions. In addition, corn supplies some important phytonutrients including several antioxidant compounds. Corn tortillas, cornmeal flour, polenta, popcorn, and fresh corn are all ways this versatile and important food is enjoyed today.

Millet

Millet is one of my personal favorites. This cereal grain is easy to cook and use, yet is often underappreciated and underutilized. Millet has a higher protein content than wheat or rice, and is rich in B vitamins and minerals. It can be cooked like rice, or you can lightly preroast it in a skillet. Millet has a soft yellow color and a great aroma, which is a bit like popcorn. It is also great when cooked as a cereal, or as a side dish, similar to rice. Millet can also be used in breads or muffins, casseroles, as a pilaf or stuffing, or in soups. An important staple for many people around the world, millet is particularly widespread in parts of North Africa and India.

Quinoa

Quinoa is another grain from Central America and, similar to amaranth, it has a much higher protein content and quality than either wheat or rice. Quinoa can be used as a cereal, a ricelike side dish, or it can be ground into flour and incorporated into pastas and other foods.

Rice

Rice is a real staff of life for countless people throughout the Far East. Similar to wheat in the West, most rice today is refined. In milling brown rice into white, the nutrient-rich bran and endosperm layers are removed, leaving the nutrient-depleted familiar white rice. Although white rice is basically an empty-calorie carbohydrate, intact whole-grain brown rice is a wonderful food for a nutrient-dense diet. Brown rice comes in many flavor varieties; it is gluten free, and for most people, hypoallergenic.

Rye

Rye is another northern European grain commonly used in breads and other baked goods. Low in gluten compared to wheat, it has good protein and mineral content, and is high in magnesium and iron. Rye's strong taste is a good indication of its rich array of phytonutrient compounds.

Spelt

Spelt, widely eaten in Europe and the Middle East from prebiblical times through the Middle Ages, was a commonly available food source by the time of the Bronze Age, and has been a part of our ancestors' diets for the past 6,000 years. Today, it is still eaten in Northern Europe, and is making a resurgence in health food circles as an alternative to wheat.

Wheat is a hybridized plant. This means that it did not exist until humans created it by crossing desirable strains of wild grasses until they developed the size and characteristics they were seeking. Spelt is a wild variety of the grains related to these wild-grass ancestors of wheat.

Spelt is known to botanists as covered wheat, which refers to how its kernels are attached. In Europe, other primitive, covered wild grasses are known as einkorn and emmer, and scientists believe that spelt was probably developed by crossing emmer with another type of wild grass.

Nutritionally, spelt is 10 to 25 percent more protein dense than typical hard red wheat. It is also believed that spelt is easier to digest than wheat and is better tolerated by people with allergies or wheat intolerances. Many products in health food stores are made from spelt flour, ranging from spelt bagels and cookies, to bread and English muffins.

Teff

Teff, a little-known grain in America, is an ancient grass that has been used in Ethiopia and other parts of North Africa for thousands of years. The smallest grain in the world, teff is extraordinarily nutrient dense, with solid amounts of protein, minerals, and vitamins. Teff makes a great porridge, and is traditionally ground into flour to make injera, the bread of Ethiopia. It is also the basis of a fermented beverage that is rich in B vitamins.

CHAPTER 22

Fiber

Nutrient density is obviously centered around nutrients. Amino acids, essential fats, minerals, vitamins, and even many phytochemicals are nutrients in the sense that they facilitate biochemical processes and build, nourish, repair, replace, and support the cells and tissues of the body. But what about fiber? Traditionally considered an inert substance, fiber has often been thought of as little more than a bulking agent, something useful for keeping the bowels moving, and not much else.

Fiber has, however, turned out to be much more complex and important than previous generations of nutritionists suspected. Research has established that various types of fiber can alter cholesterol levels in blood plasma, increase bile secretion, lower blood pressure, nourish beneficial bacteria in the colon, and even reduce the incidence of certain types of cancer. What has become clear in the past few decades is that fiber has profound implications for health, and possibly even for longevity. Whether or not a diet is dense for fiber is a relevant, important question after all.

TYPES OF FIBER

Fiber was once thought to be simply roughage; virtually synonymous with cellulose, the woody material found in the stems of plants, shrubs, and trees. It was thought to be merely the indigestible substance left over from food after the good stuff is removed.

Fiber is now classified in two broad categories: insoluble and soluble. Insoluble fiber, the type people traditionally think of, is often found in cereal grains and other foods, and consists of cellulose, hemicellulose, lignins, and waxes. As the name implies, these types of fiber dissolve poorly in water. Soluble fiber includes gums, mucilages, pectins, and sterols. Though their functions can differ significantly, both of these classes have important physiological effects in the body.

EFFECTS OF DIFFERENT TYPES OF FIBER

The insoluble fibers, particularly cellulose and hemicellulose, tend to accomplish their functions through mechanical means, often as a bulking agent, and by acting locally, such as in the colon. Insoluble fiber helps speed elimination by decreasing bowel transit time and softening stools. It also help to absorb and dilute toxins, contribute to a feeling of fullness, and reduce bacterial toxins.

The soluble, gel-forming fibers, also have direct, local influences on the digestive tract. Similar to the insoluble forms, they dilute bacterial and other toxins (including heavy metals), help lubricate the bowel, and contribute to a feeling of fullness, or satiation. But soluble fiber also has advantageous systemic effects, such as increasing bile acid production and excretion, lowering serum cholesterol and fats, and stabilizing blood sugar. Both the soluble and insoluble forms of fiber contribute to fecal bulk, help regulate symptoms of constipation and diarrhea, and improve overall bowel tone and health.

SOURCES OF FIBERS

Generally, fruits and vegetables are an excellent source of dietary fiber. Soluble fiber, in particular the pectins, comes primarily from fruit. Apples, bananas, cherries, citrus, grapes, and many other fruits supply pectin, which is often concentrated around, or just under, the skin or peel. Nuts and seeds, particularly almonds, hazelnuts, and sunflower seeds, and dried fruits, such as dates and figs, are also excellent sources of dietary fiber. On the other hand, dairy products, meat, and seafood are considered fairly poor sources.

Food sources of other soluble fibers, including the gums and mucilages, come from legumes and beans, particularly kidney and pinto beans; from oats; and from sesame seeds. Psyllium seeds, the main ingredient in such over-the-counter products as Metamucil and other bulking agents, are another excellent source. Psyllium seeds, husks, and powder can be purchased inexpensively at health food stores, and are a safe, effective remedy for constipation as well as diarrhea. Many fresh vegetables, including asparagus, cabbage, carrots, corn, green pepper, and kale, also contain high amounts of soluble fiber.

Insoluble fiber is obtained from whole-grain cereals and whole-grain products in which the bran is retained. Refined white flour always has the bran removed, which makes white-flour products essentially fiber free. This is a primary reason why nutritionists have always considered the SAD diet, with its overreliance on refined flour, a leading cause of constipation and other bowel disorders, including diverticulosis and even colon cancer. Such bowel disorders are extremely rare in populations that consume large amounts of unrefined vegetables and grains, which provide abundant amounts of dietary fiber. Other good sources of insoluble fiber include brown rice and other whole grains, oats (which contain soluble and insoluble fiber), and pears.

CHAPTER 23

Vegetables—Cruciferous and Dark Leafy Greens

Vegetables are at the top of any list of nutrient-dense foods, and the two main groups—cruciferous vegetables and dark leafy greens—are discussed separately here.

CRUCIFEROUS VEGETABLES

The group of vegetables known botanically as the cruciferous family is one of the best studied, most nutrient dense, and widely eaten of all foods groups. Named after the crosslike formation of the primary leaves, which emerge just after sprouting, the cruciferous family includes such well-known vegetables as bok choy, broccoli, Brussels sprouts, cabbage, cauliflower, kale, and mustard greens.

These vegetables, sometimes called brassicas, are a nutrient-dense source of the essential minerals sulfur, and selenium (a highly regarded mineral with known anticancer properties). In recent years, broccoli and its complex relationship with both of these minerals has been the focus of much research. Some studies have tied consumption of cruciferous vegetables with a reduced risk for certain cancers.

Much of this research has centered on the phytochemicals (sulforaphanes and indole glycoinolates) present in this family. These sulfur-containing compounds may play a role in cancer prevention by helping to break down excess estrogen, and by stimulating the production of other enzymes that play key roles as antioxidants.

Brassicas are nutrient dense in other ways as well. All members of this family are high in calcium and magnesium; they supply abundant amounts of soluble and insoluble fiber, and they are also dense for vitamin C and folate. In addition, raw and lightly cooked brassicas are rich in carotenoids (vitamin-A equivalents), chlorophyll, and plant enzymes.

Although broccoli has gotten the most attention, the other members of the cruciferous family are also nutrient dense for specialized sulfur compounds. All the brassicas are, in fact, medium-dense sources of protein, and good suppliers of the B vitamin, niacin, as well.

Brussels sprouts and cauliflower are also dense for various nutrients, including folate, niacin, protein, and vitamin C. Neither pack in the calcium that other vegetables in this family do, but Brussels sprouts do contribute good amounts of iron, selenium, and vitamin E, and cauliflower is another very good source of dietary sulfur compounds and fiber.

The brassicas richly deserve a prominent place in any nutrient-dense diet. Consistently delicious and health-promoting, these vegetables are a gift from millennia of farmers and villagers around the world.

DARK LEAFY GREENS

Many of the cruciferous vegetables are used for their greens, or tops. Bok choy, chard, kale, and mustard greens are all brassicas that make their contribution to your diet through their nutrient denseness for calcium, sulfur compounds, and selenium.

Dark leafy greens stand out as excellent sources of chlorophyll, folic acid, hyaluronic acid (important for eye health), and various cartenoids. Not only are dark leafy greens wonderful sources of many nutrients, they are also delicious, versatile, and easy to use.

Beet Greens

Beets are famous for pulling mineral nutrients out of the soil. Beet greens, or the leafy tops of beets, are an exceptional source of iron. They are quite delicious steamed or fresh, and can easily substitute for spinach in recipes.

Bok Choy

The creamy white stems of this familiar vegetable give a distinctive watery crunch to many dishes. The dark green tops of bok choy can be used in soups and stir-fries.

Chard

Chard greens can be used like bok choy, and have comparable nutrient value, being high in calcium, carotenoids, folic acid, and, when eaten raw, enzymes.

Kale

Kale is an exceptionally nutrient-dense leafy green with the most calcium of any vegetable. It is also a great contributor of folate, iron, and vitamin C, along with carotenes and a surprising amount of protein.

Mustard Greens

Mustard greens are similarly high in calcium, carotenoids, fiber, folate, iron, protein, and vitamin E. They are delicious steamed or fresh.

CHAPTER 24

Sea Vegetables—Seaweed

For millennia, coastal people have harvested extraordinarily nutrient-dense oceanic plants—seaweed—for food and numerous other uses. Sea vegetables were introduced to the general public as seaweed in the late 1960s, principally through the macrobiotic movement, a dietary approach to healthy eating brought here from Japan. A mainstay of the traditional Japanese diet, this venerable food source has maintained a discreet, low-key presence in this country ever since, though many people are now rediscovering it through sushi bars and health food stores.

Despite their low profile, these plants have tremendous nutritional benefits. If they seem a bit exotic for your taste, please take a closer look because there is real diversity in this class of foods. Besides different flavors and textures, these nutrient-dense friends from the seas can bring substantial quantities of important trace nutrients into your life.

Among the many edible seaweed species, there are two major classifications: the browns and the reds. Brown seaweeds include most of the better-known varieties. Arame, bladderwrack (fucus), kombu, hijiki, sea palm, and the kelps are all listed in this category. Red seaweed includes the commonly eaten dulse and nori.

In terms of nutrient density, all of the edible seaweeds are renowned for their concentrated minerals, derived, of course, from their ocean home. Sea vegetables are known as superior sources of the essential trace mineral, iodine, which is necessary for optimal thyroid health and functioning. Ingesting sea vegetables provides virtually all the trace and ultra-trace minerals found in seawater. Since life evolved out of the oceans, the salinity and electrolyte (mineral) balance of blood is seemingly a reflection and reminder of our earliest oceanic roots, and it makes sense that, through this connection, sea vegetables could be vitally important constituents of an optimally healthy diet. For people who live inland, or do not eat fish or shellfish, sea vegetables could play an important role in building good health.

In addition to supplying a broad range of dissolved trace minerals, sea vegetables also contain protein and vitamins, not to mention other unique plant compounds. These phytonutrients, which have developed in response to their unique growing environment, are being actively investigated for their health-enhancing properties.

Kelp, for instance, is noted for containing large amounts of alginates, or alginic acids, unusual compounds with the ability to chelate, or bind, heavy metals, such as lead and mercury, and remove them from the body. These acids can also help remove radioactive elements, or radioisotopes, such as strontium 90. In Japan, research indicates that kelp may aid in tumor inhibition and cancer prevention. Indeed, the well-known connection between soybeans and cancer-prevention may actually be related to a different component of the Japanese diet—seaweed consumption.

The palatability of seaweeds, which offer flavor, texture, and a touch of the exotic to food, makes it enjoyable to use in cooking. Many people have discovered that powdered dulse or kelp granules make a great flavoring for popcorn. One company, Maine Coast Sea Vegetables Inc., markets seaweed granules (plain and flavored with garlic) in convenient salt shaker-style containers. These are natural accompaniments to many meals, and are indispensable for the nutrient-dense cook's kitchen.

Sea vegetables are purchased dried and are easily stored. Most are quickly reconstituted by either soaking, steaming, or simmering in hot water for several minutes. The leftover water is a mineral-rich broth that makes an excellent base for soups or gravies, and can also be drunk straight as a tonic, or used as a fertilizer for houseplants or gardens.

Seaweed can also serve as a salt substitute, supplying healthy sodium in balance with chloride, electrolytes, and potassium. I serve reconstituted seaweed with fish, and in salads, soups, or stir-fries. You can also make crunchy snacks by roasting seaweed in a skillet with almonds, sesame seeds, a little oil, and tamari—a tasty alternative to low-nutrient chips or crackers.

Many types of seaweed have a mildly chewy texture. Dulse has a soft, almost buttery consistency, and a beautiful deep purple hue. Sea palm is similar in shape and color to dark green spinach fettuccini. Arame and hijiki are found in distinctive jet-black strands that stand out nicely in salads, soups, and stir-fries.

For centuries, coastal people all over the world, including the Atlantic-coast Indians, the Celts, Scandinavians, and the inhabitants of the Pacific and South Sea Islands, have all benefited from this bounty of the seas. Now, when the mineral content of the soil and food is being so rapidly depleted, it makes good sense to avail yourself of this highly nutrient-dense food as frequently as possible.

I strongly encourage everyone to include these amazing foods in their diet. Utilizing the wisdom of the oceans, and bringing the energy of the seas into your home and body may help you heal in profound and unanticipated ways.

CHAPTER 25

Fruits

Fresh fruit is an important component of a nutrient-rich diet. Fruit is easily enjoyed just as it comes from nature—unprocessed, simple, and nutritious. Uncooked fruit is a living food, supplying energy in the form of ready-to-assimilate carbohydrates. Being a whole food, fruit also supplies a spectrum of other valuable nutrients. All fruits are great sources of fiber, often in the highly beneficial soluble form (pectin is one such substance).

Fruit is also dense for enzymes and the mineral potassium. And many fruits are excellent sources of ascorbic acid, vitamin C. Antioxidant molecules, known as bioflavonoids, often accompany ascorbic acid in nature, and fruit is a great source of these. Fruit also supplies a diverse array of phytonutrients—many acting as accessory nutrients with antioxidant or other functions.

I feel that fruit is often underrated by nutrition experts. In general, fruit does not contain enormous amounts of most vitamins, minerals, protein, or essential fats, but it does supply good amounts of other nutrients. Plus, fruit is convenient, generally inexpensive, and delicious. Instead of giving us empty calories, preservatives, and other artificial ingredients, fruit helps connect us with the bounty and generosity of nature.

Interestingly, with all the conflicting nutritional claims for different foods that have been made over the years, the claims for the healthiness of ingesting fruit have remained constant. Study after study has revealed that a higher fruit intake corresponds to a reduced likelihood of many diseases, including cancer and cardiovascular disease.

However, thanks to today's agribusiness procedures, fruit is changing. Many old, or heirloom, varieties are being phased out in favor of newer varieties that may be more desirable because they travel better, keep longer, or have a more uniform appearance. Unfortunately, these are not always as nutritious, or even as tasty as older types, so it may be worthwhile to check out farmer's markets, organic varieties, and other sources.

Find and use varieties you like. For example, some oranges are too thick-skinned or seedy, too sweet, or too sour for certain tastes. I personally seek out Mineola tangelos, for example, because they are easy to peel, are very juicy with few or no seeds, and have the perfect balance of tartness and flavor for my taste buds. This is true for lemons, too. Many of the new, hybridized varieties, even the organic ones, are bred to have super-thick skins because it helps them travel and keep longer, but they have hardly any juice in them. Meyer lemons, considered top of the line in the lemon world, have paper-thin skins, are incredibly juicy, and have a hint of sweetness to round out their lemony tartness. They can almost be eaten like an orange and make the best lemonade imaginable, providing a lot of juice value for the money. They are not always available, but when they are, I stock up.

Most fruit is nutrient dense. Some of the best include blackberries, blueberries, cherries, grapes, kiwi fruit, nectarines, peaches, pineapples, and raspberries. Reaching for a piece of fruit instead of a quick-fix, empty-calorie candy or sweet is an important way to improve the nutrient density of your diet.

CHAPTER 26

Nuts and Seeds

Although the term *health nut* has been negatively applied to people who actually *care* about what they eat, the phrase is actually a compliment. Nuts (and seeds too) are a frequent staple for vegetarians and other health-oriented people because they are consummate nutrient-dense foods.

Nuts and seeds are the source of nutrients for a future generation of organisms, as are eggs (*see* Chapter 27). They are complete, self-sufficient foods containing the broad spectrum of nutrients necessary for the healthy and robust beginning of a new life. And they are renowned for their ability to keep because they must stay protected from the ravages of nature in order to remain viable until the appropriate conditions for germination occur. This is one reason why many nuts and seeds are first-rate sources of some hard-to-obtain antioxidants, notably vitamin E.

Nuts and seeds are also good sources for many of the essential amino acids in protein, and of the plant-based fatty acids, another indication of their overall ability to provide energy for the plant-to-be. These fats are the primary reason why nuts and seeds so often have an abundance of vitamin E. It is, after all, the main fat-soluble antioxidant vitamin, and is one of nature's primary ways to protect seeds from becoming rancid. In addition to their healthy oil, protein, and vitamin-E contents, nuts and seeds are good sources for many of the B vitamins, as well as for the minerals calcium, magnesium, selenium, and zinc.

Nuts often get criticized for their fat content, but most of their fats are actually the desirable ones. Lipids from *un*roasted nuts and seeds are typically high in the sought-after monounsaturated fatty acids, and are balanced with useful polyunsaturated fatty acids as well. The only really undesirable fats are the oxidized ones in roasted nuts that are damaged by air, heat, or light, and the trans fats from hydrogenated or partially hydrogenated oils. Because of the double risk posed by roasted nuts—from heating the oils inside the nuts themselves, and from the oils used in the roasting process—it is a good idea to avoid them. But raw nuts and seeds are another matter; they are highly nutrient-dense foods that are very valuable in a healthy diet.

What are the healthiest nuts to eat? The answer depends on what nutrients you want. Brazil nuts, for example, are highest in selenium, and are the single most nutrient-dense food available for that mineral. Almonds and sunflower seeds are great sources of vitamin E. Walnuts are known for their alpha-linolenic content, and sesame seeds are good sources of calcium, copper, magnesium, and zinc. All nuts and seeds are good sources of fats, and are considered heart healthy due to the fiber and vitamins they contain, plus the fact that their oils are a healthy blend of saturates, monounsaturates, and polyunsaturates. Keep in mind that nuts should be fresh and raw—not roasted—stored properly in a refrigerator or in airtight containers, and, if possible, not left out of their shells for an extended period of time.

NUTRIENT DENSITY OF SPECIFIC NUTS AND SEEDS

Eat a variety of the following nuts and seeds to increase the nutrient density of your diet.

Almonds

Among the most versatile and delicious of all the nuts, almonds are nutritionally dense as they contain fiber, the minerals calcium, manganese, magnesium, potassium, and zinc, and the vitamins B_2 (riboflavin) and E. Almonds can play a significant role in a nutrient-dense diet because they are great raw, ground up into meal or butter, made into a delicious nut milk, or sprouted (soaked overnight).

Brazil Nuts

Brazil nuts are the single best source of the important mineral antioxidant, selenium. They are also rich in manganese, magnesium, and zinc, and the B vitamin, thiamine. Similar to other tropical nuts and oils, Brazil nuts have a high percentage of saturated fats, although they are well-balanced in mono- and polyunsaturated oils. Since it is possible to get too much selenium, Brazil nuts should be eaten in moderation.

Cashews

Cashews are nutrient dense for the minerals copper, iron, magnesium, potassium, selenium, and zinc. They are also a good source for thiamine (vitamin B_1). Cashews are noteworthy in that they have the highest carbohydrate total of any nut. They are also impossible to buy completely raw because heat, or other means, must be used to separate the nut from its shell.

Hazelnuts (Filberts)

The hazelnut is another nutrient-dense nut that can be enjoyed for its taste as well as its nutritional contributions. Filberts are great sources of fiber, the minerals manganese, magnesium, and potassium, and the vitamins B_1 (thiamine), B_6 (pyridoxine), E, folic acid, and pantothenic acid.

Macadamia Nuts

Hawaiian-grown macadamia nuts, particularly rich in polyunsaturated oils, have the highest fat content of all nuts, and are also one of the lowest in overall protein content. Macadamias are a good source of niacin (vitamin B_3), pantothenic acid, thiamine, and the minerals copper, iron, manganese, and potassium. In order to reduce the breakdown and rancidity of the oils, store these nuts in the freezer or refrigerator.

Peanuts

Peanuts are technically legumes, not nuts, and therefore have a slightly different nutritional profile than most nuts. Similar to nuts, though, peanuts are high in the minerals iron, magnesium, and potassium, and are moderately good sources of vitamins B_6, pantothenic acid, and thiamine. Completely different from the nuts already discussed, peanuts have, by far, the highest levels of folic acid and niacin. Raw peanuts are also a good source of natural vitamin E. Although almost always eaten roasted (usually in low-grade cottonseed oil), they should be avoided in this form. In America, almost all peanuts are conventionally grown with a lot of chemicals and pesticides, and for this reason, I strongly advise seeking out and buying the organically grown varieties.

Pine Nuts (Pignolia)

Pine nuts, along with almonds and sesame and sunflower seeds, are among the most protein dense of all nuts and seeds. They are also an excellent source of the minerals manganese, magnesium, potassium, and zinc, and the B vitamins folic acid, niacin, and thiamine. As you would other oily nuts, it is advisable to store pine nuts in airtight bags in the freezer or refrigerator to preserve the nutritional quality of their lipids.

Pistachio Nuts

Pistachios are nutrient dense for protein, healthy oils, and several key nutrients, including the minerals potassium and zinc, the B vitamins folate (folic acid), pantothenic acid, thiamine (B_1), and especially, vitamin B_6. Though lacking the density of some nuts, pistachios are moderately good sources of calcium and magnesium.

Pumpkin Seeds

Pumpkin seeds are one of the most nutritionally dense of all seeds, and contain the highest protein content of any seed or nut. They are extremely high in iron, manganese, and potassium, and have the highest magnesium and zinc content of any seeds. Pumpkin seeds are also dense for chlorophyll, folate, niacin, and vitamin A (carotenoids). Pumpkin-seed butter is an extremely nutrient-dense way to get the benefits of this food and, taken in moderation because it is also calorie-dense, is a great alternative to conventional peanut butters.

Sesame Seeds

I consider sesame and sunflower seeds the two most nutrient dense of all the seeds. Sesame seeds have the highest overall mineral levels, while sunflower seeds have the highest levels of many vitamins. Sesame seeds are particularly dense for calcium, copper, iron, manganese, magnesium, and zinc, and are also rich in phosphorus, potassium, and the vitamins B_6, folic acid, and niacin (B_3). Tahini (sesame-seed butter) can be made from either toasted or raw sesame seeds, and is an excellent, nutrient-dense alternative to peanut butter. Halvah is a traditional Middle Eastern dessert made from ground sesame seeds sweetened with sugar and often flavored with cocoa and pistachio.

Sunflower Seeds

Along with sesame seeds, sunflower seeds are probably the most nutrient-dense seeds available. As with all seeds and nuts, sunflower seeds are best used raw because the roasting process adds heated, processed oils that detract from the original quality of the fresh seeds. In addition, heat from the roasting process may degrade some of the original vitamins and the other heat-sensitive nutritional components.

Sunflower seeds are top-notch sources of calcium, copper, iron, manganese, magnesium, selenium, and zinc. They are also a great source of vitamins B_6, E, folate (folic acid), niacin, pantothenic acid, and thiamine, and are dense for fiber and phytosterols (natural plant hormones). Sunflower seeds can be added to salads, eaten raw, ground into a meal or flour, made into a nut butter, or sprouted and eaten with salads.

Walnuts

Walnuts are a good nutritional source for fiber, folic acid, and the minerals manganese, magnesium, potassium, and zinc. One of the fattier nuts, they are considered a good source of polyunsaturated oils, and in particular, the omega-3 fatty acid, alpha-linolenic acid. To prevent rancidity, it is important to store walnuts and the other very oily nuts, such as macadamia and pine nuts, in airtight containers in the freezer or refrigerator.

CHAPTER 27

Eggs

Without question, eggs are a supremely nutrient-dense food. So, why have they gotten such a harsh reputation from some medical specialists and nutritionists? It has always fascinated me that this food is touted as one of nature's perfect foods by some, and considered a dreaded dietary risk by others. It would seem that the humble egg, a symbol of life itself to many, has developed a schizophrenic reputation.

The truth is, eggs can be both great and terrible. My dividing line is drawn according to two major criteria. The first is related to how the eggs are produced, and the second as to how they are cooked.

Eggs produced by the commercial poultry industry are among the most heavily chemicalized foods in this country. The enormous economic pressures on these producers has led them to use extremely large amounts of synthetic estrogens to induce and maximize egg production, chicken growth, and maturation rates. In addition, massive quantities of antibiotics are used as a preventive strategy and to forestall potentially devastating infections, as well as to increase growth rates. As a result, commercial chickens and eggs are loaded with residues from these agricultural chemicals.

The consequence is unfortunate, both for the birds and for the consumer, and so my solution is to avoid such foods. The egg really does have the potential to be one of nature's ideal foods, and the good news is that you can easily find this type of superior egg by buying from the many smaller producers of eggs that are either organically certified or that involve far fewer chemicals in their production. Once again, a thriving demand from informed and concerned shoppers has led to a positive response from responsible and committed farmers.

Organically raised eggs do cost more than commercial eggs, but the extra price is well worth it. As far as I am concerned, organically raised eggs are still a bargain, being a highly nutrient-dense food, and an extremely valuable part of a nutrient-dense diet.

What are eggs dense for? A whole egg is really a self-contained nursery for the production of a fully formed and functioning organism, and that means it has to be a well-rounded nutritional unit. Everything needed to fully develop a baby bird is present—from calcium to make its bones, to proteins and fats for its immune system, muscles, and nervous system, and copper and iron for its blood.

Despite the well-rounded nutritional profile, eggs are best known for several key nutrients. The protein they contain is of the highest quality—the amino acids, the subunits of protein, are present in a ratio that is close to ideal for use by the body. In fact, some amino acids that are limited in other foods are richly supplied by egg protein. Also, eggs are particularly dense in the B vitamins biotin, choline, inositol, and pantothenic acid, and also supply other hard-to-get vitamins, such as B_{12}, as well as the fat-soluble vitamins A, D, and E. Additionally, eggs are noteworthy for their valuable supplies of the minerals iron, phosphorus, zinc, and, most particularly, sulfur.

Two of the most important and useful components of eggs are cholesterol and lecithin; both are found exclusively in the yolk. Egg-yolk lecithin is a key source of compounds known as phospholipids, which are crucially important molecules with active roles in cell membranes, particularly in the brain and nervous system. Phospholipids are also involved in the production of the neurotransmitter acetylcholine in the brain, and are important for optimal brain function, including memory.

THE CHOLESTEROL STORY

Whole eggs are sometimes referred to as nature's perfect food, as they provide everything necessary to develop and sustain a new life—every egg is potentially an entire, fully developed organism and a complete, self-sustaining nursery. Yet, for years the medical profession has told people that we should strictly monitor and limit our intake of them. What's the reality here?

Those on one side of the cholesterol controversy believe this one component of eggs is a harmful, threatening substance that is dangerous to hearts and arterial systems. This view is, however, simplistic to the point of being misleading. To understand the role of the egg in health, you need to clearly understand what cholesterol is, what its purposes are, and under what circumstances it can behave differently from its intended function.

Perhaps the most vilified of all nutrients, cholesterol is actually a biologically essential molecule. The good side of cholesterol is, it is so vital to your health and well-being that the body regularly manufactures some in the liver. According to most nutritional experts, dietary cholesterol in the right form and amounts is considered extremely important for enhancing health.

Cholesterol has many crucial functions in the body. Your body uses this vital substance to manufacture several key compounds, including antistress adrenal hormones (corticosteroids), vitamin D for calcium absorption and bone density, and the sex hormones estrogen, progesterone, and testosterone. All of these are ultimately derived from cholesterol.

Where then does this idea of unhealthy cholesterol come from? Studies that isolated and fed cholesterol to test animals (rabbits) and induced hardening of the arteries prompted scientists to conclude that cholesterol is a bad molecular substance. There are at least two things wrong with these findings, and both relate directly to wholeness and nutrient density. For one, nature has intended cholesterol to be ingested as part of a larger, whole food containing other, synergistic, substances that aid in its metabolism. In a whole egg, cholesterol is not an isolated compound, but is closely aligned with lecithin, a unique substance that increases its solubility and absorption. And also, when talking about any diet, you must look at the appropriateness of the food for that person or test animal. In the case of rabbits, the test animals used, it is important to acknowledge that, in nature, these animals are strictly vegetarians and therefore *they never eat cholesterol under natural conditions.*

Another factor that needs recognition is the *form* of the cholesterol. Cholesterol in an egg yolk is protected from oxidation damage by naturally occurring antioxidants, such as vitamin E and other substances. When cholesterol is exposed to high temperatures and air, as in freeze-drying, frying, or scrambling, the cholesterol can become damaged (oxidized), and will be unusable as a source of hormones and other biochemicals. Damaged or oxidized cholesterol is the form commonly found in atherosclerotic plaques. If this form is fed to test animals, as in powdered eggs, is it fair to blame the natural form of cholesterol on hardening of the arteries? Can any really meaningful conclusions be drawn based on this kind of research?

The anticholesterol hysteria of the past several decades is slowly being reevaluated by many prominent nutritionists, scientists, and medical experts who have found that the cholesterol-lowering drugs (statins) can have alarming negative side effects, such as sexual impotency and an increased risk of heart attack; for some users it turns out that having a too-low cholesterol could be just as dangerous as having cholesterol that is too high. Many experts now believe that cholesterol is not the one-sided culprit it was previously considered to be. As usual, though, medical dogma and traditional thinking is often hard to overturn, and a large, profitable industry has sprung up around cholesterol-lowering drugs and programs, making it important for you to know the complete story on cholesterol and the real risks for heart disease.

I noted earlier that two main considerations exist regarding the healthiness of eggs. The first, how eggs are *produced,* with or without hormones and antibiotics, is discussed above. The second factor refers to how eggs are *cooked* (boiling and poaching are good, frying and scrambling are *not* good), and this may hold the key to understanding how cholesterol can pose a danger. Similar to many molecules, cholesterol is very susceptible to damage from heat, light, and oxygen. The attack on cholesterol by oxygen under the influence of the high temperatures reached when eggs are fried or scrambled is known as oxidation, which literally alters cholesterol molecules, often rendering them unsuitable for their normally intended uses, and even making them toxic. Freeze-dried or powdered eggs and similar products may contain substantial levels of this oxidized cholesterol.

For these reasons, *The Nutrient-Rich Diet Eating Plan* recommends that people mainly eat boiled or poached eggs. Boiling and poaching occur at a much lower, and therefore less damaging, temperature than frying or scrambling. Good evidence exists that undamaged cholesterol does not tend to build up to harmful levels in the body. To the contrary, in fact, there are strong indications that healthy dietary cholesterol actually works to *regulate* blood levels. When cholesterol is ingested in a healthy form, the liver does not have to manufacture as much, so a better balance can occur.

Over the years, I have counseled many people to resume eating organic, boiled eggs, often to their relief. Many people have told me how much better they felt as a result, and how glad they were not to feel guilty for enjoying a food they loved. As with many nutrient-dense foods, their instincts were correct all along.

CHAPTER 28

Dairy

Dairy in the form of mother's milk is people's first food. This is how nature intended us to get milk, directly from our mothers. Milk is the perfect food for babies and infants—nutrient dense, perfectly balanced, and full of everything needed to get the right start in life.

Somewhere along the way, though, things have gone astray. Nowhere in nature do animals drink milk past early childhood, yet today people not only drink milk into adulthood, but they consume it in enormous quantities. And most milk in America has been manipulated, processed, and changed in ways that render it a completely different substance from milk from natural sources.

Dairy can be healthy and nutrient dense, but you need to be fully aware of the different aspects of this issue. If you want to take full advantage of the best available, you should understand the promise of truly natural dairy products, as well as the perils of commercial dairy products. As with every other class of foods examined in this book, there is a broad spectrum of quality for dairy products.

The topic of dairy is complex, and requires a book of its own to do it justice. Nonetheless, in order to better understand how dairy today fits in with the principles of nutrient density, it is necessary to look squarely at the major issues surrounding this food class. The relative healthiness and safety of dairy is a very controversial subject. A lot of money is involved in the manufacturing and marketing of dairy products—the dairy industry is enormous, and very powerful. Nonetheless, it is important to consider that this beloved and heavily advertised food group may not always be good for everyone. And, on the other hand, there may still be a place for dairy—of the proper quality—in a truly nutrient-dense diet.

ISSUES SURROUNDING DAIRY

In its natural form, dairy is nutrient dense. It is certainly dense for calcium, as everyone knows, but it is also dense for protein and a good contributor of some important lipids and fat-soluble vitamins. So, since dairy is touted as a great food, and does contain decent quantities of valuable nutrients, what is the problem?

Unfortunately, that question has a number of troubling answers, the short one being *processing*. Milk directly from a cow or goat (or camel, sheep, water buffalo, or yak, depending on your cultural background) is an important food source for many people, as are the fermented drinks and cheeses made from such milk. But the truth is, virtually no one in America gets to experience fresh, unaltered milk in its natural state because it is subjected to several major processes, each of which alters its chemical and nutritional properties. Milk today typically comes from cows that are treated with antibiotics and hormones, and is then subjected to the processes of pasteurization and homogenization.

Pasteurization

All commercially sold milk today, and all products made from it, is pasteurized. Pasteurization—heating milk to the point of killing or inactivating dangerous bacteria—is certainly a laudable and worthwhile accomplishment. But pasteurization also destroys naturally occurring enzymes and proteins found in the raw milk. Pasteurized milk, therefore, is no longer equivalent to the raw milk that comes directly from a cow, goat, sheep, or other animal.

Enzymes are always present in living foods. Raw milk, as intended for the nutritional support of an infant (normally of the same species), is a living food. When left out in a warm climate, raw milk acts as a nutritious media for certain (usually beneficial) bacteria, and the end result of this naturally occurring inoculation from ambient bacteria in the environment is cultured milk products, such as yogurt or kefir. For thousands of years, these naturally fermented milk products have been enjoyed for their nutritional benefits. Many cheeses were also discovered through this process of natural fermentation and culturing.

Culturing raw milk has several benefits. Beneficial bacteria, such as lactobacillus, are known to synthesize enzymes and other compounds that may be valuable secondary nutrients in their own right. Further, such bacteria tend to digest, or metabolize, milk sugar (lactose), so cultured products tend to be lower in lactose content. People who are lactose intolerant and cannot tolerate pure milk can often enjoy yogurt with fewer adverse effects.

By contrast, pasteurized milk resists natural culturing. Instead of *going good,* commercial milk tends to go rotten if left out. Commercial milk that has been pasteurized is no longer a living food, since its enzymes have been denatured. Similar to other dead things, it becomes putrid and rots, a strong indication that pasteurized milk has vastly different properties than fresh, alive, raw milk.

Homogenization

The second major processing technology employed to alter milk from its natural state is homogenization, the process responsible for preventing cream from separating out from the rest of the milk. In fresh, raw milk, the fat globules tend to rise to the top, as they are lighter (less dense) than the rest of the milk. There the globules coalesce, making a layer of fat-rich cream, which is primarily butter fat.

Since fat tends to easily oxidize and go rancid, homogenization technology was invented to increase the shelf life of milk and improve its overall visual consistency. Homogenization makes fat globules smaller, and because of this reduction in mass, the fat tends to stay dispersed in the whole solution and not separate out into a layer of cream. This may not seem bad, but as usual, you have to pay attention to what ultimately happens when nature is manipulated. In the case of homogenization, it turns out that drastically altering the size of these fat globules also changes the nature of the milk-fat globule membranes, or MFGM. Studies are currently looking to determine if changing the nature of this membrane could have adverse effects on milk drinkers.

Naturally associated with milk fat is an enzyme known as xanthine oxidase (XO). This enzyme is widely considered an atherogenic irritant, which means it can create inflammation in the linings of blood vessels, leading to a cascade of responses thought to ultimately result in hardening of the arteries. While the size of an average fat globule prevents much XO from being absorbed into the bloodstream, it is postulated that the significantly smaller fat globules of homogenized milk allow relatively large amounts of this enzyme to be absorbed. This still-controversial theory could account for some of the atherogenic (artery-hardening) properties thought to be associated with the consumption of homogenized milk.

Hormones and Dairy

Milk has sometimes been referred to as a hormone delivery system, because it is a way that peptides and other important messenger molecules are conveyed directly from mother to baby. Important immunoglobulin complexes are found in colostrum, the *premilk* present in the first few days after birth that is richly complex with important immunoglobulins and other unique chemical compounds for the developing infant.

Because of milk's affinity for proteins, hormones, and other compounds, there is concern that adding synthetic hormones to the feed of dairy cows can have a negative effect on human health. Synthetic hormones increase milk production in dairy cows, and many scientists are outspoken in their concern that these estrogens and other hormones (such as recombinant bovine growth hormone) can pose dangers to consumers of milk and other dairy products. Genetically engineered growth hormone, for instance, is known to increase levels of the insulinlike growth factor 1, or IGF-1 in cow's milk. IGF-1 is known to accelerate the growth of existing breast cancer cells, and cause the proliferation of others. IGF-1 is strongly suspected to be a leading factor in breast cancer, and possibly other cancers, and this relationship is being actively studied. Furthermore, it has been increasingly noted that synthetic estrogens in commercial dairy products may be causing premature puberty in young children.

Dairy has been implicated in many situations of poor health. Food allergies, arthritis, asthma, eczema, and even some forms of diabetes are all thought to be related to the excessive, inappropriate ingestion of dairy. The main factors for determining if dairy is appropriate in your diet center around your ethnic background as well as the degree of processing the dairy products have undergone. Through careful selection of minimally processed dairy, it is possible to lessen the risks of dairy while maximizing its benefits.

Dairy and Ethnicity

One of the more interesting trends in nutrition is the relationship between genetic patterns and dietary needs. Dr. Peter D'Adamo's book, *Eat Right 4 Your Type,* makes a case for adopting a dietary lifestyle based largely on the different blood types. This research, while still somewhat preliminary, makes good sense. Since different populations evolved in vastly different environments and climates, with different local foods, it makes sense that over hundreds of thousands of years, natural selection would create different sensitivities among different populations.

An example of this principle at work is evident by examining different people's responses to dairy. While most Northern Europeans are able to digest milk sugar (lactose) into adulthood, the same cannot be said for people from other regions. In particular, most people of Asiatic and African descent are largely lactose-intolerant. In fact, the majority of people who genetically descend from warm, tropical, or semi-tropical climates have this trait, including native Americans and many people from the Mediterranean, Mexico and other parts of Central America, and the Middle East. For all these people, a drastic reduction in dairy products would be prudent because elevated incidences of cancer, diabetes, obesity, and other problems in these populations could well be linked to eating a SAD diet that is largely inappropriate for them, given the preponderance of dairy in the SAD diet.

The Nutrient-Dense Spectrum

For people who choose to eat dairy, or who are continuing but cutting back, it is clearly important to choose the best dairy products available. Fortunately, a spectrum of quality does exist. With dairy, making the best choices possible is vitally important. From the standpoint of nutrient-dense principles, the majority of commercial dairy products are not acceptable simply because virtually all commercial milk and cheese products, including commercial brands of cottage cheeses, ice creams, sour creams, yogurts, and other products, are made from antibiotic-contaminated, homogenized, pasteurized milk with synthetic hormones added. In *The Nutrient-Dense Eating Plan,* such products are basically unacceptable, and therefore, forbidden.

However, you can purchase certified organic milks, cheeses, and many other dairy products that do not have added synthetic hormones, pesticide or herbicide residues, or the antibiotic drugs routinely given to herds of dairy cattle. Such cleaner dairy products are now widely available through such companies as Alta Dena, Horizon, Seven Stars, Stonyfield Farms, and others.

Yet, while organic milks and cheeses are much healthier choices, they are still pasteurized and homogenized, so being organic doesn't necessarily mean completely natural. Organic dairy products definitely represent a giant step in a positive direction and are useful in your dietary evolution, but they are still not considered all that desirable on the higher tier levels.

The next step up is to choose organic products made from *un*homogenized milk. Government regulations say that all milk sold in stores must be pasteurized, but this is not true of homogenization. Most companies homogenize their milk because they believe that's what most consumers want and expect, and because it does improve milk's shelf life. Still, at least a few companies are offering organic milks and yogurts that, while pasteurized, are not homogenized. Brown Cow yogurt and Seven Stars yogurt are two nonhomogenized yogurts that offer high-quality dairy in a commercial context.

The next level of dairy to consider are products made from *un*pasteurized raw milk, which is full of enzymes, and is the form nature intended you to use. If you obtain raw milk locally, get to know the farmer and her or his degree of cleanliness and technique. Cows and goats that are well cared for and kept clean and healthy should give safe milk. However, since there is always some risk involved in buying anything fresh and local, you need to use common sense in selecting these products.

While raw milk cannot be sold commercially, some states do make allowances for the sale of certain cheeses made from raw unpasteurized milk. Perhaps the best known American maker of raw-milk cheeses is California-based Alta Dena. Organic Valley out of Wisconsin is another. As a consumer, you should be aware that these companies make both kinds of cheese, some from unpasteurized and some from pasteurized milk, so always pay attention and read labels carefully. Taking a food company for granted could mean you end up with something you didn't bargain for.

Dairy for Adults

As noted, adults of many different ethnicities can exhibit signs of lactose intolerance to varying degrees. While babies have no problem with their mother's milk, many people experience a pronounced change regarding dairy as they grow up because, by adolescence, many have lost the lactase enzyme, the one responsible for the ability to digest lactose (milk sugar). Lacking this enzyme, continued exposure to lactose (milk) poses a problem.

The bottom line here is that nature never intended people to continue drinking milk, or putting it on their cereal, past early childhood. Going against nature's intentions is often a prescription for trouble, and the people who persist in consuming milk into adulthood seem to be at greater risk for arthritis, diabetes, eczema, heart disease, obesity, and other problems than people who do not consume dairy products as adults.

Given these concerns, many people are beginning to question the milk industry's campaign to get people to drink *more* milk. Targeting minorities by using popular sports figures and other role models as spokespeople for milk ads seems to conflict with public health goals of reducing poor health in ethnic populations.

One partial solution for lactose-intolerant adults who want the benefits of dairy may be yogurt and similarly cultured milk products. Since the bacteria used to colonize and culture milk into yogurt metabolize (digest) milk sugar, most yogurts are low in lactose, relative to milk, and can often be better tolerated by those who are lactose intolerant.

Goat's Milk

In America, dairy is usually equated with milk from cows, but other cultures have traditionally gotten milk, cheese, yogurts, and other products from camels, goats, sheep, yaks, and other locally available (and cooperative) animals. Since the earliest days of agriculture and animal husbandry, goats (and sheep) have provided an excellent source of nutrient-dense food, and a slightly different spectrum of proteins and fats than cow's milk, making it better tolerated by some sensitive individuals than cow's milk. Although nutritionally similar to cow's milk in overall denseness, goat's milk is slightly higher in protein, total lipids, some minerals, and many of the vitamins.

Health food stores generally carry goat's milk cheeses and yogurts along with the usual cow's milk products. Both products are often derived from homogenized and pasteurized milk. Raw goat's milk cheeses are available, but to find them you have to read the labels carefully. I consider raw goat's milk cheeses very good quality products, and quite desirable from the standpoint of *The Nutrient-Dense Eating Plan*.

In many rural communities, people still like to raise a few goats for their milk and cheese, and whenever I relocate, I always make an effort to find a local person who produces and sells goat's milk. These efforts have nearly always been rewarded, and my diet has been all the denser for it.

I offer a word of caution, however. Pasteurized goat's milk is widely available in health food stores, but the same nutritional principles regarding pasteurized cow's milk apply to pasteurized goat's milk. Plus, in contrast to the mild taste of fresh, raw goat's milk, the taste of pasteurized goat's milk is often too strong for many.

CHAPTER 29

Green Foods

The phrase *green foods* refers to a class of highly nutrient-dense foods that are rich sources of chlorophyll, the plant-based pigment that is the direct intermediary between all life on this planet and the star it circles, the sun. Because these chlorophyll-containing foods are so closely linked to the sun, they are considered to be very low on the food chain, and eating them amounts to ingesting nutrients in a very unrefined, almost primitive state; like sea salt, such nutrients are in a unique position to nourish you at a very basic level. Although difficult to measure scientifically, the effects of these foods are easily felt by people. Many are extraordinary contributors of key enzymes and nutrients—and I consider them genuinely valid sources of nutrient-dense nutrition.

Although some people think of these foods as *supplements,* I consider them to be complete foods, just as I understand that bee pollen, nutritional yeast, and seaweed are the same intact, unaltered, and unprocessed whole foods that they are in nature. Some of these are widely used as condiments and nutritional boosters, but they are still, in and of themselves, naturally occurring, nutrient-dense whole foods.

MICROALGAE

Many green foods are forms of algae. The blue-green algae from Oregon's Klamath Lake, chlorella, and spirulina are several widely marketed types. They come in tablets and powders, and are often mixed into various vitamin and mineral formulations, or added to energy bars and smoothies as nutrition boosters.

Blue-green algae, chlorella, and spirulina, are considered among the oldest organisms on earth, and have remained essentially unchanged for billions of years. In addition to their chlorophyll, these plants are unusually dense sources of protein (60 percent by weight) and minerals, including chromium, copper, iron, manganese, magnesium, selenium, and trace minerals. Algae also contain other interesting pigments besides chlorophyll—various carotenes, an unusual blue pigment called phycocyanin, and xanthophylls, all of which are being studied for their ability to enhance the immune system. Algae are also sources of beneficial, hard-to-get lipids, including gamma-linolenic acid. Special polysaccharides from algae's cell walls (which some researchers believe can chelate and remove heavy metals), and the nucleic acids DNA and RNA are other compounds contributed by these unique plants.

ADDITIONAL GREEN FOODS

In addition to microalgae, other green foods include wheatgrass and barley grass. The young, tender sprouts of wheat or barley are composed of plant tissues undergoing rapid growth and cell division, and the result of this metabolic activity is that these sprouts have a higher enzymatic activity than at any other phase in their life cycle. Fresh wheatgrass juice, for example, is a very dense source of the important antioxidant enzymes, catalase and superoxide dismutase (SOD), which protect sensitive cells against free radicals and may help to combat some cancers and inflammation.

In addition to metabolically important enzymes, young grasses are excellent sources for some B vitamins, chlorophyll, and minerals. Chlorophyll is a complex mixture of pigments, and includes various carotenoids that can act as antioxidants. Chemically, chlorophyll is analogous to hemoglobin in higher animals, so you can think of chlorophyll as the blood of plants. The primary difference between chlorophyll and hemoglobin is that the latter has an iron ion (charged atom) at its core, while a chlorophyll molecule has a magnesium ion at its center. This is why most green plants are good sources of magnesium. All the green foods mentioned in this chapter, and especially fresh wheatgrass or barley juice, are good sources of this important mineral.

Generally available in health food stores and juice bars, these grasses can be juiced and drunk fresh, which is the best way to obtain their benefits. I consider small quantities of these juices to be extraordinarily potent, nutrient-dense foods; so potent, in fact, that they are best consumed in small quantities of one or two ounces at a time.

Many green foods marketed today as nutritional supplements are complex mixtures of several foods, with other nutrients and concentrated foods added. Barley and wheatgrass often come in dehydrated, powdered form, and are sometimes mixed with dried, powdered microalgae and other nutrient-dense ingredients. These superfood blends are easily incorporated into smoothies or other health drinks, and are a valid way to introduce high levels of nutrient-rich foods into your diet. They can be incorporated into cleansing regimes, or used to jumpstart a sluggish or toxic metabolic state, or they can be used to add to the overall density of your diet. They are also a great way to rebalance or alkalinize the pH of an overly acidic system. The SAD diet is renowned for its acidity, due primarily to its emphasis on refined carbohydrates, dairy products, and meat.

Green is the color most strongly associated with life on our planet. Ingesting adequate quantities of foods rich in this pigment makes intuitive as well as common sense. Eating generous amounts of chlorophyll-containing plants will go far in assuring that you have a good base for your nutrient-dense lifestyle.

CHAPTER 30

Nutritional Yeast

Many foods are nutrient dense. Unique among all the classically nutrient-dense foods, however, nutritional yeast (Brewer's yeast) is known for its exceptionally abundant range of high-quality nutrients.

WHAT IS NUTRITIONAL YEAST?

Yeasts are microscopically small plantlike organisms that multiply by dividing or budding. Devoid of chlorophyll, yeasts are dependent on their immediate environment (instead of the sun, like most plants) for food or energy sources. As a single-celled organism, each yeast carries its own compartment of genetic information, or DNA.

Whenever I am asked which foods are the most nutrient-dense, nutritional yeast is always near the top of my list. Yet for many, yeast presents a bit of an enigma and is therefore tremendously underutilized. While I have always known people who make use of it, far too few have taken full advantage of its powerful nutritional benefits.

There are several reasons for this. First, people do not know how to relate to yeast, and they often simply have no idea what to do with it. I tend to refer to it as a food, but many people consider it more a supplement, which could lead to confusion on how to use it to full advantage. Secondly, yeast is a bit exotic for many tastes. Nutritional yeast has inherited a reputation as a food for health nuts, just too unusual for many. People can understand that yeast might be an indispensable ingredient in making beer or bread, but what role it might play at mealtime escapes them. Thirdly, there is a mistaken view that yeasts are unhealthy or potentially bad for them, a notion that took hold as an extension of the candida hypothesis. Finally, people may vaguely think that Brewer's yeast might be good for them, but very few really understand how truly amazing this food is as a powerful source of nutrients.

YEAST AND CANDIDA OVERGROWTH

Candida albicans is the Latin name given to a species of yeast that normally colonizes parts of the human intestinal tract and other tissues, including the mouth. When kept in balance with the rest of your microorganisms, candida is a benign part of your environmental flora. However, when the ecological balance of organisms is upset (for example, through the use of pharmaceutical antibiotics), candida can take over, overwhelming the system with its aggressive growth. Metabolic byproducts of candida are thought to suppress the immune system, and may lead to an inflammatory or allergic response.

This candida hypothesis may still be unproven to the satisfaction of some, but it is widely accepted by many holistic practitioners. And since the existence of candida overgrowth has been extensively reported in the medical literature, fewer of today's practitioners are denying its existence. With each new report, it becomes almost indisputable that the overuse of antibiotics has created a climate in the digestive tract that could allow for a takeover by opportunistic microorganisms.

How often does candida overgrowth occur? Is it being properly and accurately diagnosed? How should it be treated? These may be important questions for a practitioner to ask, but they have little to do with nutrient density and nutritional yeast. In their concerns about candida, and in their haste to treat it as effectively as possible, some practitioners caution suspected candida patients to avoid all beers, breads, and baked and fermentable foods that contain yeast. Although it may be appropriate to remove carbohydrates from the diet of a suspected yeast (candida) patient, the reason for doing so is to withhold an energy source for candida's growth, since candida metabolizes (ferments) carbohydrates. Because of this restriction, people have incorrectly assumed that the problem lies with the yeast in those foods, rather than with the carbohydrates, and have lumped all yeasts together as part of the problem. Therefore, in the minds of many, all yeasts are problematic and troublesome.

As far as nutritional yeast goes, however, nothing could be further from the truth. Candida overgrowth is caused specifically by the yeast organism, *Candida albicans*, whereas the organism for nutritional yeast is *Saccharomyces cerevisiae*. There is no evidence that nutritional yeast contributes to a candida problem or makes it worse. On the contrary, the nutrients in Brewer's yeast make it an extremely valuable ally in building up resistance to such problems. As an extremely dense food, nutritional yeast helps you function better, by building up your immunity and host resistance, and by facilitating tissue repair.

THE NUTRIENT DENSITY OF NUTRITIONAL YEAST

Brewer's yeast might be the most nutritionally versatile of all foods. While other nutrient-dense foods can be high in certain vitamins, minerals, or phytonutrients, yeast supplies large amounts of a wide range of nutrients. It is an outstanding source of the trace minerals copper, chromium (190 mcg), and selenium (>60 mcg).

As the single best source of many of the B vitamins, including B_1, (thiamine), B_2 (riboflavin), B_3 (niacin), and B_6 (pyridoxine), Brewer's yeast is a nutrient-dense powerhouse. A single serving of one brand is listed as supplying 80 percent of a person's requirement for B_1, 90 percent for B_2, 50 percent for B_3, 40 percent for B_6, and 15 percent of the requirement for folic acid. In addition, nutritional yeast supplies B_{12} (5 percent), iron (10 percent), manganese, magnesium (8 percent), potassium (›600 mg), sulfur, and substantial amounts of the nutrients inositol (100 mg) and choline (›125 mg).

Yeast is also an important source of protein. A thirty-gram serving gives you a full 16 grams of protein, making it approximately 50 to 60 percent protein by weight (the rest is principally carbohydrate and fiber; yeast is a no-fat food). Yeast protein is high quality, rich in the amino acids lysine and tryptophan, which are often low in vegetable proteins. Nutritional yeast could therefore be considered an important and useful way of complementing proteins in a vegetarian diet.

In addition to protein and its constituent amino acids, nutritional yeast also supplies the biologically important enzymes glutathione and superoxide dismutase (SOD). As components of your antioxidant defense system, these enzymes are important for cancer prevention and control.

Nutritional yeast is also an unusually dense source of the nucleic acids DNA and RNA, which are the biological molecules of genetic information. DNA and RNA are composed of subunits of amino acids with highly specific sugar molecules. Yeast is more than 6 percent nucleic acids by weight; since you ingest countless microorganisms, you consume each yeast cell's nucleus and biochemical machinery as well.

USING NUTRITIONAL YEAST

Yeast is surprisingly easy to incorporate into a nutrient-dense diet. As a food, a sprinkle-on condiment, or as a supplement, yeast will dramatically boost the overall density of any meal.

Perhaps the simplest way to enjoy the benefits of yeast is to sprinkle it on as a condiment—many health-oriented restaurants and cafes now include it on the table with other condiments. Yeast has a nutty, yeasty-cheesy taste that can be quite enjoyable. I frequently spoon some onto my millet, rice, or vegetables, and it is delicious added to soups or sprinkled on salads. One of its most popular uses is as a flavoring for popcorn. Many health food stores around the country sell prepopped popcorn spiced with yeast, and sometimes with other nutrient-dense sprinkles too—granulated garlic, powdered seaweed, or spirulina, for example. Another traditional use of yeast is as a *breading* for tofu. Sautéing tofu or tempeh in a batter of yeast with a little water, or coconut or olive oil, can create a nice crunchy texture and coating that is a pleasing contrast to the creamy smoothness of the underlying tofu or tempeh.

Nutritional yeast also comes in capsules and tablets, an easy option for those who find the taste of yeast disagreeable but desire its nutritional benefits. While this option is fine, I want to stress that yeast is a nutrient-dense food, to be enjoyed as such.

Many companies make nutritional yeast and it is sometimes sold in bulk bins in health food stores as a yellowish powder or as flakes. Lewis Labs sells a mild-tasting imported version that comes in sealed cans (preserving the freshness of such a nutrient-rich food this way is a good idea). I find their yeast, consistently fresh and palatable, popular when served to friends who have never tried (or liked) yeast before. Red Star nutritional yeast is another excellent company with a proven track record. Much of the bulk yeast in health food stores comes from this company.

Even though the terms nutritional yeast and Brewer's yeast are interchangeable, most yeast sold in stores is not a byproduct of the brewing industry, but is grown expressly as a nutritional food. Due to the presence of hops, real Brewer's yeasts may have an unacceptably bitter taste. Nutritional yeast from Lewis Labs, Red Star, or other companies is often grown on sugar beets, and one of the advantages of yeasts grown on this medium comes from the numerous nutrients absorbed by the deep tap roots of the beets.

There is, as stated previously, no evidence that nutritional yeast can in any way contribute, cause, or exacerbate conditions like candida overgrowth. Besides its being an entirely unrelated species, nutritional yeast is inactivated by high temperature-drying techniques. In contrast to the live yeasts used in brewing or bread making, nutritional yeast cannot cause any fermentation or leavening. Since yeasts are considered plants, nutritional yeast is a highly recommended nutrient-dense food for everyone, vegans and vegetarians included.

CHAPTER 31

Garlic

Would you be surprised to learn that the humble garlic bulb is one of the most actively researched and studied foods? Garlic has been investigated for its potential in preventing cancer, its immune-enhancing properties, and its renowned cardiovascular support. Through all this scrutiny, this most pungent of herbs has revealed it is worthy of all the fuss that has been made over it for centuries.

Garlic is a prominent member of the allium family that also includes chives, leeks, onions, scallions, and shallots. The alliums are all related by their close relationship with the element sulfur, the yellow mineral responsible for much of their flavor, odor, and medicinal properties. It is the complex, biologically important chemistry of sulfur that intrigues biochemists and nutritional researchers investigating the health-bestowing properties of garlic and its allium relatives.

Biologically, sulfur is an essential constituent of many proteins and biochemical pathways, yet some people avoid the most sulfur-dense foods because the smell can be so powerful. This is a shame, as these people are missing out on a very important agent of health. Although researchers are still skeptical about the health benefits of some foods, garlic is not one of them. It is a pioneering food that has forged its own unique place in nutritional science, transcending the myths and folklore that have accompanied it through the ages. In fact, I would say that garlic has proven so strongly medicinal that it is hard to classify it as *just a food.* It is certainly a food, and an extremely nutrient-dense one at that, but it is also a botanical medicine, a condiment, an herb, a spice, and a prime example of Hippocrates famous food-as-medicine, and medicine-as-food statement.

In studies, there is growing evidence that garlic has antitumor and anticarcinogenic properties—its consumption is linked to a reduced risk for cancers of the breast, colon, esophagus, lung, and stomach. It offers protection to the cardiovascular and circulatory systems, and it has been shown to effectively lower triglycerides and both total and LDL cholesterol. Garlic is an effective antibiotic, killing a wide range of pathogenic bacteria in the digestive tract as well as systemically. Garlic is also effective at lowering blood pressure, and is able to inhibit platelet aggregation. And it has strong antioxidant properties, inhibiting the oxidation (free-radical damage) of cholesterol and other lipids in your blood. For all these many benefits, garlic deserves praise and a regular place in your nutrient-dense diet.

CHAPTER 32

Herbs and Spices

There is a broad range of herbs and spices with nutrient-dense capabilities, and they are a quick and easy way to add both diversity and denseness to your diet. By their very nature, herbs and spices are phytonutrient rich, since the same molecules that give them their unique flavors, aromas, and characteristics also tend to be potent antioxidants.

THE PHYTONUTRIENT ROLE OF HERBS AND SPICES

Before beginning this section, please be aware that I am talking only about whole herbs and plants. This is not about the bottles of encapsulated isolated components, such as garlic (allicin), ginseng, milk thistle, and St. John's wort, that the vitamin and supplement industries find easiest to identify (*see* Chapter 15).

The world has countless sources of naturally edible plants and other foods—one tribe of South American Indians is known to utilize more than 600 species of edible plants. But because of monocropping and the selective practices of chemical-based agriculture, the world's consumption of diverse foods has dropped precipitously.

Scientists believe that most plants evolved unique antioxidant molecules as a strategy for coping with environmental stresses, such as ultraviolet radiation and insect predation. In adapting to their unique environmental niches, these plants have created an astonishing array of phytonutrients. There are brightly colored pigments that attract beneficial birds and insects, and compounds that attract pollinators, discourage insects or other pests from devouring them, heal wounds, and prevent microbial damage. This diversity and ingenuity in the plant world can be of great use to humanity by providing an enormous range of plant-based molecules to nourish and protect the internal environment of your body.

The term *spices* really describes people's culinary relationship with certain plants, whereas *herbs* is generally more of a botanical term. Herbs often refer to the leaves of culinary plants, while spices refers to the bark, roots, or seeds of plants. Cultivated over millennia, the relationship between people and herbs and spices has not just been about taste, but also about practical convenience, for it turns out that, worldwide, every one of the thirty or so most frequently used culinary herbs and spices has measurable, distinct antibacterial properties. Three of these—allspice, garlic, and oregano—inhibit a nearly universal range of microbes.

Recent research has revealed that these antibacterial properties almost always work best when combined with other spices. This synergy is reflected in the culinary tastes of many cultures, which commonly use a mix of spices. Mexican and Latin-American chili powders are a blend of antioxidant-containing herbs and spices, such as cayenne, cumin, garlic, oregano, and paprika. Other well-known blends of herbs and spices include curries, complex blends of spices unique to specific geographic regions of India and Southeast Asia, Asian five-spice blends, and the classic French four-spice mixes. Scientists who research spices have found that those culinary plants with the strongest antioxidant properties tend to come from the warmer climates, which fits with the fact that fungi, microbes, pests, and other potential spoilers of foods and digestive tracts thrive in hot climates. Herbs such as oregano, and spices such as chilies, curries, and hot peppers, have evolved as an integral part of the cuisines of these hot-climate cultures. Worldwide, the most common herbs and spices are (in order) alliums, chives, chili peppers, lemon/lime juice, parsley, ginger, bay leaf, coriander, and cinnamon—all warm-weather plants. Other significant herbs with antioxidant activity include basil, dill, oregano, peppermint, rosemary, and thyme.

THE USEFULNESS OF TASTE

Herbs and spices help ensure that your taste buds also experience a diversity of nature's beneficial compounds. These foods may often appear to be more about *flavor* density than nutrient density, but there is a fine line here, since many of the flavors and tastes these herbs and spices carry also function as antioxidants, and carry their own information to your body.

Tastes have their own usefulness through their ability to communicate with your body's organs. A sweet taste, even independent of the insulin-stimulating sucrose molecule, can stimulate your pancreas and other body parts involved in sugar metabolism. Similarly, it is well known that bitter-tasting foods have a pronounced effect on the liver and gallbladder. Since these organs are involved in the digestion of fats, bitter-tasting substances may help alert or prepare your body for their digestion—and for centuries herbalists have employed bitter-tasting herbs for exactly that function.

Today, however, the SAD diet is responsible for a marked imbalance among the different tastes. Compared to the diets of indigenous people and what is known of ancestral diets, the diets of today are disproportionately rich in sweet and salty tastes. The bitter taste, traditionally provided by many natural foods has all but disappeared from most diets. Though not yet well studied, all these changes and their consequences will become clearer in years to come. In the meantime, steer yourself toward a more balanced approach to eating, and enjoy a variety of tastes; if you are craving certain foods, your tongue might be trying to tell you something. This is another beauty of *The Nutrient-Dense Eating Plan:* It supports the use of more diverse culinary tools to restore balance and harmony to your taste buds, as well as the rest of your body.

SEVERAL BENEFICIAL HERBS AND SPICES

The following herbs and spices have particularly beneficial antioxidant qualities that make them useful in a nutrient-dense diet.

Cayenne (Hot Pepper)

Cayenne pepper contains the phytonutrient capsaicin, which provides potent antioxidant protection. Capsaicin appears to protect the important lipid (fatty) portion of cell membranes from oxidative (free-radical) damage, thereby offering protection to the entire cell and its sensitive inner structures. Free-radical damage is thought to be closely related to atherosclerotic disease and cancer. Cayenne-containing chili powder also helps to protect intestinal tissue against ulcers, and other components of hot peppers help to improve blood flow and cardiovascular health by dilating the blood vessels.

Cinnamon

The enticing aroma and flavor of cinnamon hints at the unique qualities present in the phytochemicals of this most enjoyable spice. For centuries, cinnamon has been a culinary delight in many, generally sweet, foods and beverages.

Interestingly, much of the current research on cinnamon centers on its ability to positively influence blood sugar. With aging, the cell's sensitivity to insulin tends to decrease, a decline that can lead, in some, to adult-onset diabetes (type 2), and in others, to a cluster of symptoms widely referred to as Syndrome X, believed to be prevalent in the adult population in this country, and related to a high incidence of atherosclerosis and heart disease. Cinnamon can help to combat these conditions because it contains a group of specialized polyphenols—flavonoids—that increase the sensitivity of fat cells to insulin, making them more responsive to this hormone, thereby allowing it to do its job more effectively. When cells and insulin cooperate with each other, blood sugar problems often improve markedly.

Fenugreek Seeds

Some studies have shown that fenugreek seeds are useful in the management of insulin-dependent diabetes. They help lower blood-glucose levels and also lower LDL cholesterol and triglycerides.

Ginger

For many Americans, ginger is little more than an interesting spice, best added to certain types of cakes and desserts, but ginger, like garlic, has been extensively researched for its many health benefits. Indigenous peoples of the tropics and practitioners of traditional Indian (Ayurvedic) medicine believe ginger root (*Zingiber officinale*) to be of great benefit.

As with many medicinal/culinary herbs and spices, the strong, unique flavor of ginger is connected to the presence of specific phytonutrients, and these compounds protect the liver from toxins, and have antioxidant capabilities as well as specific properties that help to supress the enzymes contributing to inflammation and platelet clumping.

Oregano

The principal varieties of oregano, Greek, Italian, and Mexican, have higher antioxidant power than any other herbs. In comparative studies, the oregano varieties, all members of the mint family, exhibited even higher antioxidant capabilities than pure vitamin E, and were comparable to the synthetic preservative BHA in their ability to prevent free-radical damage. In another series of tests, oregano showed much higher antioxidant activity than flavonoid-containing foods, such as apples and potatoes, and had *four* times the antioxidant capabilities of blueberries, one of the most protective fruits known.

Turmeric

The bright orange-yellow pigment in the spice turmeric (*Curcuma longa*) comes from a unique class of compounds known as curcuminoids. In research, these molecules have proved to be even more potent antioxidants than vitamin E. Other studies have shown that extracts of turmeric are on a par with both steroidal and nonsteroidal drugs as effective anti-inflammatory agents. Recent studies have looked at turmeric's potential as an aid for arthritis and other inflammatory disorders, and have also found that curcumin surpasses aspirin in its ability to suppress platelet aggregation (clumping), which could be of benefit to heart patients. In addition, plasma fibrinogen levels, a major risk factor for heart attacks and strokes, have been brought down with the use of turmeric. Finally, there is evidence that the curcuminoids in turmeric also appear to offer protection to the liver, and may have antiulcer activity as well. The presence of turmeric in curry mixtures is probably a key reason why curries are such good preservatives.

Additional Herbs and Spices

In addition to the herbs and spices listed above, bay laurel, dill, rosemary, sage, sweet bay, and winter savory also have strong antioxidant properties. Studies have shown that black pepper, mace, and sage, as well as ginger (discussed above), can slow the development of rancidity in ground meat. Rancidity is oxidation that specifically occurs in fats. When meat is ground up, the exposure of the fat to oxygen is dramatically increased, speeding up the rate at which it breaks down, but fortunately, the naturally occurring components of herbs and spices can counter the tendency of these foods to become rancid.

CHAPTER 33

Salt

Salt has always been an indispensable part of the human diet. For millennia, it has been a universally valued, traded for, and appreciated commodity. Yet today, it seems that many people's relationship with salt is based more on fear and concern than appreciation. Consistent warnings from the medical profession regarding the link between salt intake and hypertension (high blood pressure) have soured many people's relationship with salt. And it is true that the fast-food industry's overuse and misuse of processed salt has received its fair share of publicity, further contributing to people's suspicions. Salt is yet another example of a normally desirable, naturally occurring substance that has been misused by processing, making it a negative food for many people. The relevant question here might be whether or not there are more nutrient-dense alternatives to standard processed table salt.

SALT TODAY

Much of the salt used in the West is quite different from that used by ancestral people around the planet for millennia. Today, salt is bleached and purified of any possible contaminants, then kiln-dried (sterilized) at very high temperatures. Manufacturers also use additives in this processing, because they absorb moisture, act as bleaching agents, prevent caking, and promote flow. Some FDA-approved salt additives include aluminum-containing salts, iodine, iron, polysorbate 80, propylene glycol, silicon dioxide, and sugar.

By law, salt can contain up to 2 percent additives. The 98 percent of the salt that remains is basically pure sodium chloride, but many people feel that the body responds differently to refined salt than to natural salts, probably because the trace minerals normally found in natural salt deposits are refined out of processed salt. Natural salts always have a slight brown, grey, or pink hue due to the presence of these naturally occurring trace elements, while sterilized, kiln-baked, processed salts are always pure white. Trace analysis on unrefined sea salts reveals they are actually a complex, subtle mixture of up to eighty different elements that are naturally found in seawater. There can be up to 2 percent of these minerals and trace elements in unrefined sea salt, reflecting the composition of ocean water.

Although such minerals are present in relatively small quantities, electrolytes and ultra-trace minerals actually work best in *low* concentrations, and although scientists have not yet isolated the functions of many of these minerals and elements in the human body, it may nevertheless be shortsighted to deny their relevance. Since people evolved from the early oceanic environment of this planet, ingesting small quantities of the concentrated essence of human origins should count for something.

SODIUM VERSUS SALT

Many people equate sodium with salt. While salt is chemically known as sodium chloride—an ionic compound made from chlorine and sodium—salt deposits in nature are always found to contain small amounts of many other mineral compounds, *which processing removes.* I feel that the balance and complexity provided by these other ions is the principal reason why the sodium in natural salt is far less likely to lead to hypertension and related problems than processed salt.

Another important factor in the development of hypertension is the overall balance in the diet between sodium and another electrolyte, potassium. For millennia, natural diets that consist mainly of unprocessed fruits and vegetables have been quite high in potassium relative to sodium, but the processing of food and the development of the fast-food industry has led to a reversal of this ratio, and people now eat much more sodium than potassium for the first time in human history.

Hidden salt that has been pre-added by the manufacturer contributes far more sodium, on average, than the amount added by people at the table from the salt shaker. This fact, coupled with the loss of large amounts of protective potassium due to processing, is the true cause of hypertension and other problems associated with excessive salt intake. Only around 15 percent of Americans are genuinely sensitive to sodium and need to severely limit their salt intake. For the other 85 percent, mineral-rich sea salt is a safe, desirable, and nutrient-dense condiment to be enjoyed in moderation. This form of salt is your friend, and can be a valuable nutritional support instead of a substance to fear or avoid.

NUTRIENT-DENSE SALTS

If you want to experience salt in its natural, most nutritionally dense state, I recommend you experiment with the following salts. The significant difference in taste and feel between these and the processed white granules every American is so familiar with will be readily apparent to you.

- RealSalt, mined from central Utah, is the remnant of an ancient inland sea (not the famous Great Salt Lake) that once covered much of North America in the Jurassic era. RealSalt has a subtle pinkish color, due to its trace minerals.

- Celtic Sea Salt is another gourmet salt, mined in a traditional manner in the British Isles. It has a coarse texture and is light grey.
- Brittany Sea Salt, Fleur de Sel, and Sea Star—all from France, the source of many high-grade salts that are sun-dried in special age-old salt marshes—are extremely high-quality, natural sea salts that look and taste far superior to conventional processed salt.

These, and many other brands of natural salt that you can find in health food stores, help show how even the smallest things can make a big difference in your diet—how the humble salt of the earth can make contributions to a nutrient-dense eating plan that is safe and effective.

CHAPTER 34

Sweets

In its natural state, as sugar cane, you can chew on a piece of cane and get its wonderfully sweet taste. Along with this sweetness comes an abundance of naturally occurring minerals, such as chromium, required for metabolizing the sugar. Cane sugar is a natural, complete, wholesome carbohydrate food, but refining the cane removes almost 100 percent of its natural minerals and vitamins. The end result is the familiar white crystals, which are incapable of sustaining health.

SWEET CONCERNS—SUGAR

Of all the warnings about the Standard American Diet (SAD), the most concern has been about the enormous prevalence of sugar consumption (the average person consumes approximately 140 pounds per year). It is also the most widely ignored concern. Sugar is ubiquitous, and yet few people realize how new this substance is to bodies and diets, especially in the quantities ingested. Except for limited quantities of natural sugars, such as honey and maple syrup (and these sugars occur only in narrow geographical ranges), sugar did not appreciably exist in the Western diet until the mid-1700s, when sugarcane plantations were created in the West Indies, mostly as fuel for the rum industry.

With the advent of cheap slave labor and mechanized technologies for refining sugar cane, there was an unprecedented sweep of dietary changes that has continued up to the present. Accompanying these changes have been enormous changes in health and disease patterns that reflect this rise in the consumption of sugar and other refined carbohydrates.

The food industry today uses sugar in an incredibly liberal and indiscriminate fashion. It is added to baby foods, baked goods, beverages, cereals, and even traditionally nonsweet foods, such as French fries, ketchup, pickles, meats, and soups. Sugar—in a variety of forms—is a part of almost everything that food processors serve people, and this is an enormously worrisome trend because sugar is anything but a nutrient-dense substance.

Processed, refined sugar is 100 percent carbohydrate in the form of the disaccharide known as sucrose. Sugar as it is found in nature (in sugar cane or sugar beets) contains both fiber and substantial quantities of minerals, but refining sugar removes virtually all of the fiber and minerals. Thus, aside from the caloric energy it provides, sugar is devoid of any nutrient value.

Ingesting large amounts of sugar may be even worse than it sounds. Metabolizing sugar takes energy which requires the presence of various nutrients to make. Since sugar does not supply these nutrients, the body has to rob its own store of them in order for this energy production to occur. Like a parasite, sugar actually depletes you of valuable nutrients, which can lead to long-term health problems. Because the metabolism of sugar results in a net loss of nutrients, refined sugar is a *negatively* nutrient-dense food and should be put in a special class of negative nutrients, along with hard liquor (*see* Chapter 37), hydrogenated oils (trans fatty acids—*see* Chapter 20), and a few other harmful substances.

There are still more ways that sugar can be harmful. Its too-rapid absorption by the body can upset your normal body chemistry. Your adrenals, liver, and pancreas respond to an influx of sugar by secreting hormones, such as insulin, to bring your blood-sugar levels back to normal. When these organs become exhausted or overwhelmed from processing too much sugar too often, however, improperly high blood-sugar levels can occur. Ultimately, if overworked insulin-producing cells wear out and shut down, diabetes can result. And there's more. Sugar is associated with increased mortality risk due to the accelerated rate of atherosclerosis (hardening of the arteries) that accompanies elevated blood sugar. And accelerated aging is also associated with the body's inability to properly metabolize large amounts of dietary sugars because elevated sugar in the bloodstream can combine chemically with protein residues to form new compounds known as advanced glycation end products, or AGEs. These molecules can lead to a loss of normal function, and often accompany the premature aging of tissue. Examples of AGEs include cataracts, a clouding of the lens in the eye, and discolorations of the skin, commonly known as liver spots. Other conditions associated with high-sugar consumption include behavioral disorders, a decrease in immunity, dental caries (cavities), headaches, high blood pressure, intestinal disturbances, and obesity—a depressing list of conditions that never need to occur.

Sugar's prominent place in the SAD means that sugar-rich, empty-calorie foods usurp an opportunity to be eating more nutrient-dense foods. According to government surveys, most people, especially children, older people, and pregnant women, do not meet even the most basic nutritional requirements. Because they fill up on sugar-laden snacks and junk foods, there's no room left for healthier, more nutrient-dense foods. And sugar's addictive nature only compounds the problem. The more you eat, the more you crave.

The candies, ice cream, and sugary snack foods that so many people love are only part of the problem. Breakfast cereals, breads, cakes, cookies, jellies and jams, muffins, soft drinks, and even commercial yogurts are just some of the high-sugar foods that many eat every day. And these are the obvious sources of sugar in diets. According to the Center for Science in the Public Interest, added *hidden* sugar accounts for more than 80 percent of all ingested sugar; so many people probably don't even know the full extent of their exposure to this negatively nutrient-dense food. Furthermore, since baby foods often have sugar added to them, the desire for this taste is inculcated at a very young age, and research suggests that some children get almost one-half of their calories from sugar.

SWEET CONCERNS—CORN SYRUP AND FRUCTOSE

The same problems with refined white sugar also exist for corn syrup and fructose, with several variations. These days, much of the sweetening power added to beverages, desserts, foods, and snacks of all kinds comes from corn syrup, or more commonly, something called high fructose corn syrup (HFCS). Normally present in fruit, fructose is a simple sugar that is commonly made from corn. Large amounts of commercially produced fructose is connected with a variety of problems associated with its overall lack of nutrient density. In addition, large amounts of fructose can induce certain mineral imbalances, such as for copper. In general, many foods associated with HFCS are heavily processed, and often nutrient-poor choices.

SWEET SOLUTIONS

No matter what is said about sugars, the fact remains that the sweet tooth is not going away. The sweet taste is, after all, a legitimate part of people's taste heritage, along with bitter, salty, and sour. The question becomes then, what are the best options available to you? What are the most nutrient-dense sugars and sweets available, and how can you best incorporate them into enjoyable but healthy eating?

Artificial Solutions

A thriving industry has grown up to cater to those who would like to avoid sugar and its calories, but not the sweet taste that accompanies them. Many authors and researchers have voiced concerns about artificial sugars, such as aspartame (NutraSweet), cyclamate, and saccharin, and I encourage you to learn more through articles, books, and websites. Suffice it to say, none of the artificial sweeteners contribute useful minerals, vitamins, or other needed components of your diet, and therefore they are not part of *The Nutrient-Dense Eating Plan.*

Sweet does not have to mean nutritionally empty. Instead, there is an alternative, more impressive spectrum of denser sugars and sweets from which to choose.

Blackstrap Molasses

When sugar cane is boiled down, pure sugar crystals are separated from the liquid residue of the cane, resulting in a thick, dark liquid which is known as molasses. These crystals of pure sugar are removed and then further refined, ultimately yielding the familiar granulated sugar we know so well. Subsequent boilings remove even more sugar, concentrating the original nutrients and phytocompounds of the sugar cane, yielding stronger and stronger molasses. The liquid of the first boiling results in a molasses that is lighter in color, flavor, and nutrient value. The thick end product, much darker in color, richer in flavor, and denser in nutrients, is called blackstrap molasses.

Compared to other sugars, blackstrap molasses is a truly nutrient-dense food, in fact the only sweetener that gives your body more than it removes. Its nutrient profile is truly impressive. Although most forms of sugar have, at best, trace amounts of vitamins and minerals, blackstrap molasses has generous quantities of calcium, iron, magnesium, and potassium. It also (depending on the quality of the soil the cane or beets were grown in) contains chromium, copper, manganese, and other trace minerals. The vitamins B_6, niacin, pantothenic acid, and riboflavin are also present in detectable quantities.

Blackstrap molasses has a strong, slightly burnt-bitter taste that appeals to some people and is a turnoff to others. I happen to love the taste and often take it by the spoonful. It has the consistency and color of chocolate syrup, and blends well with milk to make a refreshing, deliciously nutritious molasses milk. For an iron-rich, mineral-dense drink, try mixing it with chilled almond, goat, or rice milk. For added synergy and nutrient density, try blending it with carob powder. With a banana and some ice you can concoct a great nondairy, nutrient-dense shake. The taste of blackstrap molasses is a little strong for many baking applications, but its strong flavor does work well with ginger (bread, cookies, and snaps) and natural licorice. I sometimes drizzle it over yogurt to make a nutrient-dense sundae. Blackstrap can also be combined with less intensely flavored sweeteners, such as barley malt or rice syrups.

Evaporated Whole Cane Juice

Marketed under the trade names Sucanat and Rapadura, evaporated sugar-cane granules (whole cane juice sugar) offer a more nutrient-dense alternative to white or brown sugar. Due to their strong similarities to conventional sugars, these products are good transitional foods if you are gradually moving through the tiers toward an increasingly dense diet.

Are these products truly nutrient-dense foods? I would have to say they are not, because they are still little more than simple sugars. Still, it is important to give them credit for containing substantially higher levels of many nutrients than commercial sugar. Although minerals are not present in nearly the same concentrations as molasses, whole cane juice does contain appreciable levels of calcium, iron, and potassium, and the trace minerals chromium, copper, and manganese. Small, yet detectable amounts of some B vitamins are also present, which are completely undetectable in conventional sugar. Nutritionally, evaporated whole cane juice lies midway between the void of white sugar and the denseness of blackstrap molasses.

When using transitional foods such as this, keep in mind that nutrient density is a journey, and there are all kinds of stepping-stones to use on your way. By making intelligent choices, you can continually increase the density of your diet, moving into new areas of growth and exploration, while working within your personal comfort level.

Honey

Honey (along with fresh ripe fruits) was probably one of humanity's very first sweeteners, a gift from the relationship of bees and flowers. Although honey does not have a strong nutritional profile, I still believe it deserves a place in a nutrient-dense diet. It is a strong sweetener (even sweeter than sugar), but is metabolized a little more gradually and gently because it contains more fructose than regular sugar.

Even among honeys, a spectrum of quality exists. Honeys come in a wide variety of colors and flavors, according to the flower sources used by the bees. Therefore, due to the differing phytonutrients conferred by different plants, the nutritional properties of different honeys will vary slightly, and according to some, different types of honey can have different effects. Alfalfa, alpine, buckwheat, clover, desert flower, orange blossom, tupelo, and wildflower honey are just a few of the many fine varieties available today.

The method used to process honey has a distinct influence on the final product. Most commercially available honey has been substantially heated prior to packaging. This heat-treated honey remains in a liquid state because the heat applied during processing deactivates certain enzymes, thereby preventing the honey from crystallizing. From a marketing point of view, this is desirable—the honey looks nice, keeps well, and is easy to use.

Raw honey, on the other hand, is a vastly different product. Because it is unheated, it is much thicker, and has a different nutritional profile from heat-treated, liquefied honey. Raw honey also commonly contains small amounts of other bee byproducts, such as pollen, propolis, and waxes, each with their own special properties. And, most important, since they are not subjected to heat treatment, the original enzymes in raw honey remain fully present and active. In this way, raw honey is denser in trace phytonutrients and active enzymes, and much more vital than commercially heated honey (not unlike the difference between fresh, raw cow's or goat's milk, and the pasteurized, homogenized variety). Truly raw honey is less common in stores than heated, liquefied honey. A good source for an exceptional product is Really Raw Honey, Inc. Their website is: www.ReallyRawHoney.com.

Stevia

Although stevia is relatively new to health-conscious Americans, many people around the world have been exposed to this small, unassuming herb for years. Stevia grows prolifically in warm climates, and is popular in Japan and in South American countries, such as Brazil and Paraguay.

Extracted from its powdered or dried leaves, the compounds in stevia that are responsible for its sweetness are unique because they are noncarbohydrate. This is favorable for two reasons. First, being noncarbohydrate, the phytocompounds that give stevia its sweetness have no calories. Second, since it is not a sugar, stevia does not elicit an insulin response, which makes it safe for people with diabetes.

Stevia is a mystery to many people. Used for hundreds, if not thousands, of years in South America and Asian countries, it would seem to have a safe track record. And, since it is noncaloric and safe for anyone with diabetes, it would appear to be the perfect no-calorie sweetener. Nonetheless, the Food and Drug Administration (FDA) is being ultracautious when it comes to stevia, ostensibly protecting the public from any potential dangers that could arise from the abuse or overuse of this herb. But, given the enormous lobbying power and clout of the sugar industry, it makes you wonder who these regulatory agencies are *really* protecting—the American consumer, or the sugar and artificial-sweetener industries.

ADDITIONAL SWEET SOLUTIONS

For the health-conscious consumer looking for ways to ease off commercial sugar, there are still more options. While none are as nutrient dense as blackstrap molasses, other sweeteners can offer legitimate ways to transition from a less-dense diet to a denser one. And, as with evaporated whole cane juice, having options offers more creative freedom as you explore new ways of nourishing yourself and your family.

Agave Nectar

Agave nectar is a relatively new sweetener that should rapidly gain popularity as people become more aware of it. Agave nectar—extracted from the agave plant, which is also the traditional source for tequila—resembles thin honey, and has a clean, sweet taste. Although it does not offer much nutritionally, agave nectar is an excellent sweetener for tea and other beverages. It dissolves faster than honey, is very stable, even for baking, and does not solidify the way honey does. In addition, agave nectar is higher in fructose than normal sugar, is sweeter than sugar, so less is needed, and should appeal to vegans who do not wish to use honey.

Barley Malt Syrup and Brown Rice Syrup

Barley malt syrup and brown rice syrup are also good options. These sticky sweeteners have the consistency of honey or molasses, but with less intense sweetness than corn syrup, honey, molasses, or sugar. They can be used for baking and other purposes. Barley malt syrup has a wonderful malty flavor, while brown rice syrup has a distinct butterscotch taste that many people love. Neither syrup is very nutritious, but both are richer in complex carbohydrates than ordinary, simpler sugars, and therefore they get absorbed in a more gradual, less stressful way for the pancreas.

Birch Sugar

Birch sugar, derived from the sap of birch trees, is different from other sugars because its sweetness comes from the molecule, xylitol, which is unique for several reasons. First, since xylitol has a low glycemic index relative to ordinary sugar, it will not produce the hypoglycemic effect (low blood sugar) associated with normal sugar intake. Second, xylitol has 40 percent fewer calories than regular sugar. Finally, since xylitol cannot be used by cavity-forming bacteria, it will not contribute to tooth decay. Birch sugar comes in a granulated form, and is indistinguishable from ordinary table sugar.

Date Sugar

Date sugar, made by pulverizing and powdering dried dates, is another option for nutrient-dense enthusiasts. Date sugar is a good alternative for baking and other culinary applications because whole dates are an excellent source of soluble fiber, and contain the minerals calcium, magnesium, and potassium. Date sugar is less sweet than regular cane or beet sugar, and is particularly good in granolas and muesli-type cereals.

Maple Syrup

Maple syrup, the concentrated sap of sugar-maple trees, is a true gift of nature in the minds of many. Organic maple syrup is a wonderful flavoring and a real treat, but as with the other sugars mentioned, it is not a particularly nutritious food. Nonetheless, maple syrup does contain relatively high levels of the minerals calcium and potassium, and some phytocompounds in the form of flavonoids.

CHAPTER 35

Chocolate

The plant world has been very kind to humans. In the chemical laboratories that are the plants of the world, tens of thousands of interesting and useful molecules have been synthesized to supply everyone with antioxidants, minerals, vitamins, and a wide array of other essential nutritional substances. At the same time they are providing benefits for people, these molecules are also performing important functions for the plants themselves, attracting pollinators through color and scent, acting as protective antioxidants, repelling pests, and protecting plants from climate change, predators, or other environmental stressors, among other functions.

THE COCOA PLANT'S GIFT TO THE WORLD

The world has taken advantage of these plant compounds for clothing, dyes, fiber, medicine, and nourishment. But what probably means the most to people are the aromas, flavors, and textures that these substances possess. Take chocolate and its parent, cocoa, for example. It has captured the hearts (and taste buds) of people everywhere and is, in fact, the most craved food in the world. Cocoa, the powdered spice from the pod of a tropical tree, began as a sacred beverage used ceremonially by the native people of South and Central America, and its cultivation spread throughout the tropics in response to the near-universal demand for this *food of the gods*. Recent figures indicate that today the average American ingests approximately twelve pounds of chocolate a year (I consume a lot more).

Is chocolate nutrient dense? The answer lies in understanding both the makeup and the type of the chocolate discussed. Most chocolate contains a lot of sugar, which is an *anti*nutrient-dense substance. The wide range of chocolate products in the marketplace—chocolate-flavored drinks, cocoa powder, frostings, milk- and dark-chocolate candies, puddings, syrups, and so on—often contain a wide range of additives, including hydrogenated oil, that affect nutrient quality.

So, is chocolate a health food? Certainly the chocolate and candy industries would love you to believe it is. Cocoa powder, which *does* contain high-quality, potent antioxidant substances, might offer beneficial effects for problems, such as cardiovascular health. But in order to benefit from them, you need to understand which chocolates contain the densest sources of these nutrients and a minimum of the bad stuff.

The antioxidant molecules from cocoa solids are flavonoid phytonutrients. And the specific flavonoids found in chocolate are procyanidins, chemically related to similar molecules found in other antioxidant-rich foods—berries, black and green teas, cherries and other purple-red fruits, legumes, red wine, and other notable health foods. What is remarkable about the procyanidins found in cocoa solids (the unsweetened raw material of chocolate) are the diverse ways in which they can protect the blood vessels, heart, and platelets of your cardiovascular system.

Cocoa solids have the important ability to inhibit the oxidation of circulating fats in the bloodstream. Oxidized (rancid) fats are leading suspects in hardening of the arteries, and are why antioxidants, from vitamin C to vitamin E, have been credited with reducing the risk of heart disease from free-radical oxidative stress. Studies have also shown that the flavonoids in cocoa can raise the levels of HDL, the protective form of cholesterol. Other studies have demonstrated that platelets become less sticky and fragile after eating cocoa solids, diminishing the likelihood of platelets clumping together and forming clots. This is important because the tendency of blood to become sticky and clot directly increases the risk of heart attacks, strokes, and other ailments. Further, chocolate is nutrient dense in the key minerals copper, iron, and magnesium. A single, high-quality dark-chocolate bar will supply approximately 10 percent of the recommended daily value (RDV) of iron. The density for magnesium runs even higher—a single high-quality dark-chocolate bar can have from 50 to 100 milligrams of magnesium. Chocolate is also dense for the amino acids phenylalanine and tyrosine, which are important neurotransmitter precursors.

Chocolate contains other, nonnutritive, compounds as well, and these substances, such as phenylethylamine, theobromine, theophylline, and others, may contribute to some of chocolate's renowned psychoactive effects. Related to caffeine, which chocolate contains in small amounts, these agents may be responsible for boosting energy or elevating a person's mood.

Chocolate can definitely have a place in a nutrient-dense lifestyle, but it is important to discriminate between its different grades. The denseness or quality of chocolate is directly proportional to the percentage of cocoa solids it has, as this is where the flavonoids and other nutrients are found. Since most chocolate is a mixture of cocoa solids, sugar, and other ingredients, such as fats (cocoa butter), lecithin (an emulsifier), and flavorings, it is important to have the highest levels of cocoa solids and the least amount of the other items.

The best chocolates never contain artificial flavors and colors, hydrogenated oils, or preservatives. Milk chocolates always contain dairy, and have a lower percentage of cocoa solids than dark, bittersweet, or semisweet chocolates. To get the most cocoa solids and the least sugar, I recommend chocolate bars with a cocoa content of 55 to 70 percent. As usual with all nutrient-dense foods, simple is best. The best chocolate bars have the fewest ingredients. These usually include cocoa liquor, which consists of crushed cocoa beans (sometimes referred to as cocoa mass), cocoa butter, lecithin, sugar (optimally, unrefined), and vanilla. Natural flavorings, such as orange, mint, pieces of fruit, or various nuts are often added as well. Chocolates such as these are a wonderful and acceptable part of most nutrient-dense diets, and there are some great chocolate producers—Chocolove, Dagoba, Green & Black's, Newman's, and Rapunzel, to name a few—putting out some delectable nutrient-dense delights.

As I have said, *The Nutrient-Dense Eating Plan* is not designed to be an austerity test. Food (and eating it) is one of the great joys of life. There is no reason why a superb healthful diet cannot include the great pleasures of life, and a mouthful of delicious dark chocolate certainly qualifies as one in my book.

CHAPTER 36

Beverages

If the often-repeated truism, you are what you eat, is the heart of this book's eating plan, it is equally true that *you are what you drink*. You may think of food as the main contributor to your daily nutrient intake, but your daily liquid consumption can easily swing the balance of your diet for better or for worse.

The body consists primarily of liquid. Though the numbers vary according to your age, body type, and other factors, between 55 and 65 percent of the body's makeup is water. Most of the nutrients in your body are found in solution, and food has to be liquefied by mastication, saliva, and digestive juices before it can be absorbed through your intestinal lining and into your bloodstream. Rapidly absorbable carriers of nutrients—juices, teas, and water—fulfill this function.

With today's eat-on-the-run lifestyle, many people drink, rather than eat, their meals. Super-sized sodas, meals-in-a-can, coffee-to-go, and various fruit-flavored juice drinks have become staples for many who do not seem to have the time or inclination to sit down to a *real* meal. Unfortunately, most of these beverages fail the nutrient-density test.

So, how *can* you find the most nutrient-dense beverages in this fast-paced world? The truth is, there are many drinkable nutrient-dense options available. Similar to other aspects of creative eating, you just have to be mindful and a little proactive. As you explore these options, you will see how easy it is to move beyond the soda and coffee mentality. And, as you begin to become more nutrient replenished, the need for that quick-fix energy boost in the form of liquid caffeine or sugar will tend to diminish.

WATER

Water is the basis of life. It is the universal medium within which all the body processes work. The great irony, though, is that many Americans drink very little water.

From a nutritional standpoint, it is possible to think water has a nutritional density of zero. After all, water does not provide protein, fat, carbohydrates, or vitamins. Culturally, our idea of pure water is water that is free of contaminants, minerals, and taste. For many, water is a means to an end, used to add flavorings to, mix with alcohol, or dunk a tea bag in—fine for boiling pasta or steaming vegetables, but of little use alone.

As a physician and nutritional counselor, I have always found it strange when someone says they don't *like* the taste of water. I am uncomfortable with such a statement because it seems unnatural—water is, after all, the most natural thing in the world. To not *like* the taste of water is to me a sign that a person's taste buds and normal instincts are off-base. It is also an almost sure sign that the person has been brainwashed by artificial flavorings and sweeteners, such as aspartame (NutraSweet), MSG, or saccharin.

Of course, there is the strong taste of tap water coming out of faucets or water fountains in this country. Chlorine, along with other substances such as fluoride, gets added to municipal water supplies to sanitize them, yet this treated water is sometimes so unpalatable that it seems unfit to drink. Chlorine levels in treated water are known to fluctuate widely, depending on when the chlorine is added, and depending on local standards, which may differ from town to town.

Apart from the issue of taste, some scientists have raised serious concerns about the consequences of a lifetime spent drinking chlorinated, fluoridated water. Chlorine is known to chemically combine with naturally occurring organic (carbon-based) compounds found in reservoirs, leading to the creation of new chemical species, known as chlorinated hydrocarbons, which are known to be carcinogenic. Because of these concerns, the public has been bombarded with a lot of confusing messages. People *want* to believe that their water is safe. After all, if you cannot trust *water,* what can you trust?

When I was growing up, the idea that tap water could be unsafe was ludicrous, as was the idea of paying for water. Water was free, and the idea of shelling out good money for bottled water seemed ridiculous. Today, far fewer people find that idea ridiculous. The bottled-water industry is the single fastest-growing segment of the bottled beverage industry. Like most people I know, I routinely buy bottled water, and cannot conceive of *not* buying it. Instead of resenting the fact that I have to pay for water, I am grateful that there is good, clean, unadulterated water for sale. As with many Americans, for me chlorinated tap water is simply no longer an option. Pure, clean water is the cornerstone of any good diet and lifestyle, even if it does not supply vitamins or other nutrients.

Much has been written about the importance of being well hydrated and I will not repeat those arguments here. Common sense, as well as medical science, should tell you that good water is vitally important to your health and well-being. Being underhydrated can aggravate or lead to numerous problems, such as bladder infections, constipation, depression, fatigue, headaches, or joint pain, to name a few.

Not all bottled waters are the same. While some people may disagree, I feel strongly that the best waters are artesian or mineral, not distilled. Distilled, purified waters are clean and safe, but the problem is, they do not contain any naturally occurring minerals. Purified waters start out as treated municipal waters, and are highly processed to remove any impurities, including chlorine. The result is like *any* processed product, with no *life* left. I realize this is not something that can be easily measured, but given a choice, I'd rather drink *living water* that comes directly from a certified pristine aquifer or spring.

Such waters have small amounts of dissolved minerals, and intuitively feel better to me. Several brands of spring or artesian water actually contain significant amounts of naturally occurring calcium, fluoride, magnesium, and silica, as well as other minerals, making spring water denser than the purified, distilled waters. My personal hierarchy of water quality has artesian spring water at the top, then distilled water, with tap water at the bottom of the list.

BLACK, BRONZE, AND GREEN TEAS

Teas are extracts of specific plants or herbs infused in hot water. Hundreds of plants all over the world are consumed in this way, and can make important contributions to the overall denseness of your diet. Teas can energize, relax, or stimulate you, boost your immune system, supply you with antioxidants, and support you in innumerable other ways. Teas will not give you macronutrients, such as carbohydrates, fats, proteins, or vitamins, in any appreciable amount, but teas do provide an opportunity to ingest small yet potent amounts of various phytonutrients.

Camellia sinensis, known simply as tea, is perhaps the most widely consumed beverage in the world, and has been extensively studied for its beneficial properties. In both its black and green forms, tea contributes the phytochemical compounds known as catechin polyphenols. These molecules are biologically active, and studies have shown a wide range of benefits, including antibacterial properties, antioxidant capabilities, cardiovascular conditions, platelet stickiness, reduction of the risks for cancer, strokes—and even lessening cavity-forming bacteria on teeth. Other studies have linked tea consumption to an improvement in bone density, a lessening of inflammation in inflammatory bowel disease, and the ability to lower cholesterol and triglyceride levels.

In addition to its flavonoid content, camellia sinensis is also a good provider of naturally occurring fluoride and the essential trace mineral manganese. Many consume black tea for its caffeine, but tea only contains about half the caffeine of coffee, which makes tea a good way to wean yourself off a coffee habit that may have gotten out of hand. For many, tea provides the morning jump-start they need without that jittery feeling that can result from drinking too much coffee.

Tea drinkers can easily moderate the amount of caffeine they get by the type and strength of tea they brew. Black tea is the strongest, and includes Assam, Ceylon, and Darjeeling varieties—English Breakfast or Irish Breakfast are blends of these. Earl Grey is black tea flavored with bergamot. Bronze teas, such as oolang, are lower in caffeine than black, but higher in the desirable polyphenols. Green teas have the lowest amount of caffeine, and are highest in antioxidant flavonoids. All three, black, bronze, and green, are derived from the same plant, camellia sinensis, but differ because of the degree of fermentation allowed to occur during processing.

HERBAL TEAS

The world of tea seems evenly split between black tea drinkers and those who favor herbal teas. Both have their virtues, and both have a place in a nutrient-dense lifestyle.

Herbal teas really run the gamut of the plant world. *Diversity* is a key principle of nutrient density, and the diverse world of phytonutrients is richly represented by the broad range of options available to the herbal tea drinker. The phyto-laboratories of plants provide a rich array of compounds (antioxidants, flavors, and pigments) that have biologically active properties. Chamomile, echinacea, ginger root, ginseng, kava kava, lemonbalm, licorice, mints, nettles, sage, and valerian, to name a few, are widely available in bulk, custom blends, and tea bags. Although there are rare exceptions, herbal teas are safe and useful drinks for most people. Herbal teas can aid digestion, energize you, help you relax or sleep, quell nausea, and soothe frazzled nerves. Chai teas, currently popular, are blends of black tea, herbs, and spices, such as anise, cinnamon, cloves, nutmeg, and pepper, which are believed to offer unique synergistic benefits.

YERBA MATÉ

Yerba maté, or maté as it is more commonly known, is the national drink of millions of people in Argentina, Paraguay, and Uruguay. Maté, with its unique taste, deserves special mention as a nutrient-dense beverage because it contains comparatively high levels of minerals and other unique phytonutrients, including antioxidants. A traditional herbal medicine of the tropical rainforest regions, maté promotes mental clarity and wakefulness without the speedy jitteriness of caffeine.

JUICE

Fruit juice, one of the most widely consumed beverages in the United States, has the potential to be nutrient dense and healthful. Unfortunately though, the vast majority of juice is highly processed, pasteurized, and often spiked with corn syrup, fructose, or other sweeteners.

There are, however, nutrient-dense options. The densest juices are, by far, the fresh, raw juices. Like all living plants, freshly juiced fruits and vegetables are concentrated sources of enzymes, sensitive molecules that can stimulate white blood cells, among numerous other functions. Advocates of raw (living) diets are outspoken proponents of what they call *enzyme nutrition,* diets that are super-dense in plant enzymes, which provide them with tremendous energy and vitality.

Most Americans eat few raw foods. With the exception of the occasional salad or fruit, most food is cooked and devitalized. Fresh juices are probably the quickest way to get substantial quantities of potent nutrients into your body. Whether you juice up a couple of organic oranges or a grapefruit for breakfast, down a glass of fresh carrot juice, or grab a shot of wheatgrass juice at the health food store's juice bar, live juices can jump-start your diet and supply you with a healthy serving of relatively easy-to-assimilate nutrients.

Juicing has several notable qualities. Juicers break down the cell walls of fruits and vegetables, making it incredibly easy to absorb the nutrients, particularly beneficial for people with compromised digestive systems. Fresh juices can give you generous amounts of phytonutrients—the amount of carotenoids found in a single glass of carrot juice, or in a blend of carrots and other vegetables, will probably exceed your intake from all other sources combined. But remember, fruit juice can also supply a lot of fruit sugar, too. Consider diluting some of the sweeter ones with spring water.

A good number of books have been written on the subject of juicing. Many fruits and vegetables juice up readily and can be custom designed to meet anyone's needs. And in terms of nutrient density, fresh juices are consistently found near the top of the list. Antioxidants, chlorophyll, enzymes, minerals, pigments, vitamins, and a host of other phytonutrients are all easily swallowed and absorbed when you drink freshly juiced plants.

Bottled Juices

While bottled juices are definitely inferior to fresh juice in terms of enzymes, there are advantages to pasteurized juices. I always recommend organic varieties that are 100 percent juice. Too much of the juice on the market today contains high-fructose corn syrup, or increasingly, grape-juice concentrate. This may sound like a healthy sweetener, since it is derived from a natural source, but it is basically pure dextrose (glucose), and adds calories, but no nutrients—it is really no better than regular white sugar. And, since it is derived from white grapes, it contributes none of the antioxidant pigments found in the red and purple varieties.

I recommend using some bottled fruit juice for the highly pigmented antioxidants found in colorful fruit. The Knudsen brand, for example, offers Just Blueberry, Just Cranberry, and Just Tart Cherry. These unsweetened juices are dense sources of antioxidant pigments and potassium. The Just Cranberry offers 15 percent of the recommended daily value of potassium per serving, while providing low levels of carbohydrates and simple sugars. The Just Tart Cherry contributes 8 percent of iron, and a very generous 410 milligrams of potassium per serving. All these juices provide large amounts of potassium relative to sodium, and restoring a healthier potassium to sodium ratio is thought by many nutritionists and biochemists to be crucially important for maintaining health (*see* Chapter 33).

Other Juices

In recent years, other types of juices have become available in the marketplace. The Odwalla company, for example, offers flash-pasteurized technologies to bring consumers high-quality, fresh-squeezed-style juices with excellent nutrient density. These refrigerated juices are found in health food stores around the country, and increasingly in many grocery stores. Anthocyanin-rich berry blends, antioxidant-rich blends, carrot juice, fresh citrus juices, smoothies, spirulina or chlorella-fortified green drinks, and others are now readily available, considerably increasing your nutrient-dense beverage options.

AMAZAKE

If you are relatively new to health food store products, you might be unfamiliar with amakaze. (You might be unfamiliar with it even if you do frequent such stores.) Originally from Japan, amazake is made from sweet brown rice that is enzymatically broken down to release natural sugars from the rice's carbohydrates. It tastes like a shake, and is often flavored with almonds, cinnamon, dates, vanilla, or other natural flavors. Some manufacturers, such as Grainaissance, fortify amazake with alfalfa, blue-green algae, spirulina, or barley or wheatgrass. Amazake is filling and offers a somewhat nutrient-dense answer to the question, "What should I drink?"

NONDAIRY MILK

Many people either cannot drink cow's milk or choose to avoid it, but still want a beverage with a milky consistency. Alternative milks, from soy, almonds, rice, and oats offer delicious, innovative ways to have your milk and drink it too. The easiest way to get these is to purchase them ready-made. Since the demand for dairy alternatives is so high, all health food stores and upscale food markets now carry a wide selection of dairy-free milks, from the old standard of soy milk to rice milk and almond milk. Consistency and flavor vary from brand to brand, so I always encourage people to try a variety of types until they find one(s) they like. The nutrient density of these milks is not that great, but they are becoming increasingly important options for many people's diets. And they can also serve as useful stepping-stones

Almond Milk

Making almond milk is actually quite easy. The only equipment you need is a blender. Soak a handful or two of almonds in cold water (overnight is fine, but even a few hours will work.) The almonds will begin to come to life, plumping up and softening, as they absorb water. After rinsing out the soak water, simply throw the almonds in the blender with enough water to give you the consistency you desire. If you like, strain the milk though a cloth or clean rag. That is really all there is to it. This almond milk has all the wonderful nutrition of the nuts, including B vitamins, fiber, flavonoids, good fats, magnesium, and proteins—and the flavor, too.

for transitioning to an ever-denser diet. But be aware that many experts have voiced concern about consuming too much soy, including soy milk, due to the presence of phytoestrogens (plant hormones).

In Chapter 34, blackstrap molasses was discussed as a truly nutrient-dense food, supplying generous quantities of such minerals as calcium, chromium, iron, and potassium. One of the best ways to incorporate molasses is to mix it, like chocolate syrup, in rice or almond milk. Chilled, this is a delicious energy drink, which also tastes great when spiked with a dash of carob powder, cinnamon, or vanilla. I usually just spoon it in and stir, but you can also make a great shake by throwing it in the blender with some ice cubes and a banana.

Most of the commercially available alternative milks are good substitutes for commercial cow's milk, but are not very nutrient dense. You can, however, increase the density considerably by making your own nut milk. Homemade almond milk is the easiest and most nutritious of all the dairy alternatives (*see* Part 4, Nutrient-Dense Recipes).

RAW MILK

Most states and municipalities have laws governing the sale of raw, or unpasteurized, milk. Many communities, however, still have families that milk their own cows or goats and supply it to friends or neighbors. I have often obtained raw milk this way, and have always revered it as a real gift, unsurpassed as a fresh, living health food full of enzymes and vitality. I especially love chilled, fresh goat's milk, and drink small amounts of it, as I would a glass of fresh carrot juice or some other living, vital drink.

As with any unpasteurized product, raw milk should be treated with respect, as it could contain dangerous or disease-causing microbes. I personally have never gotten anything but a wonderful feeling of healthiness from drinking it, but for legal and medical reasons, I suggest you exercise good judgment and common sense if you find you have access to such a food. Make sure it was produced under sanitary conditions, and stored properly (immediately refrigerated, in a sterilized, tightly sealed jar).

In reading about the many healthy beverages available, I hope you are beginning to see how a little creative substitution can help you to break out of the habits of nutritional inertia. When you open your eyes to the richness of choices available, you will find that you can use every opportunity, whether drinking, eating, or snacking, to increase the denseness of your diet. And see, too, how easy it is to turn to a nutrient-dense eating lifestyle.

CHAPTER 37

Alcohol

Along with refined sugar, alcohol is usually considered a source of empty calories—the polar opposite of a nutrient-dense substance. And, as with sugar, alcohol requires the presence of stored nutrients for its metabolism, using up and ultimately depleting certain B vitamins and minerals, so that alcohol contains the same negative nutrient density as sugar—it takes more than it gives back.

However, the relationship between alcoholic beverages and health (or lack of it) is more complex than that. A spectrum of quality seems to exist in every category of food, and alcoholic beverages are no exception. Studies show that, even within this class, a continuum of density exists. To be sure, most alcoholic drinks do you no real good, except to possibly relax you and allow you to unwind. And, of course, alcohol can be extremely detrimental to your health, affecting your liver, nervous system, pancreas, and even your immune system, not to mention creating serious hazards on highways and in homes. For too many, alcohol abuse is a serious, tragic problem.

Yet there is another side to alcohol. Many people seem to have a need to experience what alcohol provides, and societies have always made allowances for this social (and sometimes religious) need, as evidenced by the sacred place that fermented drinks have held in virtually all cultures and times. Whether it is beer and wine in European and Mediterranean societies, sake in Japan, barley chang in Himalayan countries, or various fermented alcoholic drinks in tribal African societies, all underscore the nearly universal appeal of fermented beverages.

The difference is that today there is an unprecedented scale of commercial production and availability of alcoholic beverages. And the truth is, the vast majority of these drinks are terribly unhealthy. So where does that leave people? What, if any, benefit might alcoholic beverages offer to offset the damage alcohol ingestion can cause?

RED WINE

For years, researchers theorized that the most likely explanation for the "French paradox" was red wine. This phrase is used to explain the baffling fact that some cultures (France, Italy, Spain) traditionally consume a high-fat diet, yet have a very low rate of heart disease, which goes against traditional thinking on the association between a fatty diet and atherosclerosis. This is especially true since the French diet is not only high in fat, but also has high amounts of saturated fats from butter and cheeses—the very fats most strongly thought to cause heart and vascular disease. (*See* Benefits of the Mediterranean Diet in Olive Oil section of Chapter 20.)

While scientists suspected that the low rates of heart disease in the French were likely due to wine consumption, it took time to figure out precisely why wine confers this protection. Initially, researchers assumed it was the alcohol (ethyl alcohol) itself, but studies showed that was not the case. This became clearer when research revealed it was only red wines, and not white, that are associated with this reduced risk. When studies showed that red grape juice was similarly protective, it became obvious that the protective factor was not the alcohol, but the grapes themselves.

Red (but not white) grapes are rich in the phenolic flavonoids known as anthocyanins. Anthocyanins are pigments responsible for the purple-red coloring of many berries, grapes, and similarly pigmented fruits. And, as discussed in Chapter 13, these anthocyanins are actually potent antioxidants.

The French paradox story shows that certain antioxidants can retard the onset and progression of atherosclerosis by slowing down the oxidation of fats, particularly the bad LDL cholesterol. Other studies have confirmed these findings, and have also shown how these compounds can even inhibit platelet stickiness, another important risk factor for heart disease. From all this, it is evident that anthocyanin molecules give red wine a definite health advantage over white wines. In fact, studies show that, compared to red wines, the whites are not merely neutral, but actually *increase* the susceptibility of lipids to free-radical oxidation, while reds reduce the oxidation.

Further studies have led researchers to suspect that there may be more benefits to some alcoholic beverages than just the anthocyanins. In addition to these pigments, red wines contain other phenolics, including catechins, flavonols, and tannins, all of which are biologically active phytochemical compounds with antioxidant capabilities. Then too, red wines contain generous amounts of magnesium, which is a well-known cardioprotective mineral.

Does all this mean that red wine is a health food? I would not go quite that far, but numerous studies *have* borne out that moderate consumption (one to two glasses a day) lowers your odds of getting a stroke or even arthritis. And epidemiological (population) studies of different countries reveal that women in Greece, Portugal, and Spain have half the breast cancer rates of women in the United States, although they consume approximately four times the amount of wine that American women do. In another study recently published in a prestigious medical journal, moderate alcohol consumption produced favorable effects on insulin and blood sugar values.

It should be noted that some people believe there are at least three differences between organic wines and the conventional variety: sulfites, other agricultural chemicals used in conventional grape production, and cost. There is no question that organically produced wines are often more expensive. From a health standpoint, the major issue seems to be problems from added sulfites, which are strong antioxidant preservatives that are frequently added to processed foods and wines to extend shelf life and appearance. A sizable minority of people are sensitive to sulfites, which can result in asthma attacks, headaches, skin problems, wheezing, or other symptoms.

Some have pointed out there is no such thing as a sulfite-free wine since sulfites occur naturally and are usually detectable in organic wines as well as conventional ones. But the real point is that the levels of sulfite in organic wines are far lower than the levels typically added to wines made from conventionally grown grapes. I have found that many people who seemingly cannot drink red wine because it gives them a headache or hangover do fine when they try a glass of organic wine.

The other issue concerns conventionally grown grapes themselves, because grapes are one of the more heavily sprayed crops. Moreover, the natural sugars in the grape skins help the pesticides and other sprays adhere more strongly to the grapes than to some other crops. Since the way grapes are grown is chemically intensive, it stands to reason that wine is potentially a heavy source of these sprays in a wine drinker's diet.

BEER

Many people might be surprised (and happy) to learn that beer is a *potentially* nutrient-dense food. In many cultures, fermented beverages are thought of as important foods that provide abundant amounts of vitamins, minerals, enzymes, organic acids, and protein, along with the more obvious effects of alcohol. Historically, it is thought that both beer and bread arose from the preparation of grain-based gruels, or porridges, that were allowed to ferment from yeasts, either by accident or intentionally. Yeast, of course, is an essential element for the successful development of both beers and breads. Fermentation is the process by which yeasts feed on carbohydrates, and yield byproducts, including ethyl alcohol.

Grain-based porridges have traditionally been staples throughout the temperate and tropical world. When porridge is allowed to ferment, the growing yeasts add amino acids, minerals, and vitamins to the mixture. Fermenting is a good way to improve the absorbability of the grain's nutrients and a good way to preserve the nutritional value of the food (or beverage). Yeasts are wonderful sources of many important nutrients (*see* Chapter 30), being particularly rich contributors of the B vitamins, including niacin, thiamine, and riboflavin, and important amino acids, nucleic acids, and other factors.

Research has confirmed that some beers resemble red wine in inhibiting platelet aggregation (stickiness), a risk factor for such cardiovascular conditions as heart attacks and strokes. It is widely believed that the flavonoid components of beer are primarily responsible for these beneficial effects, an idea reinforced by the finding that, in at least one study, flavonoid-dense dark beers were much more effective than light beers containing fewer of these antioxidants.

Japanese scientists have found that some varieties of stout beers from around the world are able to inhibit the induction of certain cancers in laboratory test animals. In another study conducted in Israel, researchers found that moderate beer drinking lowered total cholesterol by 25 percent, and LDL cholesterol by more than 27 percent.

As far as the nutrient density of beer goes, certain beers (stouts) are considered good sources of iron. In general, small-batch microbrew beers are far denser for nutrients than the highly filtered, pasteurized, and processed commercial beers. Such microbrews are much closer to the dense, traditional brews of the past, and many even have residues of yeast at the bottom of the bottle, a testament to their naturalness. Commercial breweries, on the other hand, add numerous chemicals to their beers, such as clarifying agents, foam (head) stabilizers, and so on. The ancient tradition of fermenting grains to make natural alcoholic beverages has, like so many others, become a chemical-based industry.

ETHANOL

Most alcoholic beverages are basically empty calories and ethanol, which itself is a controversial topic in the health world. The general consensus seems to be that small amounts can have beneficial effects on cardiovascular health. However, once that moderate threshold is exceeded, the negative effects of excess alcohol quickly take over.

URETHANES

Lastly is the almost unknown issue of urethanes. Although they have received little attention in the media, their presence in distilled drinks is significant. A suspected carcinogen, urethane is a highly toxic byproduct of fermentation and distilling, and its levels are increased by distilling techniques, such as heating. Because of this, some types of alcoholic beverages are higher in urethanes than others, particularly (cooking) sherries and bourbons. Urethane levels are hard to predict, and can vary widely, but very high levels have been found in fruit brandies and many types of sake (rice wines). To its credit, the distilled spirits industry is working with the FDA and other government agencies to try and get the levels of urethanes down. In the meantime, due to its extremely toxic nature, I recommend avoiding bourbons, brandies, sherries, whiskey, and commercial pasteurized sakes.

SUMMARY

The nutrient-dense diet strongly favors a diverse diet based on sound principles of commonsense nutrition. It also demands a certain level of responsibility and expects people to be able to make sensible decisions based on their knowledge of the pros and cons of different foods. Alcoholic beverages are no different. While alcoholism is a serious personal and social problem, it should be acknowledged that most people *can* drink responsibly. For those individuals, *The Nutrient-Dense Eating Plan* advocates organic red wines, and microbrew beers as the most nutrient dense and healthiest alcoholic beverages. Within those categories there is a lot of room for choices, as both classes of spirits are credible sources of nutrients, in particular antioxidant flavonoids. Unpasteurized microbrew-style beers are also decent sources of folic acid, other B vitamins, and small amounts of different minerals.

PART 3

Applying Nutrient Density in Daily Life

CHAPTER 38

Overcoming Obstacles

Everyone faces obstacles. You may wish for utterly consistent, smooth sailing throughout your journeys, but the reality is there will always be bumps in the road, challenges, and occasionally, setbacks. How well you face up to these, and how skillfully you can overcome them and not lose sight of your goals is the real measure of your commitment to health. Being successful in your endeavors depends upon your tenacity and your ability to anticipate, and then respond to, challenging situations.

Food obstacles are basically of two types: outer or inner. Outer obstacles are the challenges you face from situations, people, or events that are outside you. They include such things as not having the right foods available, not having the money to buy what you want, or having a family that is not supportive of your food choices.

Inner obstacles are the challenges that originate from your own attitudes. When making a dietary transition, most obstacles fall into this category. Inner obstacles include such things as a dislike of shopping, a lack of confidence in your own cooking skills, or no motivation. Your inner obstacles are the hardest to deal with because your mind tends to call the shots, which is why I emphasize awareness of your state of mind, as well as your motivations and attitudes. *The Nutrient-Dense Eating Plan* is not just about changing how you eat; it is also about changing how you think and feel about food.

Change is never easy, and for many, dietary changes present a particularly interesting challenge. Everyone may want to be healthy, or at least have a healthier lifestyle, yet people frequently undermine themselves or sabotage their own efforts, often reverting back to comfortable old patterns they know are not in their own best interests. What can you do to improve your own personal success rate? Even more relevant, how can you succeed at implementing a nutrient-dense eating plan when other diets have failed?

The Nutrient-Dense Eating Plan teaches that successfully improving your diet begins with insight and honesty about your motivation and sincerity. Seeing exactly which changes make you uncomfortable, and understanding why, can significantly improve your chance of success.

OBSTACLES/SOLUTIONS

The following is a brief list of some common patterns and problems people can face when confronted with the opportunity of changing their diets. Suggested solutions are also included.

Fears or Dislikes Shopping

This obstacle may seem a bit silly if you have no problem with grocery stores. Although I personally enjoy hunting and gathering quality food, I know many people who find shopping a bore, a waste of time, even intimidating. I think this sometimes stems from being uncertain about food, as in not knowing *what* to buy, or *why* or *how* to prepare it. Disliking shopping for food may therefore be traced to a larger feeling of ambivalence, or a lack of confidence about food. It certainly makes sense that you won't get enthused about procuring food if you're not sure what to do with it.

The solution to this obstacle is pretty obvious. I have seen, firsthand, many people warm up to shopping once they feel more comfortable with good food. In order to approach shopping with some degree of enthusiasm, it is first necessary to generate some heartfelt connection with good food itself. If you love good food, it stands to reason you will love seeking it out and bringing it into your world. If you are ambivalent about food, or fear it (that cultural eating disorder again), then you will feel the same about shopping for it. Comfort begins with familiarity. Therefore, the best solution to this obstacle is to become empowered, through familiarity, with nutrient-dense foods in all their manifestations.

Budget Concerns

Many people encounter sticker shock when they see the prices of organic and other health-oriented items. Their concern is extremely valid, especially when people are used to paying less for subsidized, commercial and fast foods. However, there are a lot of long-term hidden costs associated with poor-quality foods, including a higher risk of medical expenses, and time off work due to poor health.

We cannot put a price on health, feeling good, and having the energy to really enjoy life and live it to its fullest. But these are the promises of a really healthy diet and many people (myself included) are willing to pay more to improve our chances.

However, there is another, more practical side to this question. A nutrient-dense diet does not *have to* cost significantly more than conventionally grown, less-dense foods. Many savvy shoppers have learned that nutrient-dense staples, such as beans, lentils, rice, and sunflower seeds, are inexpensive and can supply them with maximum nutrition for minimal expense. And, in general, the bulk items available at many health food stores cost less than their packaged counterparts. Other cost-saving ideas include buying through co-ops, gardening and trading home-grown food with neighbors, and stocking up on sale items. Furthermore, as your nutrient-density level goes up, you buy fewer unnecessary and less-dense items. Money that used to go for candy, chips, cookies, sodas, and low-quality meats and dairy can now be used to purchase much higher-quality food. (*See* Chapter 39, Cost Analysis.)

Lack of Confidence in Cooking Skills

I have counseled many clients and patients who feel they are not capable of cooking healthy meals, a lack of confidence that often comes simply from a fear of the unknown. But, as you will see in Part 4, the recipe section, nutrient-dense cooking is actually the easiest way of all to cook. I seldom measure anything because good-quality ingredients are generally more forgiving, and because I like to emphasize simplicity in my meals.

Kitchen Equipment

In the kitchen it is important to feel inspired. Kitchen utensils and other equipment can help you feel supported in your efforts to prepare delicious, nutrient-dense food. Fortunately, your kitchen only requires a few essential items:

- A set of decent quality pots with lids for cooking rice, steaming vegetables, etc.;
- A set of cast-iron pans or similar good-quality cookware for sautéing;
- A blender and/or food processor for grinding nuts, making smoothies, and so forth;
- Nice cutlery—important and useful.

These are the basics. Of course, it is always good to have other favorite items on hand, such as colanders, garlic presses, a nice tea pot, strainers, a vegetable steamer, and any other equipment you find personally useful. Most cooks seem to find they use only a handful of items most of the time, so let your budget and experience guide you. Quality kitchenware can last a lifetime, and you can always add to your kitchen as time and budget allow.

With a little time and practice, anyone can master the art of throwing together quick and easy meals and snacks that are delicious and nutrient dense. For people raised on instant, precooked, or microwaved meals, nutrient-dense cooking is actually an empowering, uplifting experience—basic cooking skills, such as soft-boiling an egg, poaching fish, or cooking perfect brown rice, are actually easily learned skills.

Lack of Kitchen Preparedness

This is an interesting obstacle. I have known a number of people who would not cook or spend any quality time in their kitchen. Eventually, I realized it *is* hard for many people to be motivated if they feel unsupported, equipment-wise. This really hit home when I saw one friend who *never* cooked turn into a kitchen whiz after she received a beautiful set of new pots and pans. Since then, I have noticed a similar pattern—old, beat-up, poor-quality cookware often leaves people uninspired to cook. Nutrient-dense cooking does *not* require a lot of fancy gadgets or high tech equipment, but it is nice to feel surrounded by quality, both in food and in the *means* to prepare it.

Availability of Fresh, Nutrient-Dense, Organic Foods

While this is not a problem in any sizable city or town, there are still numerous places in America where health foods are not yet widely available. Solutions to this obstacle include co-ops, farmer's markets, mail order, online ordering, and shopping expeditions to nearby big cities.

Motivational Obstacles

A lack of motivation to change your diet for the better is a major inner obstacle because, without the motivation or desire to better your situation, there is really very little you can accomplish. A lack of motivation signifies that there may be little understanding of the connection between what you eat and how you feel, or the long-term consequences of an unhealthy, suboptimal diet. It can come from a fundamental lack of self-worth, the feeling that maybe you are not *worthy* of being healthy. Or, it can come from a fear of failure, and a basic lack of confidence in your ability to succeed at dietary change.

If you think at the outset you are not going to be successful, then there is little reason to get motivated. Therefore, the real solution to this obstacle is the confidence-boosting knowledge that transitioning to a more nutrient-dense diet is doable, easy, and fun.

Laziness

What is normally called laziness is often a lack of motivation combined with a too-hectic lifestyle. The nutrient-dense plan is perfect for time-crunched individuals. With a minimum amount of forethought and anticipation, a person can easily make better, denser choices for foods, even on the run. Quick snacks, premade deli-type foods, and other ready-to-eat whole foods are available these days at health food stores and supermarkets in every major city.

Not Eating at Home

While this may not seem like much of an obstacle, the truth is, many people do not eat at home or cook for themselves, and therefore have less control over what they are eating. Their nutritional fates are left in the hands of the restaurants they frequent.

The solution to this obstacle is obvious. People trying to adopt a nutrient-dense lifestyle need to change their restaurant selections to more accurately reflect the quality of food they expect, and they need to learn how to order the densest foods and meals on the menu. (*See* Chapter 44, Dining Out.)

IN SUM

The obstacles I have listed are hardly insurmountable. In each case, a little creative application can take care of them. Most of these obstacles lie within your mind—ambivalence, laziness, or lack of motivation or willpower are the principal prescriptions for failure—but if you are truly enthusiastic about the idea of reclaiming your health and taking back responsibility for yourself, then there is no limit to what you can do. These two core ideas—enthusiasm for a great diet (and great health) and the desire to feel personally responsible for your situation—are the keys to making *The Nutrient-Dense Eating Plan* work for you.

CHAPTER 39

Cost Analysis

Whenever I give a talk on nutrition and healthy eating, someone inevitably raises their hand with a comment or question concerning the higher costs of healthy and organic food. My first instinct is to respond with "tell me something I don't know." But I do empathize with these sentiments. It is hard enough to eat healthily without having to also worry about higher prices. But understanding the bigger picture, such as the hidden costs of eating poorly and the hidden benefits of eating healthily, can help you resolve any problems you may have concerning healthy organic food by putting the whole question in larger perspective.

At the outset it must be acknowledged that you do, in fact, pay more at the market for unadulterated, clean, minimally processed food. While this may seem counterintuitive (why pay more when less is done to it?), it is actually what you should expect: premium food *should* fetch a premium price. What skews people's expectations is that the market is flooded with cheaply made food products. Unfortunately, these low-quality, mass-produced foods cut corners by relying on cheap, synthetic materials for their appearance and nutritional content.

The real issue here is about priorities, not dollars and cents. If standards concerning your body are in place, then food needs to be recognized as an extremely high priority; you *should* spend as much as you can spare to ensure that you consistently nourish yourself densely. Fortunately, there are many ways to shop and cook nutritiously and economically at the same time. Later I shall examine several strategies for cutting costs while shopping wisely.

Why *do* some foods cost significantly more just because they are grown organically? The answers involve how food is produced, how it is subsidized, and who controls the market and the media through advertising—all aspects of a complex web of food production that ultimately translates into consumer prices and food availability. The hard truth is that food is not just about agriculture and nutrition; it is also about agribusiness, economics, and politics. In particular, much of it is about the heavy-handed influence of the chemical industries that manufacture the antibiotics, herbicidal agents, hormones, pesticides, synthetic fertilizers, and agricultural or veterinary chemicals and drugs.

My personal view is that part of the price I pay for organically grown food is a *reward tax,* a thank-you to the land and the farmers who grew the food in a sustainable way. I also believe it is important to show with your dollars exactly which food, and which agricultural system, you think is worth supporting. If paying more for better food communicates to the powers-that-be that you support a cleaner environment with fewer chemicals in the ground, water, and air, then it is well worth it. I am far less comfortable paying lower prices for a product from a company that shows disregard for the health of the land, or the possible consequences to future generations. I would rather pay much more for food with a less questionable background.

There are other hidden costs behind much of the cheaply produced food that most of America consumes. An obscenely high percent of the gross national budget goes for healthcare costs that studies say are mostly unnecessary. Good nutrition and other sensible prevention strategies could save this nation countless *billions* of dollars now spent on treating cancer, diabetes, heart disease, obesity, and other diet-related diseases. Conventional food may be relatively inexpensive at the checkout line or fast-food restaurant, but an enormous price is being paid in healthcare costs and human suffering. The only real beneficiaries are the pharmaceutical, medical, chemical, and agricultural interests.

More and more, science is connecting the dots between what people eat and disease risk. Biochemistry, cell physiology, genetics, and population demographics are some of the fields where nutritional insights are occurring at a dizzying pace. The big picture reinforces the notion that natural, clean, and safe is the best policy. Even if it does cost more initially, a nutrient-dense diet is imperative in order to regain health, as individuals and as a nation.

You can start rather simply. It is important not to resent the higher costs of higher quality, more expensive food. Transition slowly, utilizing the tiers and adding new foods as your budget and enthusiasm allows. Any progress is good. As you build up your nutrient-dense staples, the goal of having a totally nutrient-dense kitchen gets closer and closer, and doing it gradually should not put too much of a strain on your budget.

I say all this because how you talk to yourself is important. If you resent the higher costs of good food, then you give yourself a convenient excuse not to try something new. On the other hand, if you let yourself really enjoy expanding your nutritional and culinary horizons, then nutrient-dense eating will be an uplifting, enriching experience, and well worth the cost. The old-style thinking has been, "How can I cut corners and spend the least amount possible on food?" The new-style thinking I advocate is, "How can I get the most nutrient-dense, high-caliber food as practically and reasonably as possible?"

There are numerous ways to maximize your food dollars without sacrificing nutritional principles. Buyer co-ops are one great way to get health foods at a significant savings, usually at close-to-wholesale prices. They accomplish this by:

- Buying in bulk, such as case lots and minimum orders that are split among co-op members;
- Circumventing the markup of stores;
- Direct shipping to co-op members.

Another strategy for reducing spending is bulk buying in stores. Many health food stores offer items in bulk, so you can buy exactly as much or as little as you want. Because bulk items are seldom individually wrapped, the savings on packaging are passed on to the buyer. Many staples, such as dried fruits, granola, nuts, and various legumes and whole grains, are sold this way. Many nutrient-dense foods sold this way—beans, brown rice, lentils and other legumes, millet, rolled oats, and split peas, for example—are surprisingly inexpensive. Making these the centerpieces of meals is a nutritionally sound, economical way to stretch your food dollars.

Smart shopping is an art, so look for sale items and stock up on bargains when you find them as another way to keep your expenditures more balanced in the long haul. And remember, when you transition into healthier eating, you won't be spending money on old foods, such as candy, chips, and soda, so that money is freed up for higher-quality foods.

Certainly, many foods on the nutrient-dense list *are* substantially more expensive than their conventional counterparts. But by shopping carefully, and becoming more familiar with nutrient-dense foods and their preparation, I think you will find that the gains with *The Nutrient-Dense Eating Plan* far outweigh any losses, and in the long run, you will not be paying substantially more than you spend on the SAD.

CHAPTER 40

Instinctual Shopping

Our paleoancestors were consummate foragers. They climbed trees for bird's eggs or honeycombs, dug roots, gathered fruits, nuts, and seeds, harvested grains from wild grasses, fished, hunted, and generally learned to read the signs of nature for evidence of abundance.

Today, people largely do their hunting and gathering in the supermarket aisles, across the table at the farmer's market, or by scrolling down the items offered for sale on various websites. Yet creative and economic shopping is still an art, even if it looks far different from the ways of our ancestors.

How do you shop for high-quality food these days? Advertisements scream out from packages, shelves, and magazine pages, telling you what to buy and why it will make your life better. Hunting and gathering in a fast-food world is a challenging, but not very relaxing experience. But, there is a better way that is more in keeping with the principles of *The Nutrient-Dense Eating Plan*. I call this *instinctual shopping*.

Instinctual shopping means ignoring the hype and the advertising, and learning to listen to your inner voice. Instinctual shopping means learning to trust yourself, and your own body's knowing what it wants and needs. Instinctual shopping also means it is OK to have fun. Fun is often missing from the modern shopping experience. From the harried looks and hurried demeanors of people who are grocery shopping, it certainly does not look like a fun experience. Instinctual shopping provides an opportunity to get closer to your food and its origins. Shopping, after all, is where the relationship with food *usually* begins. If you shop with the right frame of mind, you are more likely to select food that will nourish and honor you, a potentially joyous activity.

Purchasing your food in a more conscious fashion is more intimate and personal, allowing you to find the most appropriate foods for your needs, and foods that are more in touch with the seasons, your personal cycles, and your particular tier level. You will also be less prone to buy foods that undermine or sabotage your efforts at nutrient density, and you will find it easier to make effective transitions.

Instead of dreading shopping as a chore, I encourage you to approach it as part of the adventure and excitement of transitioning to a healthier diet. When you begin to appreciate the goodness of good food, you may even come to experience a bit of the sacredness that bringing good food into your life can signify. I remember being at a health food store in Paonia, Colorado, the day that a large shipment of food came in off the distributor's eighteen-wheeler. The excitement of the employees as all this great, wholesome food was brought in and unpacked was beautiful to behold. You could tell this food was appreciated, for it was all destined to bring health, happiness, and creativity to the people of the community. Experiencing that moment reminded me how food does connect us back to the hunting, gathering, and foraging of our distant ancestors, people who were appreciative of, and grateful for, nature's bounty.

GUIDELINES FOR SUCCESSFUL INSTINCTUAL SHOPPING

Use the following guidelines to develop a more relaxed, rewarding, and enjoyable shopping experience.

- Do not shop when you are in a bad mood, pressured, or in a hurry. Relating to food is best done when you feel calm and centered.
- Notice what you notice. In other words, slow down enough to see what catches your eye. Are certain colors calling you? Bright orange carrots, emerald green broccoli, purple cabbage, or vivid red-yellow mangoes might be trying to tell you something. Perhaps your immune system is asking for more antioxidants, or your blood vessels are looking for a good scouring. If your eyes linger on the eggs, you could need more protein, or adrenal support. Wherever your attention goes, pay attention to it. It is probably not by chance. Tuning in to these apparently random connections is an important aspect of instinctual shopping.
- In connection with this, learn to trust your innate sense of knowing what your body wants. Do not censor perfectly good, healthy foods simply because they do not fit your preconceived notions of what you should buy.
- Dare to be bold. Try a new brand or a new variety of produce, or that nutritional yeast or cod-liver oil you have been reading about. You do not have to wait for the perfect time, or the formal entry to a new tier to try something new. If you are curious about some nutrient-dense food, consider that an invitation to check it out. Throwing caution to the wind and trying something new can only add a little color and excitement to your diet and your shopping trip. Remember, the heart of *The Nutrient-Dense Eating Plan* is diversity. The worst that can happen is that you may not like what you bought.
- Slow down. Many people rush through their shopping. Remember, every experi-

ence in your life can be infused with quality. Shopping is not a chore to get over with, but a sacred act. It is how you get nourished. Also, when you slow down, even a little, you notice more, and you will be more in touch with your inner knowing.

- Become more intimate with your food. Nutrient density is about cultivating a *relationship* with food. Really feel that cabbage. Is it nice and dense, solid? Smell your produce. It should inspire you to take it home. If something does not make you want to cook with it, leave it behind.
- Do not guilt buy. That is, do not buy something because someone or some book tells you that you should. Instead, buy food because it appeals to you and makes intuitive sense, or because it has genuinely aroused your curiosity.
- Shop with the seasons. The quality of food often fluctuates with the seasons. Apples are harvested in the fall. If you are purchasing them in spring or early summer, you know they have either sat in storage since the previous autumn, or have been shipped from a faraway place, such as New Zealand. Since really fresh produce is the best, this is less than optimal. Many other foods, such as avocados, pomegranates, and some citrus, are only available for short periods of the year, so when they are, take advantage of them. When they are not, make do with other foods.
- Get to know your favorite varieties. This is really important. There is frequently an enormous difference between varieties, so when you find your favorite varieties, stock up. There are different varieties of bananas, citrus, olives, raisins, and practically anything else you can think of. Since *The Nutrient-Dense Eating Plan* is about enthusiasm for great foods, make sure you find varieties that inspire *your* taste buds.
- Which brings up the next point. Always stock up when you find a winner. When our ancestors foraged, they would gorge on different foods as they came into season. Whether it was the annual salmon run or the ripening of wild berries, people knew instinctually to take advantage of nature's bounty. Long-distance transportation, shipping, and storage technologies have erased some of this effect, but with local fruit and vegetable harvests, you can still take advantage of seasonal availability to enjoy nature's abundance *when the time is right.* Many studies have shown that nutrient levels tend to be highest in freshly picked produce. This is also in keeping with macrobiotic principles, and is generally an economically sound way to shop.
- Know your brands. Certain companies, often smaller, organic companies that occupy specific niche markets, definitely hold higher standards of food quality,

integrity, and nutritional potency. Finding your favorite companies and developing a trusting relationship with them is important for shopping comfort.

- Expand your options. The first thing I tell someone who wants to change his or her diet is that you have to start by changing your shopping habits. Increasing your options means finding stores that have large offerings of helpful alternatives. If you are accustomed to shopping at a conventional grocery store, try exploring a natural foods market. You will be amazed by the variety of choices. If you live in a small community or do not have a natural foods market nearby, seriously consider other options. Try organizing a shopping expedition to the nearest big town once or twice a month, or consider ordering online or from a catalog. Perhaps you and some friends could set up a buying co-op. Remember, you are limited only by your imagination and your motivation.
- Splurge occasionally. Within the limits of budgets and common sense, it pays to reward yourself with an occasional healthy, but indulgent treat. Remember, food should be fun. If a treat is what it takes to keep you shopping healthily, go for it.
- Learn to read labels. It can be frustrating to buy something, only to discover later that you were misled by a label that made the product seem healthier than it really is. Learning how to quick-scan for unwanted ingredients, such as MSG or other additives, is an important skill that can make your overall shopping experience more fun, quicker, and more rewarding. Feeling confident in knowing exactly what you do and do not want is an important part of instinctual shopping. (*See* Chapter 45, Label Reading.)
- Shop with a friend. Food shopping is a personal matter; it involves you and your family's needs. However, shopping with a friend can sometimes lead to valuable feedback or new ideas you might not have considered on your own. But, if your friend distracts you from your reason for being in the store, or pushes her or his own agenda too hard, this might not be such a good idea.
- Anticipate your needs. If you are planning ahead and know what upcoming meals you are going to have, make sure you have all the necessary ingredients on hand.
- Prioritize. Remember, *The Nutrient-Dense Eating Plan* is centered on nutrient-dense staples. Prioritize your shopping to maintain a good core stock of these staples, and then supplement them with more exotic or interesting foods that might not get used as often, but that enhance the culinary appeal and nutritional quality of your basic foods.
- Strive for a well-rounded, well-stocked kitchen. The key to enjoying cooking is having everything on hand when you need it. Versatility and diversity are central

points of this plan. Nothing dooms a diet, or tempts you to reach for a quick fix or some convenient snack or junk food, more than having nothing healthy, convenient, and satisfying to eat on hand.

- Speaking of snacks, be sure to include them. Enjoy discovering snacks that meet the dual criteria of being satisfyingly fun *and* nutrient dense.
- Relax, breathe, enjoy. This is the most important guideline of all. If you find shopping is a stressful experience, then you should try and make peace with it. The whole idea of *The Nutrient-Dense Eating Plan* is to reprogram your mental tapes about food. This starts with shopping. Ideally, instinctual shopping should be a calm, nurturing, meditative experience. Shopping is where your relationship with food begins. Take your time, get to know the food, and allow it to speak to you. If you can cultivate a healthy dialogue with the food you buy, you are already on the way to increasing the density of your diet, and the quality of your life.

CHAPTER 41

The Nutrient-Dense Tier System

Knowing what to eat, and why, is vitally important if you are to feel empowered and capable of nourishing yourself. Yet this knowledge takes you only halfway. In addition to knowing *what* to eat, you need to learn *how* to eat healthily. The nutrient-dense tier system shows you exactly how to do this.

Although many people wish to improve the density, or quality, of their diets, they may find it impractical or unrealistic to simply span the distance from their present dietary situation to one that is nutritionally correct and perfectly dense. Improving their diet in manageable steps can help them progress at a more comfortable pace, thereby ensuring success. Using a stepwise approach removes much of the intimidation that some experience at the prospect of making radical changes to their lifestyle, and in particular their diet.

Instead of the daunting idea of achieving an *ideal* diet, making changes in tiers, or steps, empowers individuals by giving them the opportunity to go at their own pace, respecting their comfort level and allowing them to commit to improvements as they feel ready. In my experience, through years of counseling patients, I have seen this approach work much better than trying to impose a whole program on people. If you feel heard and empowered, you can negotiate changes with enthusiasm instead of dread.

Most people have very good intentions when it comes to their diets. Yet, good intentions often fail to translate into meaningful, lasting changes. I have counseled many people about this over the past several decades, and always find it fascinating to see how easily people can get stuck in their dietary habits. Dietary habits and preferences can become incredibly entrenched, and since people strongly identify with their dietary habits, the very idea of changing their diet can be threatening.

Are you one of these people? I think a lot of guilt, and even anger, can build up in people who get fed up with being told *what* to do, and then get left alone to figure out *how* to do it on their own. When I sat down to write about *The Nutrient-Dense Eating Plan,* I knew the most important part was going to be telling people how to go about implementing change in a *doable* way.

CHANGE AND CULTURAL INERTIA

Telling people what to eat, and why, is the easy part. Most people know much of this information on some level anyway. The harder part lies in overcoming ingrained or counterproductive eating patterns, many of which stem from what I call *cultural inertia.* As previously discussed, cultural inertia refers to the subtle cultural influences people experience from birth that keep them stuck in the dominant belief systems of our culture. People are bombarded with advertising and other influences throughout their lives, and so grow up in a culture where specific brands of food products, and even restaurants and stores become a part of their lives, with a presence that is familiar and comforting.

Questioning the health and safety of some of these cultural icons may mean breaking with the values and beliefs of family, friends, loved ones, and social circles. Some may accuse you of being ungrateful or unnecessarily skeptical, or a health nut.

The nutrient-dense tier system was designed to help you deal with these issues. The tiers offer concrete ways to implement the principles of nutrient density at a comfortable, safe pace, showing you specific ways to improve your diet in manageable steps, while maintaining your individuality. Because everyone is different, the tiers offer a spectrum of ways to transition to a healthier, more nutrient-dense diet.

PRIORITIES

The tiers work because they embody a system of priorities to help you avoid the possibility of feeling overwhelmed by the amount of nutritional information coming at you. Prioritizing what is most important, most feasible, or most relevant to you is important if you are to get serious about making meaningful and lasting changes. Without clear priorities, a needless amount of time may be spent spinning your wheels. And, if you try to make changes prematurely, you may find yourself backtracking, losing valuable time and energy in the process.

By prioritizing your steps, the tiers streamline the journey, making you a more efficient traveler. Faced with the pressures of modern life, convenience and ease become a priority. But, if changing your diet seems like a hassle or just another obligation, it probably won't happen. I have heard too many people say it is just too much trouble or too complicated to eat healthy, but why should this be? After all, we have to eat anyway, so if the goal is to be healthy, full of energy, and feeling our best, then doesn't it make sense to eat the best-quality food available? To me, the answer to this is obvious, but for others it may not be so simple. For those people, the tiers work because they allow transitions to occur as slowly as necessary for comfort and confidence.

I have also noticed that some people who learn about nutrition can begin to feel guilty about their less than perfect diets. Guilt is a very negative emotion, and can paralyze more often than it motivates. In teaching people how to eat healthier, I try to stress the positive and encourage people to lose the guilt and look forward, not backward. No one has a perfect diet, and everyone has made numerous dietary mistakes in the past. Give yourself a break. It's always possible to begin anew, and start fresh with your next meal, or your next shopping outing.

By adopting the appropriate tier, you can give yourself a slight challenge, an opportunity. Instead of focusing on the faults in your diet, the tiers can give you concrete evidence of how well you are doing. And they can motivate you to go further and extend your commitment to improve yourself.

HOW THE TIERS WORK

Here are some frequently asked questions, and my answers to them.

- **What are the tiers?** The tiers are progressive steps in *The Nutrient-Dense Eating Plan* that guide you to a higher level of nutrient intake.
- **Are there rigid rules to adopt?** Tiers do *not* have fixed, rigid rules that are forced on you. I want to emphasize that tiers allow you to go at your own pace, with your comfort level respected. You commit to specific improvements *that you choose* when you feel ready.
- **Do the tiers narrow options by limiting what you can eat?** Tiers do not narrow your options because you can substitute a more healthy choice every time you decide to lose an unhealthy choice.
- **Are the tiers hard to follow?** The tiers are explained clearly and simply, making them easy to put into practice.
- **How do the tiers help the transition from a less dense diet to a denser one?** The tiers help the transition by showing you what to eliminate, stage by stage, and how to increase density through creative substitution. To me, a tier provides a sense of perspective. It is mile marker and a viewing platform where you can pause and assess where you have come from and where you still need to go. When you feel firmly grounded in one of the first tiers, you develop a sense of comfort and confidence. You can take pleasure in the fact that you have created some healthy new boundaries for yourself, and this confidence can inspire you to jump up to the next tier.

THE SPIRIT OF THE TIERS

Please do not look at the tiers as a set of fixed, rigid rules that are being forced on you. Rather, the concept and spirit behind the tiers is designed so you can cocreate your relationship to the tiers as your journey progresses. What I will do in the following pages is provide suggestions and guidelines; the final decisions, however, are *always* up to you. The real point of this section is to help guide you in making your own priorities. Remember, the most important point of *The Nutrient-Dense Eating Plan* is to reconnect you with the pleasures and appreciation of good food. The tiers are here to make your journey smoother, more pleasant, fun, and easy to implement, not to create more anxiety, pressure, or stress.

Eating healthy should be a natural process and ideally should feel freeing and liberating, not restrictive or punishing. Many people already carry guilt and other associations regarding food; hopefully, the tiers will give you a different, happier outlook.

TIER ONE

The first tier is vital to your long-term success. Tier one establishes the credibility of the nutrient-dense system, and reveals several principles that will be useful as you move through subsequent tiers. It is crucial that you get off on the right foot, and it is important at this point not to lose confidence in your ability to make real changes. It is better to take a couple of successful baby steps and build your confidence, rather than take on too much and feel bad about your inability to carry through. Trying to accomplish too much too fast creates a very real risk of failure.

To this end, in tier one you set *achievable* goals and strive for consistency and self-accountability. It is here that you learn how to read labels, and generally become more diligent and mindful about food. Your antennae are up, and you are alert to any encroachments on the boundaries you have drawn for yourself. When you take this tier seriously, you can find a sense of delight and confidence in the wholesomeness of your commitment.

The most important aspect of tier one is to level the playing field by eliminating as much of the obviously bad stuff in your diet as possible. This is your great opportunity to get clear about your priorities and commitment. By taking your first tentative steps toward establishing a decidedly healthier diet, you get to confront your fears, attachments, and resistance. Having decided, for example, to eliminate a certain additive or artificial ingredient, you have to deal with the fact that some of your favorite comfort foods may contain this item. In this first tier, you begin to face the reality of what changing your diet really means, namely having to let go of some old, unhealthy, friends.

This can be sobering as you realize that changing your diet is not going to be just smooth sailing. Although ultimately rewarding, these changes can be hard work, which you get to taste with the very first tier. Still, since you will be making these changes in steps, you should not feel overwhelmed or compelled to be nutritionally perfect all at once.

Since the first tier's primary function is to get you started on the right foot, it is important to get rid of unnecessary baggage and travel as lightly as possible. This means eliminating the principal zero-density foods containing hydrogenated oils and aspartame. It is important to eliminate these because, to borrow an analogy from gardening, in order to grow a beautiful garden, you must begin by first clearing away any debris, rocks, or weeds that choke the site to be cultivated. The hydrogenated oils and the excitotoxins, such as aspartame and MSG, are ubiquitous nutritional poisons that hold you back from achieving the level playing field necessary to begin moving toward your goal of super health. From a practical standpoint, this tier can actually eliminate a number of foods that are nutritionally mediocre or subpar. Hydrogenated oils, in particular, are found in many foods that are overprocessed, nutritionally questionable, and generally of poor quality, so when you eliminate hydrogenated oils, you also jettison any foods that contain them.

It is vitally important to get in the habit of checking labels and of not taking the safety of your food for granted. Reading labels is important because it is an implicit part of your assuming responsibility for what you buy, serve, and eat. Instead of thinking of label-checking as a chore, view it as simply part of the process of being a conscientious shopper.

Success with this tier produces several key results. A sense of accomplishment at the beginning should encourage and motivate you further. And this tier introduces you to the skills you will be using in later tiers: label reading, more careful shopping habits, thinking ahead, and creative planning with respect to dining, meal planning, or outings.

Clearing Out the Debris in Tier One

Most of the tiers involve a blend of removing some negative items and adding some positive foods. Tier one is an exception because I focus more heavily on elimination of the most obviously detrimental foods. In subsequent tiers, there will be plenty of time to add nutrient-dense foods. First, however, you must clear some of the debris from your path.

In tier one, you confront your attachments and addictions. More than a few patients have come to me in tears at the prospect of giving up their diet sodas, but many have also come to see there is life after aspartame. One of the mantras I use is that nutrient density is not about deprivation. It might first appear that way, but in tier one you begin to realize that giving up your cherished notions of what you *think* of as beloved comfort foods is not as hard as you feared. As you move forward, you will see that waiting around the corner is a whole world of healthy foods ready to take the place of nutrient-weak junk foods. Tier one begins your journey by sending a strong message regarding what is, and what is not, acceptable regarding the food you put into your body. The fulfillment of the promise of nutrient density lies ahead in the tiers to come.

TIER TWO—CREATIVE SUBSTITUTIONS

Since it is up to you to go at your own pace, when and what to cut out is your decision. Although I urge people in tier one to eliminate aspartame and hydrogenated oils, it is your choice whether or not to eliminate one, both, or neither of these substances.

The second tier builds on tier one by introducing the concept of *creative substitution,* a principle used throughout the tier system to find foods to fill the void left by the foods you eliminated. Creative substitution is central to improving the nutrient denseness of your diet, first, because it fosters diversity, and second, because whatever is removed from your diet gets replaced with something more nutrient dense. Creative substitution encourages you to think creatively. Moving through the tiers allows you to experience a continual refinement of your diet by introducing new foods, expanding your nutritional repertoire, and increasing your exposure to alternatives for lower quality foods. Creative substitution can bring exciting new options and the opportunity to break out of old ruts and habits. And it helps you to not feel deprived by providing similar, but better—healthier, tastier—versions of what you are leaving behind.

Tier two shows graphically that, if you are ready to walk this path of a nutrient-dense, healthy way of eating, you must do more than simply deprive yourself of old attachments; you must create the positive atmosphere of substituting denser foods for ones that are less dense. Creatively substituting better quality foods helps create this atmosphere, and should give you a sense of optimism for your success, and enthusiasm for your future.

A sense of enthusiastic engagement is, I think, important for the long-term success of this endeavor. Performing a task from a sense of duty is a recipe for failure. Why do something if it's no fun? You should enjoy what you are undertaking, and adding enthusiasm for the adventure of dietary change along with your commitment to a healthier self *is itself healing.*

I think it is important to dovetail tier two with tier one as soon as possible because, in the second tier, you continue to build on the principles that began with tier one. Understanding how important it is to eliminate obvious sources of trans fats, such as margarine and shortening, was a great start, and now, in tier two, you become even more aware of their ubiquitous presence. You continue the process of transitioning away from such foods in earnest, and you actively seek out healthier, nonhydrogenated alternatives. This is where you actually begin the process of creative substitution, which marks your progress from tier one.

At this point, your creativity, resourcefulness, and open-mindedness will either kick in or be severely challenged, especially if you live in a place that does not boast a large, well-stocked health food store. You might have to stretch a bit more and investigate such options as buyer's clubs, co-ops, farmer's markets, health food catalogs, or Internet buying. Sometimes these challenges are a blessing in disguise, because they reveal the depths of your commitment and enthusiasm. If you can successfully weather such inconveniences, then you truly are on the path of reclaiming your diet, your power, and your health.

Get Milk . . . Out . . . in Tier Two

Dairy is often an emotional and controversial subject. To this day, a dear friend of mine in her late forties refuses to give up her daily milk (and cheese) habit, even though she has severe asthma and multiple allergies. She is aware that many studies have investigated a likely relationship between dairy and these conditions, but milk is an important comfort food for her.

Nutrient density is clearly not all black and white. While many of the commercially raised dairy products in this country are not of good quality, there are other, more nutrient-dense options available. By using creative substitution, you can find a place in the nutrient-dense diet for quality dairy products, especially in the transitional phases.

With tier two you begin to deepen your commitment to nutrient-dense principles. The nutritional awareness you are developing in the grocery store and kitchen at this stage can also begin to translate into other aspects of your life. At some point, the realization dawns that certain fast-food restaurants, for example, pervasively use hydrogenated oils. Therefore, you may find yourself changing some of your dining-out experiences in order to achieve more consistency in your diet and principles.

Curtailing your reliance on fast food is also important in helping you break the cycle of dependency that such places foster. Reclaiming your diet means you are ultimately seeking to reestablish a fundamentally healthier relationship with food yourself. In tier two, you may not be ready to sever ties with many of your favorite eating establishments, but you do start to understand more deeply that really enjoying food, including taking pleasure in its preparation and cooking, is an important step in establishing this healthier relationship.

For some, this will not be a big sacrifice, while for others it could represent a major shift in eating habits. One couple I know have what they jokingly refer to as a condiment refrigerator, containing horseradish sauce, ketchup, mustard, relish, and numerous other condiments, but no real food, because all their food comes from restaurants, takeout places, and fast-food joints. They simply *never* cook at home, and they are not alone. These days, many people no longer have an intimate con-

Working the Tiers—One Family's Story

Recently, I began working with a family that consisted of a businesswoman, her husband (a family practice doctor), and their four children. We began with tier one, eliminating from the house the ever-present diet sodas and tubs of margarine. After the trauma of these changes sank in, we began looking at the formidable process of identifying other packaged sources of hydrogenated oils, such as cookies, cereals, and the like. Because of the extent to which hydrogenated oil-containing products pervaded their freezer, refrigerator, and pantry, and because so many people's comfort levels were being challenged simultaneously, it was important to stay at the tier one level for several months.

Throwing out the diet soda was the first signal to everyone that changes were afoot. However, because we could discuss trade-offs and compromises (for example, diet sodas out and regular and alternative sodas in), even this radical change was met with relative acceptance. And substituting butter for margarine wasn't really an issue, because everyone could accept that real butter tastes much better. This is where we stayed for a while, on the plateau of the first tier, while the logic of these moves set in.

When the time felt right, however, we began to zero in on the next phase, which marked the family's entrance into tier two. Got milk?

nection with their food. It is designed, prepared, cooked, and presented or packaged by others.

As you move through the tiers, the idea is to encourage you to assume more and more responsibility for your diet. In *The Nutrient-Dense Eating Plan*, you don't have to cook *all* your own food, but at this stage an increasingly hands-on approach will give you a more intimate familiarity with the quality of what you ingest.

So, in tier two, you further clean up your act. If in tier one you gave up diet soda but continued to drink regular soda, at this point you may choose to stop drinking *any* form of soda. Similarly, if you gave up margarine and shortening previously, at this stage you may choose to deepen your commitment by giving up virtually *any* product containing hydrogenated oils.

This tier is where you begin to actually work with substitutions. Higher quality foods, such as almond butter, replace hydrogenated peanut butter, while rice or almond milk can fill in for cow's milk. Other changes at this level could include transitioning to higher quality desserts, and exploring more organic options.

The kids in my friends' family drank *a lot* of milk. Along with each meal, a tall glass of milk would be the inevitable accompaniment. But what I saw the two boys and two girls drinking was liquid antibiotics, liquid hormones, and a homogenized, dead food. I also saw something else: premature puberty, weight problems, asthma, and poor immunity in the form of lots of colds and sick days home from school.

Milk does seem to be an addictive food. Knowing this, I could not, in all fairness, ask these kids to give up their milk. Instead, at the tier two stage, we simply began to buy healthier milk.

Without exception, all four children immediately preferred the taste of the organic, whole milk over the commercial brands they had been drinking. It was like a revelation: something inside their bodies (or at least their taste buds) sensed this was more wholesome. Good milk became the first major crack in the campaign to up the dietary ante of these all-American kids.

These first two tiers show how we can begin with just a few good steps in the right direction. The important factors are (1) don't go too far, too fast, and (2) have palatable substitutes available (real butter, whole organic milk). Respecting people's comfort zones and individual ability to handle change is of the utmost importance. Everyone likes to feel in control especially when things are changing. And no one, including kids, likes to be dictated to or bossed around.

One other significant change needs to be mentioned here, and that is eliminating commercial (nonorganic) chicken, meats, and pork, as all are products of highly chemicalized industries, which utilize some of the highest levels of hormones and antibiotics applied to any foods. The creative substitution here would be organically raised meat of all kinds, which can play an important role in a nutrient-dense diet.

Tier two also encourages you to take a more proactive stance toward a healthier diet by urging you to expand your intake of eggs, fresh fruits, nutrient-dense salads, vegetables, and possibly a few unfamiliar new foods, such as flaxseed oil, tempeh, or tofu. This tier also encourages you to expand your cooking skills, so you become more comfortable with poaching or soft-boiling eggs, or learning how to cook a whole grain, such as brown rice or millet.

There is nothing magical about the creative substitutions you can implement to increase the denseness of your diet. Like most nutrition, it is common sense. When you learn about processing, for example, it just makes sense to begin substituting whole foods that retain their mineral and vitamin content for refined, processed foods.

Here are some typical creative substitutions you can make:

- Almond butter or organic peanut butter for commercial peanut butter;
- Almond or rice milk for cow's milk;
- Brown rice or millet for white rice or regular pasta;
- Butter or coconut oil for margarine;
- Canned sardines for canned tuna;
- Haddock, halibut, or wild salmon for chicken;
- Fresh fruits for canned or frozen fruits;
- Fresh vegetables for canned or frozen vegetables;
- Herbal iced teas, juices, sparkling waters for soda;
- Honey, or agave nectar, blackstrap molasses, maple syrup, stevia, or Sucanat for sugar;
- Microbrew beer or organic red wine for other alcoholic beverages;
- Organic dark chocolate for milk chocolate or other candies;
- Organic eggs for commercial eggs;
- Organic meats for commercial meat;
- Organic yogurt for commercial yogurt;
- Whole-wheat flour for white flour.

By now, the big picture should be coming into focus. While tier one connected you with the principle that "the journey of a thousand miles begins with the first step," the subsequent tiers carry you forward, solidifying your commitment and reminding you that you are on the path for the long haul.

TIER THREE

Tier three represents the next level of adherence to nutrient-dense principles. After most of the weakest links have been eradicated, you can commit even more deeply to the nutrient-dense path, forging new ground while checking for any gaps still remaining in your diet. Ideally, you should never feel deprived or limited, so as you eliminate certain foods, go ahead and simultaneously discover credible, higher quality substitutions that allow you to feel your diet is getting better and better. This is important. If you do not experience a continual process of refinement, and the sense that you are moving in a direction of more options, higher quality food, increasing diversity, and a more entertaining and interesting diet, then something is wrong. If you start to stagnate, you will not be inspired to continue your adventure, and having a sense of adventure and excitement is critical to the success of adopting a new eating lifestyle—after all, who wants more drudgery or boredom in their lives?

Learning curves encompass both time and effort, and that is why the tiers are set up in relatively small increments. *There should be absolutely no stress* involved in this process. If it does not feel right, then you are probably not ready for the next step and should not even attempt it. If you trust yourself and the process, however, then you will know when you are ready for the next tier. As you traverse through levels of increasing density, any sense of deprivation is important to acknowledge. If you give something up and feel a void in its absence, then you should respect that feeling and find a healthy way to fill it. Voids are actually desirable, because the truth is, each one gives you an opportunity to fill it with something denser.

This is getting to the heart of the transition process. It is also the point at which you (hopefully) become more comfortable with reading labels and find yourself becoming more sophisticated and savvy with each shopping excursion. Suddenly, that loaf of wheat bread does not fool you with its nice pastoral scene and natural-looking sheaves of grain on the label. You notice instead that it still feels suspiciously soft, like the whiter *air* breads, and you discover that, in fact, it has the same dough conditioners as the common white breads. As you may also notice, there is ordinary enriched, bleached or unbleached flour listed along with the whole-wheat flour and accompanied by caramel coloring to give it that earthy, natural look. Next, you pick up a loaf you've never purchased before and you can immediately feel the difference. It is heavier and denser, and the ingredient list is much shorter. No white flour, no caramel coloring, no dough conditioners or preservatives, just whole-grain flour, a little salt, some yeast, and a bit of oil. You may not know how it will fly with the other family members, but you're willing to give it a chance. Tier three's experimentation can be fun. And there *should* be unknown outcomes because that's exactly why you're experimenting in the first place.

I often emphasize to clients that, at this point, it is all right to go slowly, choosing your battles wisely. Since change can be unsettling, try just one or two new items each time you shop rather than chucking everything familiar and going for the quick overhaul. This is especially true if you are shopping or cooking for others besides yourself. It is also more compassionate and respectful to remember that others may be less enthusiastic than you are about some of these changes, as is often the case with kids, and the occasional spouse.

Another tip to facilitate the process at this tier level is to shop for nutrient-dense treats and rewards, a practice that can help put fun back into shopping for food. I believe every major shopping expedition should include at least one nutrient-dense treat or new, fun food along with the staples. This approach is also a painless way to expand your repertoire of foods, and upholds the idea that food is really a constant reminder of the celebration and bounty of life.

Treating yourself is easy and a great way to avoid boring ruts, or taking yourself and your diet too seriously. A really good-quality dark chocolate bar, for example, can help satisfy your very normal craving for an occasional sweet. And, instead of the usual empty calories, you get a food rich in antioxidants, phytonutrients, and other valuable compounds, so you do not compromise your nutrient-dense values. Also, the rich, semisweet quality of dark chocolate means there's less temptation to binge and devour more than you need. (I have seen many people treat this chocolate with more respect and restraint than less-dense candies.)

Similarly, if you, your spouse, or your friend enjoys an occasional beer, why not surprise him or her with a nutrient-dense microbrew? Many large health food stores have beer and wine departments, featuring hard-to-find organic brands. I can guarantee that your proposed dietary changes will fall on much more receptive ears when you pull a yeasty lager, rich in B vitamins and minerals, out of the grocery bag, along with the rice milk and tofu. This sends a message that you are not entirely abandoning good times or becoming some sort of strange health fanatic. This is important, because your partner might be intimidated or worried by seeing you changing your usual patterns. Besides, it's a lot more fun to have the support of loved ones, rather than their negativity, sarcasm, or skepticism.

The possibilities for treats are endless, so stretch out and experiment. For example, if you have given up your favorite hydrogenated oil-containing cookies, discover which nutrient-dense options exist. Doubtless there are healthier versions and brands, without hydrogenated oils, which approximate the taste and style of your original favorites. Giving new foods, tastes, and yourself a fresh chance to delight and surprise you is the essence of tier three.

People's expectations can color their actual experience in a way that prevents them from appreciating what they do have. Taste is known to be more in the mind than in the taste buds; so for example, if your mind expects carob to taste like chocolate, you will be disappointed because carob is *not* chocolate. But if you let carob just be carob, you might find it's pretty good on its own. I call this *respect.* Foods, like people, deserve to be judged on their own merits, and it isn't fair to compare them to something else.

This can be a particularly difficult problem for children, who can easily get set in their ways and expect their food to look and taste exactly the same each time they eat it. This is due in part to the uniformity of fast-food and restaurant chains whose success is largely based on their stated ability to give you the exact same burger and fries, no matter where or when.

The next major step is cutting out as much of this predictable, processed fast food as possible. You will find that, after a period of being away from chemical additives and taste enhancers, artificially manipulated foods begin to taste exactly like what they are—unnatural. This marks the beginning of reclaiming your taste buds and your health, which, along with a more adventurous spirit of experimentation, is the essence of tier three.

At this tier, you can further raise the stakes and look more seriously at organic alternatives. These foods are exemplified by fresh produce, nuts, meats, seafood, and whole grains and are foods that are simple, straightforward, and honest, and grown without artificial fertilizers, chemical colors, herbicides, hormones, or other additives.

Meals and snacks also become simplified at this tier level. Dessert can simply be some nice fresh fruit, perhaps a fruit salad. A snack could consist of some raw almonds, or some crisped seaweed, or half an avocado with a dollop of humus and a drizzle of flax oil or a sprinkle of nutritional yeast. Or, a smear of almond butter or tahini on a slice of whole-grain bread with a few drops of blackstrap molasses might prove satisfying. We could call this process *grazing*.

Leftover brown rice or some millet could be warmed up as a base for a snack as could a slice or two of raw-milk organic cheese. Some cold (or warmed) leftover salmon, eaten with a handful of fresh salad greens and a drizzle of flax or fresh wheat germ oil, could similarly serve as a quick yet nutritious and satisfying snack. Sprinkle on some sunflower seeds or add a slice of red onion, and the nutrient denseness goes up even higher. At this point we may find the lines blurring between a snack and a meal.

The beauty of such foods is the quickness and ease of their preparation. These and literally hundreds of such possibilities are open to you. Freed from the tyranny of prepackaged, predictable designer products, real food, with its own simple appeal, begins to beckon in its place.

Having firmly entered the sphere of the third tier, you are starting to demonstrate a deep commitment to nutrient-dense principles. Food that does not measure up has far less appeal, and instead, you seek quality and, more important, begin to *expect* it. You have crossed some invisible threshold and are in the full swing of treating your body with increasing respect. As a result, at this level you should start to find it much easier to abandon many commercial products such as those containing hormones, in particular, beef, dairy, pork, and poultry. On the other hand, your intake of quality protein, such as safe, organic (if possible) meats, should increase, and you should delight in discovering such foods.

Further changes reflect your deepening awareness as well. Almost all white-flour products, hard alcohol, and even coffee are usually eliminated or limited at this point. In the meantime, you should continue to add increasing amounts of interesting, nutrient-dense foods. Fresh juices, sea vegetables, soaked nuts, sprouted breads, umeboshi plum vinegar, and many other foods can be added as circumstances, availability, and curiosity dictate. By the time you are firmly established in tier three, you are well on your way to a strongly nutrient-dense diet.

TIER FOUR—THE FINAL FRONT-TIER

Tier four, what I cornily call *the final front-tier,* helps you complete the journey by encouraging you to tighten up your ship and inspiring you to find further examples of nutrient denseness. In this final level, you learn to trust the process and goodness of nature even further.

Arriving at this tier means you have already given up most poor-quality food and have eliminated unnecessary additives, oils, and any food sources of aspartame or hormones. Assuming you ate them, you have even begun to stop relying on organic processed foods, such as tofu hot dogs or veggie burgers. Now you are primarily eating whole foods—beans and lentils, brown rice, millet, and quinoa, and lots of fresh vegetables and fruit. You have substituted almond butter or tahini for commercial peanut butter, rice or almond milk for cow's milk, and you are eating hormone-free eggs, fish, and meats instead of commercial animal products. So what remains to be done?

Because *The Nutrient-Dense Eating Plan* describes a process more than a destination, every tier involves an ongoing commitment to discovery: experimentation and an open-minded approach to shopping, cooking, and eating is always encouraged. This final front-tier is therefore not final in the sense of ending your learning. Instead, you continue your journey in this spirit of ongoing discovery as you fine-tune and more fully round out your nutrient-dense kitchen.

Dry goods and other staples are what make a kitchen feel well stocked, and you can really pack nutrient density in with a wide variety of nutrient-dense condiments and other essentials. In tier four, you learn to pay attention to the little details that make a big difference, and which also ensure that you do not let your standards slide. You don't want to lose the gains you've made because, in this final front-tier, you are striving for an even higher level of nutrient-dense consistency.

Condiments are a great way to add nutrient and flavor density. If you have heretofore neglected this aspect of your diet, this tier is a perfect time to change that. The unique flavors of herbs and spices come from different combinations of nature's own chemical compounds, and supply nutrient density by adding diverse biomolecules, which carry multiple messages to the body.

Another aspect of eating densely at this stage is honoring the shifting availability of foods as the seasons change. Personally, I have noticed my cravings and desires change with the seasons, and I consider this another opportunity to keep my diet

Checking-In after Tier Four

My friend Ashley, who lives on the East Coast, invariably calls me every few months to ask, "So, what are you into *now*?" She always wants to know what is new, exciting, and fresh in my nutritional and culinary world, to inspire her with new ideas, but her query always makes me stop and think about *my* process, and gives me a chance to reflect on what has newly inspired me as well. To me, the tiers are all about this ongoing discovery where learning never ends. This is especially true when it comes to the possibilities of a new taste, or a new source of higher quality nutrition.

I deeply appreciate it when people like my friend Ashley show a genuine desire to discover something fresh. I am more than delighted to share with her my excitement over discovering bliss balls (see page 265 for recipe), blueberries, coconut butter, raw foods, sardines, sea vegetables, or whatever else is my latest nutritional culinary inspiration. And, I'm equally delighted to know she will try these things out for herself, and report back to me on what has worked for her, and what has not.

diverse and dense. The freshness of the summer and fall produce provides an abundance of antioxidants, enzymes, and live foods unparalleled at any other time of the year. Similarly, around the time of autumn's first frosts, I often begin craving amaranth, brown rice, millet, oats, or quinoa. This principle of eating foods that are seasonally available is borrowed from macrobiotics, where it is a highly developed culinary and nutritional principle. I do not necessarily follow macrobiotic principles rigidly, because the trans-seasonal availability of foods has meant that high-quality, nutrient-dense foods are available year round, but I do believe it is generally appropriate and wise to be in sync with nature's cycles and your body. Overall, the level of sophistication you bring to these later tiers is often a reflection of your ability to listen to your body, the song of the seasons, and the many other subtle messages continually available from your environment, even if the environment is the produce aisle of your store.

In this tier, you can also add little touches to reinforce the denseness of your diet. Frequenting the juice bar when shopping at the health food store is, I feel, one of the many little things you can do to increase your diet's consistency. Similarly, you might increase your intake of dulse, kelp, nori, or other sea vegetables, or begin incorporating nutritional yeast into your meals more regularly. This tier is also the time to increase your intake of higher quality fruits that are particularly dense in terms of pigments and antioxidants, such as fresh blueberries, blackberries, cherries, kiwis, and raspberries.

Many Americans come from a dietary background high in starches and other carbohydrates. If you reduce the amount of bread and pasta you eat, you make room in your diet for more complex, dense grains such as amaranth, brown rice, millet, and quinoa. The final tier can also reflect a commitment to increasing the density and quality of your protein. Buffalo, elk, lamb, nutrient-dense egg salad, poached or baked halibut or salmon, sushi, and venison are all excellent sources of quality protein. If you are recovering from injuries, surgeries, or wounds, have an active or stressful lifestyle, or if you are pregnant or nursing, your requirements for protein are significantly increased.

Foraging for Food—Remembering Place

Any thorough immersion in the denseness of your diet at level four implies an open-minded and adventurous spirit. Understanding the role of food in your life can take you deeper into an appreciation of the larger web of life, and could lead you to participate more in the natural world. Foraging for at least some of your food is a rewarding activity that could provide you with a renewed sense of your place in the world.

Common outdoor weeds are an easy way to celebrate the joy of nature's bounty. Chickweed, dandelion greens, edible mushrooms, lamb's-quarter, nettles, and purslane are just a few of the wild edibles that anyone can easily learn to identify and enjoy. Edible wild plants are available in spring, summer, and fall, and can bring nutritious diversity to your salads and other dishes. Equally important, you may find an interesting connection with the distant past when you seek out, pick, and eat locally grown, wild plants. Something inside you gets nourished, and the wild place inside you gets the chance to grow a little denser in the process. This is true soul food, and is not something you can ever purchase in the grocery store.

INTEGRATING YOUR DIETARY CHOICES WITH THE TIERS

At some point, many people question the relevance or safety of their diet, and often accept some newer fad or style of eating: some decide to become vegetarians, and some may investigate a macrobiotic diet, while others may plunge into an all-raw diet. These steps are more like leaps, but people tend to consider them part of their evolutionary process.

Are these diets compatible with a nutrient-dense diet? *The Nutrient-Dense Eating Plan,* as you have learned by now, does not dictate a particular type or style of diet, except to tell you to avoid certain toxic substances (hydrogenated oils, aspartame, hormones). Instead, the focus has been on giving you the freedom to choose what you eat by empowering you with the knowledge of the relative strengths and weaknesses of specific foods. Since everything you eat is ultimately your choice, the goal of nutrient-dense eating is to make sure that your choices are conscious and are based on information rather than on advertising and marketing campaigns.

But, to answer the question above, the principles of nutrient density create endless possibilities. You can follow a nutrient-dense ovo-lacto diet, a nutrient-dense raw diet, a nutrient-dense vegan diet, or a nutrient-dense anything diet. You can be in the Zone (the Zone diet) and be nutrient dense, or you can be in the Zone and not be very dense. The choice is yours. And the same goes for virtually any of the popular diets out there. As I have stressed all along, the only constant word in nutrient density is quality. Exercising your options in a nutrient-dense way disallows only one thing—junk.

Customizing your personal ideal diet is really the final front-tier. And, as with any frontier, it is a dynamic, changeable thing. Stresses come and go, and changes do occur in personal lives, so it is only fitting that your diet could change, too. As your experience, knowledge, and body change, so too should your diet. This signifies a deep respect for change itself, and implies a healthier mindset because it means you are less stuck in your ways. Holding on to a rigid or narrowly defined diet could hold you back and malnourish you in unintended and unanticipated ways. (Think back to my friend who continues to drink milk and eat cheese and other forms of dairy even though her body has been telling her for years that it is miserable). The final fron-tier is the discovery of your own flexible nature, characterized by an ongoing commitment to discovering new and more nutrient-dense foods and creative ways to incorporate them into your life.

I hope by now you have a good idea of the freedom and flexibility available to you. Transitioning to a more nutrient-dense diet should be fun, and should also respect your personal needs and pace. There is an enormous amount of room here for any combination of steps, and my outline of the tiers should be used as examples and crude guidelines, not as the last word. If this book has done its job, you should feel sufficiently comfortable with the material to take the steps you feel ready to take. It is *your* journey. The opportunity to make it a fantastic, fun, healthy, and rewarding one is ultimately yours alone. That is the promise—and the beauty—of *The Nutrient-Dense Eating Plan.*

CHAPTER 42

Guidelines for Navigating the Tiers

Successfully working with the tiers is the heart of *The Nutrient-Dense Eating Plan*. All the knowledge and good intentions in the world will be of no help if you do not learn to walk the talk. Many people have read all the latest diet and health books, but when it comes time to actually shop, cook, or dine out, everything they've read seems to fly out the window.

The tier system is different because I show people how to actually change their diets. Getting there from here is the core of this book, and I can only trust that people will find the information practical and useful for the long haul. There have already been enough temporary fixes and fad diets that end up accomplishing little. My purpose in writing this book is to provide a guide to help people really accomplish their goals.

In the final analysis, eating healthy is very *doable*, yet it continually amazes me how easily people let themselves get sidetracked, or talked out of a healthy diet. Deeply ingrained habits, a lack of confidence, or social pressures seem the biggest obstacles, but if you are really interested in improving your diet, and therefore your health, it can be done. All it takes is direction, enthusiasm, and willpower.

Here are some guidelines to help you develop your own successful nutrient-dense eating plan.

Firm Resolutions

Do not invite failure. Tackle only what you feel capable of accomplishing, and make sure you are mentally up for the challenge. Find a balance between moving forward realistically and pushing yourself too hard. Go at your own pace, but be honest with yourself, if you are holding back too much. Do not rush, but do not get stuck either. When you are *sure* you are ready, make a firm mental resolution and promise yourself that you will stick with it. Make sure you have a strategy in place that you know will work. Remember, you are choosing to do this for *you*.

Attitudes

Attitudes are everything. Since you can change yours, make sure you are approaching the changes in your diet with the *right* attitudes. The best attitude to have is enthusiasm. If you enter the tiers with dread, you are guaranteeing yourself a miserable time. The other prescription for disaster is guilt. Lose it. You will enjoy the process a lot more and make the journey more fun if you approach *going denser* with a sense of adventure and optimism. If you view the adoption of a nutrient-dense diet as an opportunity to broaden your culinary horizons, you will navigate the tiers with ease.

Resources

Remember, nutrient density is about *quality*. Improving your diet means changing a little, or a lot, of what you eat, so take stock of your resources and make sure you have consistent access to sources of good food. Almost every major city today has large health food markets, but in large regions of America, people still do not have access to vital shopping resources. If this is true in your community, try to locate a good farmer's market, or check Appendix A for a list of companies that will ship anything you need or will provide you with a location nearest you for purchase. You may also want to plan a weekly or monthly shopping trip to the nearest good-size town to stock up on staples and other essentials.

Essentials

It is important to stock up on essentials. A good variety of nutrient-dense staples is required to successfully go through the tiers. A well-stocked kitchen is a *prepared* kitchen, and is necessary for hassle-free, nutrient-dense eating and meal planning. In addition to staples, it is important to have nutrient-dense snacks and ready-to-eat munchies, such as fruit, on hand.

Challenges

It is important to anticipate challenges. Don't be blindsided by challenging situations, such as an office party, that bowl of candy on the boss's desk, or that sudden out-of-town trip. Being prepared means anticipating times when the only food available to eat will be pure, 100 percent junk food. Learn to eat before you go, and learn to be mobile with good food that travels well and works for you. Stock the refrigerator at work with good things. If you drive a lot, consider a minicooler for the back seat of your car. Almonds, walnuts, or other nuts, fruits, hard-boiled eggs, seaweed, many raw or cooked vegetables, and other nutrient-dense foods keep surprisingly well for a day or more. If you travel out of town, you can always pack a little extra nutritional insurance. In new cities, or on business trips, visit the local health food market. (On arrival in any new city, I always check the yellow pages to find the nearest oasis.) Regional variations and specialties found in traveling can often give you fun, new food ideas and inspiration.

All of the above items are good tips for minimizing failure and increasing the ease with which you can navigate the tiers. Having a healthy, positive outlook and attitude, anticipating challenges by being proactive and prepared, not being overly ambitious and biting off more than you are ready to chew, having a well-stocked kitchen and the backup of reliable sources of food, are all sensible and important precautions that will reduce any stress or anxiety involved with dietary changes. If you are genuinely serious about your health, then these precautions will not be a burden, and you will be able to implement them effortlessly. Adopting a nutrient-dense diet really is a joy and a privilege, and approaching it with this attitude, you cannot fail.

CHAPTER 43

Working the Tiers

The most important part of *The Nutrient-Dense Eating Plan* is its respect for the unique needs of each individual. While there are definite guidelines to this plan, the important thing to remember is that *you* always have the last word. In order to eat healthily, it is essential to feel in control and empowered, so *you* can make the decisions you feel are best for you. This, in my opinion, is the only way the changes you make will be effective—and lasting.

I have already shown how moving through the four tiers is a journey of increasing nutrient denseness. In this section, I want to show you how to design your own personal tier system incorporating your own needs and insights. You can use my ideas and suggestions at your discretion. Because this plan is set up to help you eat healthily for the rest of your life, freely adapting the concept of tiers to your own changing lifestyle is crucial to your long-term success.

TIER ONE

In the first tier, my suggestion was to start slowly by not adding much to the diet, concentrating instead on eliminating the most obvious offenders, namely aspartame (NutraSweet) and hydrogenated oils (particularly hydrogenated oil shortening). Taking tier one a little further is completely up to you. Some people feel comfortable omitting other counterproductive foods at this level (milk or other dairy, for example). Others might cut out wheat products, particularly if there is a suspected allergy or intolerance to gluten.

Tier one is primarily about omitting negative foods, but it can also include the addition of a few nutrient-dense foods. Rather than go too fast, though, it is better to add only a few basic items at this level, but again, this is a matter of personal choice. You might want to add a nutrient-dense grain like brown rice or you might want to try some flaxseed oil, just to boost the variety and nutrient density of your salads and the quality of the oil you use. Another very basic way to increase your nutritional density right from the start would be to add more fresh fruits and vegetables to your diet, and to increase the amount of water you drink.

In addition to adding a few new items in tier one, you may feel comfortable making a few simple substitutions. This makes good sense in order to lessen any sense of deprivation. Substituting honey for sugar, whole-wheat flour or bread for white, and butter or olive oil for margarine, are all appropriate changes to make at this stage.

TIER TWO

In tier two you might want to build on the housecleaning you started in tier one. If you only tackled margarine in the first tier, here you might want to become more aware of hydrogenated oils by carefully checking the labels of everything you buy, and of what you currently have in your pantry. Similarly, when you go out to restaurants, you might want to check the individually wrapped packets of butter before you spread it on your bread or dinner rolls. Also at this level, you may choose to address hormones in your diet by eliminating inorganic chicken, dairy, and pork.

Tier two is also an excellent time to begin practicing basic cooking skills, such as preparing brown rice, millet, or other whole grains. Feeling a bit daunted is normal—almost everyone I know was intimidated the first three or four times they tried, but it's easy once you get the hang of it. Boiling or poaching eggs, or poaching fish, is another easy, useful skill in cooking for optimal nutrition.

In tier two, give yourself more leeway in making substitutions. If you started out slowly in tier one, you may now decide to try almond butter instead of peanut butter, brown rice instead of white rice or pasta, more fish and seafood instead of chicken, pork, or veal, more organic produce instead of conventional produce, non-homogenized organic yogurt instead of your old brand, and sugar-free natural juices instead of colas.

Tier two is a great time to begin adding almonds and other nuts, berries, flaxseed oil, high-quality fruits and vegetables, tempeh, and other nutrient-dense foods. You might also want to begin transitioning to healthier desserts, giving yourself the opportunity to try natural licorice candy, organic dark chocolate, and sorbets.

TIER THREE

Tier three is your time to up the ante on your level of nutritional integrity. If you have not done so already, you could now get acquainted with such nutrient-dense super foods as blackstrap molasses, nutritional yeast, sea vegetables, and the denser oils, such as coconut, flaxseed, and high-quality olive oils. By this level, you should be eating a high percentage of whole, natural, unprocessed foods (preferably organic if available and affordable), and you should be confident that you have eliminated almost all sources of hydrogenated oils from your diet.

Tier three is a good time to become more conscious of hidden MSG in commercial salad dressings, ketchup, some condiments, and other packaged convenience foods. Also, at this level you should be cutting back on bottled, pasteurized juice drinks. If you have not yet done so, you could aim for a mostly wheat-free diet, eliminating breads, pastas, and other flour-based foods. Needless to say, by now all animal products should be organic whenever possible and affordable. And sugar use should be minimal at this point.

TIER FOUR

By tier four, your diet is quite nutrient dense, but it is important to keep adding interesting new foods whenever possible. Experiment freely with raw honey, raw sea salt, and a wider diversity of teas and grains. Begin adding carob, raw dairy (if available), sesame seeds, and wild game. This is the time to become more consistent with your intake of fresh raw juices, sea vegetables, yeast, and the other nutritional heavyweights. Explore wild edibles and eat more fresh produce in general. If you have never been totally wheat free for any length of time, now might be an appropriate time to experiment with eliminating wheat.

YOUR OPTIONS IN THE TIERS

Pick and choose from these according to your priorities. Incorporate them when it feels appropriate.

What to Eliminate

Eliminate all hormone-containing meats (beef, chicken, pork), all hydrogenated oil-containing products, aspartame and other chemical sweeteners, commercial salt, commercial salad dressings, ketchups and other prepared condiments, margarine, nonorganic eggs, nonorganic milk and dairy (or all dairy), shortening, peanut butter, wheat flour and bakery products.

What to Increase or Substitute

Increase or substitute consumption of almond and rice milk, beans, berries, cherries, and other fruits, blackstrap molasses, coconut butter, fish and seafood, flaxseed oil, cod-liver oil, fresh juices, healthy desserts and candies, herbal teas, herbs and spices, lentils, nuts and seeds and their butters, nutritional yeast, olive oil, organic eggs, organic products in general, real butter, sea vegetables, spring water, whole grains (amaranth, brown rice, millet, quinoa), and vegetables.

SAMPLE GAME PLAN FOR THE TIERS

The following is a sample game plan for working the tiers. Feel free to adopt a different version based on your needs and readiness.

Tier One

Eliminate

- Aspartame-containing products, including sodas
- Margarine, hydrogenated oil shortenings

Substitute

- Herbal teas, juice, water for soda
- Butter or olive oil for margarine

Add

- Fresh fruit—increase to at least one to two servings a day
- Fresh vegetables—increase to at least one to two servings a day

Tier Two

Eliminate

- All commercial chicken
- All commercial (nonorganic) milk
- All sodas
- Canned and packaged soups (MSG)
- Fast-food restaurants (limit to one visit a week)
- Hot dogs, luncheon meats, salami
- Hydrogenated peanut butter
- Hydrogenated potato chips

Substitute

- Almond butter or nonhydrogenated peanut butter for commercial brand peanut butter
- Dark chocolate for other candy
- Honey for sugar when possible
- Organic chicken or seafood for (commercial) chicken
- Organic (nonhydrogenated) chips for commercial brand potato or corn chips
- Organic cow's milk for commercial milk
- Rice, soy, or almond milk for commercial milk

Add

- Another daily serving of fresh (organic) fruit
- Another daily serving of fresh (organic) vegetables
- Brown rice (cooked)
- Flaxseed oil
- Organic free-range eggs (one to four servings a week)
- Raw nuts (almonds, sunflower seeds, walnuts)
- Salads (at least three a week)
- Tofu or tempeh at least once a week
- Various herbal and black teas

Tier Three

Eliminate

- All commercial beef and pork products
- All commercial dairy products (cream cheese, hard cheeses, ice cream, yogurt, etc.)
- All fast-food restaurants
- All packaged and canned products containing partially hydrogenated oil
- Coffee (or limit to one cup a day)
- Flaked or puffed cereals
- Hard alcohol, commercial beer
- White-flour products

Substitute

- Black or green tea for coffee
- Eggs, oatmeal, or brown rice for breakfast instead of flaked cereals
- Fresh flaxseed oil for commercial salad dressings
- Fruit for most desserts
- Organic dairy (nonhomogenized raw milk cheeses, yogurt)
- Organic (hormone-free) beef, buffalo, lamb, or venison for commercial meat
- Organic red wines and microbrew beers for other alcohol
- Soy or rice-based ice creams or sorbets for commercial ice cream
- Whole-wheat, 100 percent rye, or sprouted-grain breads for white bread

Add

- Coconut butter
- Halibut, sardines, wild salmon
- Fresh carrot or other raw juices (occasionally)
- More fresh vegetables and fruits
- More nuts and seeds and nut and seed butters (pumpkin seed butter, tahini)
- Sea vegetables
- Spices and herbs
- Umeboshi plum vinegar

Tier Four

Eliminate

- All non-raw dairy
- All nonorganic produce (if possible)
- All packaged and prepared foods
- All wheat products

Substitute

- Amaranth, brown rice, millet, quinoa, and teff for pasta
- Fresh vegetables for packaged
- Organic produce for nonorganic, whenever possible and affordable

Add

- Blackstrap molasses
- Cod-liver oil
- Fresh berries, cherries, kiwis, mangoes, and other high-quality fruit, (organic if available and affordable)
- Nutritional yeast
- Sea salt (high quality)
- Wheatgrass juice (occasional)
- Wild edible weeds and plants (chickweed, dandelion, lamb's-quarter, nasturtium flowers, nettles, purslane)

CHAPTER 44

Dining Out

Now that you know how to go through the tiers, what about dining out? For many, one of the most pleasurable activities can become a baffling or frustrating experience, when your diet changes. Eating out, or course, puts you, quite literally, in the hands, and at the mercy of, the restaurateur. Quality of food, preparation techniques, additives, and hidden ingredients are all taken out of your hands, and you are left to hope for the best, trusting the reputation of the restaurant in question.

Sometimes this is actually desirable, as eating out is an opportunity to relinquish your personal kitchen responsibilities or obligations. The opportunity to have *someone else* prepare and serve your food can be a wonderful experience, an opportunity to relax and let go, while enjoying the results of someone else's creativity. You also get a chance to appreciate a wider range of foods and preparation styles, thereby increasing your exposure to a broad range of cuisine, and inspiring you to expand your repertoire.

Yet dining out can also be a maddening, frustrating experience. If you are earnestly striving to achieve some measure of consistency in how you nourish yourself, the loss of control that eating at a restaurant represents may mean you have to suspend your new standards, at least for an evening. While not that big a deal to some, for others it can be an upsetting experience. I have seen otherwise mature, sober people completely lose it when faced with menus that fall short of their expectations.

Everyone has their own level of comfort and ability to handle challenges, but I feel it's not worth losing peace of mind over things you ultimately have little control over. Granted, it is true that food can push people's buttons like nothing else because it represents the most basic level of needs—our very survival. Control over what and how we eat is fundamental to a personal sense of empowerment and autonomy.

So, the question remains: How can you best retain your nutrient-dense values when dining out? How can you enjoy the experiences and benefits of dining out without compromising the core values of nutrient density and sabotaging your best efforts to maintain an optimally healthy diet? Fortunately, these questions are easily answered once you really understand which foods are nutrient dense, and which are not.

The most obvious starting point for nutrient-dense dining is restaurant selection. In any major town or city, there is an enormous spectrum of dining choices, so selecting restaurants that offer high-quality food within your budget is becoming less of a problem all the time. One big plus resulting from the surge of interest in healthy eating and organics is the growing number of restaurants that are more conscious of what they serve their patrons. Happily, there is a steady stream of new restaurants (and established ones as well) that are making changes to their menus and upping the nutrient-dense quality of their offering. European-style restaurants, green restaurants, vegetarian restaurants, and even raw- or live-food restaurants are increasingly arriving on the scene. Many of these establishments employ highly renowned, talented chefs who are creating names for themselves due to the consistently high quality of their meals. This is a comparatively new phenomenon that should make nutrient-dense restaurant-goers rejoice. And to supply staff for these new-style natural cookery restaurants, several excellent culinary arts schools around the country are training and producing chefs of a very high caliber.

Anyone who dines out regularly knows that American cuisine is changing rapidly, reinventing itself with amazing frequency in an effort to keep up with, and in some cases lead, the public's tastes and desires for something new. And what is definitely new is the desire of increasing numbers of people to consume food that is delicious, high quality, and healthy.

Not every community has access to such enlightened eating yet, but this does not mean you should forgo the pleasures of eating out (I go out to eat whenever the chance arises.) The real art of dining out lies in learning to make the best choices from the available options, and fitting your menu selections into whatever tier you are in. The main idea here is that dining out should give you the entertainment, good company, and relaxation of a pleasant meal without totally throwing your eating plan out the window. This, in my experience, is an achievable, realistic goal.

As always, your ability to achieve denseness in dining is dependent on two conditions: the availability of good food, and the specific choices you make. You do not always have control over the first. You do, over the second. The availability of good, healthy food depends on the particular restaurant. If you get to choose the restaurant, and are in a city or area with a broad selection of choices, there is probably no problem. You merely select from any of the restaurants that offer good, fresh, wholesome food. The presence of fresh salads, good seafood, and (possibly) organic meats; an abundance of nicely prepared fresh vegetables; and the use of good-quality olive oil, fresh herbs, and other offerings, all mean you can easily have a fine meal.

The net effect of the upscaling of the American dining experience is to bring ever healthier and more wholesome foods into the mainstream of American palates. Macrobiotic restaurants, Mediterranean-style cuisines, and sushi bars, to name a few, also resonate nicely with nutrient-dense principles.

Today, there is an unprecedented array of dining options, so it is easy to enjoy fine dining without sacrificing nutrient density. I have enjoyed innumerable such meals in Asheville, North Carolina; Boulder, Colorado; New York; San Francisco; Santa Fe; and many towns and cities in between, leading me to believe that it has never before been so easy to get a great meal that qualifies as highly nutrient dense. Since quality is always emphasized in the nutrient-dense diet, fine dining can be a nutrient-dense experience.

BASIC GUIDELINES

When eating out, there are a few basic guidelines to keep in mind in order to optimize the nutrient denseness of the experience. Most of these are obvious, but since what goes on in restaurants is largely behind the scenes, it becomes important to inquire about a few things just to know where you stand.

First, I often inquire whether butter or margarine is used because margarine is cheaper than butter, and many restaurants still believe that margarine is somehow healthier than butter, and that the majority of their patrons will prefer it. The presence of margarine, particularly in the little pats that come with bread or rolls, is a sign to me that a restaurant is not of a very high caliber. Many vegetarian restaurants still prefer margarine over butter, since it does not come from animal origins, as butter does.

When ordering an entrée, my general rule of thumb is to opt for the fish. For me, red meat and chicken are unacceptable due to the unmistakable presence of antibiotics, chemical steroids, and other compounds. Organic meats are fine, but are mostly unavailable—the rare exception would be specifically health food–oriented restaurants. Fish, therefore, especially wild salmon and several other ocean-going fish, are the cleanest, best sources of protein, and also supply you with the important essential fatty acids. When available, halibut is my favorite. Contemporary American, continental, French, Japanese, Mediterranean, and other cuisines, all offer nutrient-dense, fish-based dishes of high quality. If buffalo, lamb, or venison are on the menu, I will often opt for one of those, as they tend to be raised with few or no chemicals. Another good protein entrée choice is soy-based tempeh, available at health food restaurants. Whole grains also contribute to the protein density of many entrées.

Although chicken is touted as heart healthy, and is the overwhelming choice of most Americans eating out these days, under *no circumstances* will I order it from a restaurant unless it is free range, or organic. Commercially raised chicken in this country is a horror, subjected as it is to an unbelievable array of chemicals. Commercial poultry is also thought to be one of the leading causes of salmonella, which is often the undiagnosed cause of food poisoning. I have spoken with many people who had food poisoning or gastric upset after eating out, and in almost every case, the person had eaten chicken.

My guidelines for nutrient-dense dining out are simple. Aside from looking for high-quality protein, I usually choose minimally prepared vegetables, such as steamed or sautéed, and look for any exotic or rarely eaten foods or specialties that would add diversity to my usual diet, along with the opportunity to enjoy some new tastes and nutrients.

This brings up another point. Many ethnic restaurants are excellent and wise choices for dining out. Compared with the SAD diet, ethnic cuisines are often nutritionally dense, as for example the turmeric-based curries of Indian cuisine, which contain effective antioxidants. Southeast Asian, Indian, and Middle Eastern cuisines are also recommended because they tend to be more vegetable based (more phytonutrients), make liberal use of spices and herbs, use little or no dairy, and frequently have better meat options (lamb instead of beef in Greek and Near-Eastern food).

Since you can get unhealthy foods from any nationality, avoid overcooked, heavily charred or broiled foods, fried foods, and too-sweet desserts wherever you find them. Also, keep in mind that very few ethnic restaurants serve organic ingredients. And no matter what the nationality of the restaurant you are frequenting, you should always avoid fried foods. Just because you are at a Japanese restaurant, for example, does not somehow make the tempura magically healthy. It doesn't matter what vegetable or type of seafood is surrounded by that crispy batter, deep-fried foods are always composed of overheated oils and are not good for you, just as French fries are not—opt for the baked potato instead. This may be stating the obvious, but it needs to be said because a basic principle of nutrient density is avoiding fried oils. It is amazing how common sense at home can fly right out the window when you sit down and order from a menu.

In addition to avoiding bad oils, including salad oils, at restaurants, I consistently weed out heavily sauced or cheese-laden dishes in my menu selections, especially when they are made from conventional sources of dairy.

But let's get real. You don't always have control over where you go to eat. Someone else could be picking the restaurant, or you could be in a small town with a limited range of options from which to choose. This is a common scenario. What then?

Sometimes there are no satisfactory answers, so do the best you can and let your standards slide for the occasion. This is the price we pay for living in a society where the SAD is still the norm. When faced with this dilemma, I choose the best of the worst. What else can I do? I once, however, found myself at a restaurant with a large group of friends where there was literally nothing on the menu I felt I could eat. I knew everything would be made with hydrogenated oils, and there was no salad on the menu, so I settled for water and a slice of lemon, as I made conversation and waited to go home and eat. That exception felt right to me because I was staying true to my personal values. Abstaining when everyone around me was eating was a little hard, but just looking at their food choices made me glad I was not joining them.

One point regarding this issue is that *I never let on about not eating due to the quality of the food.* Basically, I attributed my lack of appetite to not feeling well because I feel strongly it is not a good idea to make anyone feel bad. Anything negative I might have said about the food could have been taken personally by whoever had selected the establishment, or by those who ate and enjoyed the food there. Food should serve as a force to bring people together and give pleasure, not divide, and so I usually keep my views to myself unless asked. If our personal views on diet get thrown around carelessly, then food can become a source of pain or guilt, which is the opposite of what food can and should be.

Usually though, there is something on a menu that is, at worst, neutral, and can be counted on to fill you up. It can be a salad, a baked potato, or guacamole, which probably won't meet your usual nutrient-dense requirements—the salad and the potato won't be organic (and the latter could be genetically modified), the guacamole will come from a mix with who-knows-what in it, the bread or rolls will probably be made with hydrogenated shortening, and the water will likely be chlorinated tap

Healthy Muffins?

Some years ago, during the bran craze, bran muffins became very popular in restaurants all over the country. Today, many restaurants, particularly those that specialize in breakfasts, offer a choice of toast or a muffin. Because of the old connotation of bran muffins, many people still order them thinking they are inherently healthy. But the vast majority of muffins sold in restaurants today are *not* healthy, as they are made with margarine or hydrogenated shortening and are usually loaded with sugar. Flour-based baked products, such as muffins, get eliminated in the later tiers of nutrient density, but until this resolve takes a firm hold, the lure of a freshly baked muffin with breakfast is a temptation many cannot resist. Interesting, isn't it, how certain foods can get a reputation for being healthy, even when they're not?

water—but sometimes you just have to choose the best of the worst. You'll survive, in any case, and hopefully resolve to make up for it at the next opportunity.

Like all of us, on occasion I find myself staring at a menu, looking for something—anything—that might be remotely inoffensive. Sometimes I find something and other times I simply wait until I can get to a health food store or a better restaurant to satisfy my hunger and nutritional needs.

The truth is, I feel pretty lucky to be able to eat, most of the time, reasonably close to the standards and values I have set for myself. However, when I see how so many people in this country eat, and their lack of awareness of what it is doing to them, I shudder. I find it truly sad that so many people are literally eating themselves to their premature graves. Ignorance may be bliss, but I cannot help but feel the price so many Americans are paying for their eating is unfortunate and unnecessary.

This is, of course, exactly why I have written this book. In the meantime, I will continue to eat as healthily and consistently as I can. I know that, as more people wake up and raise their nutritional standards, more options become available to them. When I look at the big picture today, I feel encouraged because there are more health food stores, more farmers' markets, and more healthy restaurants than ever before.

CHAPTER 45

Label Reading

Label reading is an indispensable skill that should be developed by anyone who wishes to achieve some degree of autonomy over the packaged hype and promises of food advertising. Being able at a glance to get a handle on a product's real nutritional strengths and weaknesses is empowering for the nutrient-dense shopper. I constantly stress the importance of personal responsibility in your diet, and part of that is knowing exactly what you are purchasing. *The Nutrient-Dense Eating Plan* is definitely not in the ignorance-is-bliss camp; with nutrient density you are trying to become an ever-more-conscious eater.

Label reading is dreaded by some and an automatic reflex for others. I read labels the way many people pick a cantaloupe, checking it carefully for ripeness, soft spots, and the fruity sweet smell that lets you know how ripe it is, and what its sugar content is. Labels can instantly tell you what the nutritional strengths and weaknesses of a product are, and if it is really what you are looking for. If I pick up a product and am initially unsure whether or not it is something I want to take home, I just read the label. You can't always tell the nutritional quality of a food by its appearance alone. Sometimes packaging or presentation can fool you. Some apparently healthy foods contain partially hydrogenated vegetable shortening; there is usually no sure way to tell without checking the label. More than price, appearance, or packaging hype, labels tell you what you need to know about any given food.

As I have stressed throughout, the main rule of thumb in label reading for nutrient density is that less is more. The fewer ingredients, the better. This simplicity means that the contribution of nutrients should be from the principal food itself, not from added substances. Lots of fancy words and chemical-sounding names usually indicate synthetic or added ingredients. Learning to be comfortable with label jargon can be like learning a new language. Some additives, such as monosodium glutamate (MSG), do not always have to be labeled. The Food and Drug Administration (FDA) permits manufacturers to use the terms *natural flavoring, spices, vegetable protein,* or other code words to indicate the presence of glutamates. It makes you wonder if they are trying to keep you informed, or in the dark, about what is in your food.

Unless specifically stated otherwise, *all* margarines are composed of hydrogenated oils, and Crisco and other vegetable shortenings are also always made from hydrogenated oils. As with additives, hydrogenated oils have a variety of names, including *partially hydrogenated vegetable oil or shortening, shortening, vegetable oil,* or *vegetable shortening.*

Navigating changing terminology can also be challenging. As of now, the term *organic* has a specific legal meaning. Organic standards require food to be grown or raised without antibiotics, herbicides, hormones, pesticides, and other synthetic compounds. However the pull of commercial interests puts these standards under constant threat of attack, with various bills and federal measures that would weaken organic standards constantly being introduced in Congress. The *USDA Organic* standard for meat, for example, allows meat from livestock raised on nonorganic feed to be labeled as organic. The USDA has also mandated that foods get labeled according to the percentage of organic ingredients used in them. *One hundred percent organic, organic, made with organic ingredients,* and *less than 70 percent organic content* all contain varying levels of organic ingredients.

Other potential issues for shoppers concern substances that do not require any labeling at all. Recombinant bovine growth hormone (rBGH) is present in commercial dairy products, but a federal ruling that favored the biotech industries responsible for this drug decreed it unnecessary to list these synthetic hormones. Even worse, organic companies trying to inform customers that their products are rBGH free were threatened with lawsuits by Monsanto, the manufacturer.

The bottom line here is that everyone who wants to maintain a high standard of eating has to remain aware and vigilant. All these discouraging facts make it imperative that you, the buyer, educate yourself as best you can, and give your full support to those companies you feel you can trust.

When reading labels, it is also important to know that ingredients are listed in order of prevalence. Sugars are often broken up into different kinds to appear less abundant than they really are, but when lumped together, these sugars would be the number-one ingredient in many foods. Corn-syrup solids, dextrose, glucose, high-fructose corn syrup, and sucrose are all sugar, and are all empty-calorie, nutrient-devoid nonfoods.

Whenever possible, purchase foods and goods in bulk, or in their purest, most unprocessed and natural state. These foods seldom require labeling, as it is pretty obvious what is in them. Boxes and packages frequently contain unnecessary anti-caking agents, flow agents, fungicides, and packaging preservatives. Besides, with bulk you can buy as much or as little as you choose, and the price is generally better.

Another labeling word to be wary of, *enriched,* is usually found in connection with cereals, pasta, or wheat products. Enriched flour may sound good, but it actually indicates refined carbohydrates no longer in their original, more nutrient-dense state. Enriching food simply means that small amounts of synthetically made vitamins and a couple of minerals have been added back; however, enriched foods are never as nutritionally complete as the original version was.

Labels can be extremely helpful and honest guides, alerting you to the presence of both desirable and undesirable ingredients in items you may consider purchasing. At the same time, you should be aware that labels can also serve to conceal or confuse you, if you do not know what you are reading. It is up to you alone to understand exactly what you are buying and putting into your body, if you are to be an informed, nutrient-dense shopper. The label-reading workshop in Appendix C can help you with this.

PART 4

Nutrient-Dense Recipes

CHAPTER 46

About the Recipes

The following recipes emphasize simplicity, ease of preparation, and nutrient-dense ingredients. As a result, this section may differ slightly from other nutrition books. For example, exact measurements have been intentionally minimized because I want to encourage you to explore and find your own culinary voice. Depending upon your taste, curries can range from mild to extremely hot, precise spices can vary considerably, hummus can be thin, thick, garlicky, lemony, spicy, mild, chunky, or smooth. One friend of mine makes a killer hummus with loads of cilantro that I love, and another close acquaintance of mine hates cilantro with equal passion.

Instead of telling you what to do, the recipes here are intended to guide you in learning to prepare nutrient-dense meals with confidence. Numerous tips and suggestions are given with each recipe, and nutrient-dense variations are offered to stimulate your imagination and give you plenty of options, so you feel supported.

The following recipes do not assume you have an extensive background in cooking. Instead, they emphasize the basics, which you can build on. Soft-boiling an egg (how do you keep them from cracking?), cooking a perfect pot of rice, creating variations of nutrient-dense salad dressings, skillet dishes in twenty minutes, joyous fruit salads and smoothies, lamb pilaf, great lentil soups, almond-butter sandwiches, enriched tuna salad, blackstrap almond-milk drinks, truly great breakfast cereals, guacamole, hummus spreads, deviled eggs, and more are each clearly explained. Each recipe emphasizes one or more exceptional food, and will remind you of the nutrients you are highlighting by serving that particular food.

I often joke that my diet is actually recipe-less. Most of the foods you will find here are what I call *nonrecipes.* Instead of strict guidelines, their preparation relies on what I call creative common sense, which comes from trusting yourself and the ingredients at hand. Improvisation is the heart of this kind of creative cooking and will allow you to prepare food that is far more *in the moment* than any recipe found in a cookbook.

A good example of this improvisation is a specialty I call *one-skillet dinners,* which grew out of a bachelor's need to reduce time and cleanup. The basic tool is a cast-iron skillet, in which a succession of food is sautéed together, with the flavors, textures, and colors all combining to make a versatile, delicious, and entertaining presentation.

Since there is far more emphasis on quality than quantity, you will tend to find general guidelines on amounts of ingredients rather than exact measurements, with some notable exceptions. (For a beginner, it is important to get the proportions fairly close to ideal when preparing, say, brown rice.) It has been my intention throughout this book to convey a relaxed, trusting attitude toward food, and this recipe section continues that pattern. I believe that the actual preparation of food is where our most intimate relationships with it occur, and I sincerely hope you too will come to appreciate this truth.

Most of all, I want you to learn to relax with the recipes and have fun with them. In the long run, this approach will teach you more about cooking than slavishly following a recipe to the letter ever could. Instinctual cooking is a vital skill I hope to convey to you here.

In addition to my own selections, I am offering recipes from friends whose tasty preparations and unassailable nutrient-dense qualifications make them naturals for inclusion. One of these friends is Garima Fairfax, an amazing person, whom I originally met when we were both on the faculty at the Rocky Mountain Center for Botanical Studies, a school for the study of herbalism in Boulder, Colorado. Knowing that her approach to food is 100 percent aligned with nutrient-dense principles, I asked her to contribute to this recipe section. I think you will find her recipes delicious, innovative, and nourishing (and, unless otherwise noted, commented on by her). Her cookbook, *Kitchen Botany*, can be ordered by writing Garima Fairfax, at PO Box 631, Lyons, CO 80540.

Another friend who contributed recipes at my request is Amalia Friedman, an herbalist and creative whiz in the kitchen. Her recipes, too, apply nutrient-dense principles and rely on fresh, high-quality foods, herbs, and other condiments. Both women cook primarily with organic ingredients, and will tell you it makes all the difference in the outcomes. They also make frequent, liberal use of nutrient-dense dips, dressings, and sauces, which are great for adding nutrition, taste, and texture to meals, snacks, and side dishes. Amalia warned me, however, that she never measures or refers to a recipe, so you should use your own best judgment in juggling the proportions of the ingredients. And have fun doing so, she adds.

The keys to enjoyable cooking are to have plenty of nutrient-dense ingredients, condiments, spices, and herbs on hand, to have all the kitchen tools and good-quality cookware necessary, and to have a relaxed and easy-going attitude as you approach cooking. Above all, feel free to improvise.

It is my belief that, over time, familiarity with foods of exceptional quality will lead to a deeper confidence in your ability to use nutrient-dense foods effectively. My role as a teacher, and the role of this book, is to help you appreciate and respect these wonderful foods and ingredients.

Always feel free to improve, and don't forget to add the most important ingredient of all—a little bit of yourself. If you can taste the love and creativity you bring to the food, you cannot go wrong. And remember: There are no nutrient-dense police. Whatever you're in the mood for, prepare it and enjoy. Just make it the most nutrient-dense version possible.

CHAPTER 47

Recipes

BREAKFAST

Basic Soft-Boiled Eggs

Two or three organically raised soft-boiled eggs at breakfast is one of the best ways I know to start a day. If you have never attempted to soft-boil an egg, you may be intimidated at the prospect, but if you are curious to learn the old-fashioned art of soft-boiling eggs (the healthiest way to prepare eggs, as the lower temperature will not oxidize, or damage, the cholesterol), the method outlined below should help.

FRESH ORGANIC EGGS

First, to prevent eggs from cracking when you place them in boiling water, run them under warm or hot water for ten to twenty seconds before carefully putting them in your pan (a slotted spoon can facilitate this). Cold eggs just out of the refrigerator will crack when inserted into boiling hot water, so this prewarming under hot water helps.

There are two schools of thought regarding soft-boiling eggs. You can put them in the pan of water and gradually bring them to a boil, or you can use a spoon and place them in the already boiling water. In either case, with a little experience, you will soon be able to gauge how long they need to cook before you fish them out. After you do, using the slotted spoon, quickly place the eggs under cold running water for ten seconds, so you can comfortably hold them in your hand. Then, holding each egg (one at a time), give it a good strong whack in the middle with a knife or the edge of a teaspoon, and break it in two halves by pulling it apart. Using a small spoon, you should easily be able to scoop out the contents of each half. Eat with broken-up whole-grain toast crumbled in it and a little sea salt and pepper, or drizzle it with oil, and there you have it.

Preparation time: There are several things to keep in mind in order to get perfect, soft-boiled eggs. First is the altitude you live at. At higher elevations, such as in the Rocky Mountains, water boils at a lower temperature, which means the water you are boiling your eggs in is not as hot, and so they will therefore need to cook longer. Also, keep in mind that if your eggs come right out of the refrigerator, they will take longer than eggs that have been left out for a while. There is also the question of how you like them. To me, perfect soft-boiled eggs have completely cooked whites and still-runny yolks. Other people prefer yolks that are almost completely cooked (closer to hard-boiled). So the time can range from three minutes for room-temperature eggs at sea level to seven or eight minutes for refrigerated eggs at 8,000 feet.

Options: I typically sprinkle nutritional yeast or powdered sea seasonings, such as powdered kelp or dulse, on my eggs. Often, I drizzle fresh flaxseed or wheat germ oil, or a teaspoon of melted coconut oil over them.

Nutrient density: Eggs eaten with the above options will get your metabolic furnaces humming and help you resist midmorning blood-sugar crashes. Because this combination of protein and healthy oil can boost your metabolism, I believe it can contribute to weight loss and energy production. Eggs are particularly dense for all the essential amino acids, and for the vitamins A, D, and E, and the mineral sulfur. They also contain lecithin and, when not oxidized, good cholesterol.

Poached Eggs (or Fish)

I love poached eggs. But when I recommend poaching eggs or halibut (I love poached fish, too) as a healthy way to prepare these foods to an audience, I often notice blank faces. In this age of microwave ovens and precooked food, many younger people are not being raised to experience this very basic cooking technique. Therefore, even though this is not really a recipe, I still think it important to describe what poaching is, for the benefit of any of you who have not tried this easy cooking method.

ORGANIC EGGS

Basically, poaching means simmering or floating your eggs (or fish) in a pan of water, with a tight-fitting lid. The idea is that the food is cooked from below (the boiling water) and above (the steam). This is a great way to keep food moist and flavorful, and does not require the use of any cooking oils. Poaching is quick and easy, and because it uses a relatively low temperature, does not tend to degrade nutrients. Eggs can also be floated on the water in poaching cups, which you can buy at any kitchen store.

Preparation time: 3–4 minutes (approximate) for the eggs.

Options: Crumble some seaweed on top.

Nutrient density: Same as soft-boiled eggs.

Garima's Breakfast Smoothie

This really delicious protein-rich smoothie will keep your energy level up all morning. Once you make it, you'll want a version of it every day.

8–12 OUNCES UNSWEETENED JUICE, SUCH AS APPLE OR CONCORD GRAPE (FRESH IS EVEN BETTER)

ONE BANANA OR OTHER FRESH FRUIT IN SEASON

1–3 TEASPOONS SPIRULINA POWDER

1 TEASPOON BREWER'S YEAST

1 TEASPOON LECITHIN GRANULES

1 TEASPOON BEE POLLEN GRANULES

1 TABLESPOON FLAXSEEDS, FLAX OIL, OR PUMPKIN SEEDS

A PINCH OF KELP POWDER

Blend until smooth.

Preparation time: 5 minutes to throw everything together in the blender.

Options: Use ¼ cup unhomogenized yogurt also.

Nutrient density: This balanced smoothie supplies an abundance of vitamins and minerals, including B vitamins, essential fatty acids, chlorophyll, and trace minerals.

Garima's Rose Hips Jam

Time does all the work with this tasty jam. All you have to do is stir and enjoy.

¼ CUP DRIED SEEDLESS ROSE HIPS

¾ CUP PURE, UNSWEETENED APPLE JUICE

Soak the rose hips in apple juice overnight. Give the mixture a good stir in the morning, and add more juice if it's too thick. That's it. You're done. Serve on toast with almond butter.

Preparation time: 6–8 hours, or overnight (soaking time).

Options: You can also use apple-raspberry juice or a similar juice blend.

Nutrient density: This jam is very high in vitamin C and bioflavonoids.

STARTERS

Soaked/Sprouted Nuts

Place a handful of raw, whole (no pieces) almonds, pine nuts, sesame, or sunflower seeds and soak in a bowl or jar of fresh water. Rinse and change the water a couple of times for a day and drain, storing in the refrigerator.

Danielle's Basic Hummus

Hummus is one of those delicious, nutritionally dense, and versatile foods that can be used as a dip with vegetables, as a sandwich spread, or as a side dish. A staple of Middle Eastern fare the core of its nutrition revolves around the chickpeas (garbanzo beans) and the tahini (ground sesame seeds). The following recipe comes from Danielle, a natural-foods cook at a health food store in my hometown. Her hummus is exceptionally tasty, but I am purposely omitting precise proportions because I want you to develop your own style and confidence. Danielle's hummus has a beautiful, soft golden-yellow color due to the turmeric and a gentle combination of ingredients which complement each other nicely.

GARBANZO BEANS*
TAHINI
GARLIC
LEMON JUICE
CUMIN
SEA SALT
PEPPER
TURMERIC

**Canned or cooked in pressure cooker until tender*

Puree all ingredients together in a blender or food processor.

Preparation time: 10–20 minutes.

Options: For added density, add fresh herbs such as dill or cilantro. Flax oil and powdered sea vegetables are also good additions.

Nutrient density: Hummus is nutrient dense for calcium, good fats, and protein. Depending on what additional ingredients are used, it can also be a good source for other nutrients and phytochemicals.

Garima's Carrot and Celery Sticks with Tofu-Tahini Dip

Slice up a bowl of carrot and celery sticks and serve with the following dip.

8 OUNCES FIRM FRESH TOFU

2 TABLESPOONS TAHINI (SESAME BUTTER)

2 TABLESPOONS FRESH, SQUEEZED LEMON JUICE

1 TABLESPOON MISO PASTE

2 TABLESPOONS SPRING WATER (OR MORE, FOR THE RIGHT CONSISTENCY)

1 TEASPOON EACH FRESHLY CHOPPED CILANTRO, CHERVIL, DILL, AND PARSLEY

¼ TEASPOON GROUND CUMIN SEEDS

1 CLOVE GARLIC, MINCED

Combine all ingredients in a food processor or blender.

Preparation time: 10–20 minutes, depending on your speed in the kitchen.

Nutrient density: Calcium, protein, and phytonutrients.

SOUPS

Amalia's No-Dairy Cream of Broccoli Soup

This soup has interesting ingredients that make eating it an adventurous pleasure.

SEVERAL CUPS OF SUNFLOWER SEEDS*

ONIONS

GARLIC

LEEKS

BURDOCK ROOT, CHOPPED

GHEE OR COCONUT OIL

BROCCOLI, CHOPPED

**Soaked in spring water for a few hours*

Sauté the onions, garlic, leeks, and chopped burdock root in some ghee or coconut oil. When almost tender, add a little water and simmer broccoli in the pan until tender. Blend together in a blender or processor. Separately, blend the soaked sunflower seeds with enough water or cooking juice to make a thin mixture. Add to the already blended ingredients and blend together.

Preparation time: 25 minutes approximately.

Options: Add a little miso or Amalia's almond-yeast mix.

Nutrient density: Though dairy free, this soup compares favorably in calcium density, thanks to the broccoli and sunflower seeds.

Garima's Creamy Black Bean Soup

This is perfect for cold winter nights when you just want to curl up by a fire and enjoy a thick rich soup. You can soak the beans in the morning, make the soup later in the day, and enjoy it the same night, or you can make it right up to the point of adding the pumpkin seed butter and any condiments, then refrigerate it and enjoy it the next day—soups and stews can be even better on the second day. However you want to do it, though, you can't beat this soup for hearty deliciousness.

2 cups dried black beans
1–2 pieces kombu (seaweed)
2–3 cups sweet winter squash, baked
1 onion, chopped fine
2–3 cloves garlic
Sea salt, unrefined
Pumpkin seed butter

Soak the beans for a few hours or even overnight. Drain, rinse well, and cover with spring water or vegetable broth. Add the kombu and bring to a boil, reducing the heat and simmering until the beans are soft. Meanwhile, bake the squash at 350°F (I bake squash whole with a hole poked in the side because they are difficult to cut raw.) When a knife inserted in the side of the squash comes out easily, remove from the oven and allow to cool. Cut in half, scoop out the seeds, and spoon the squash pulp into the cooked beans. Stir thoroughly to mash the squash. Add the onions, garlic, and sea salt. Simmer ten minutes more. When serving, add a spoonful of fresh pumpkin seed butter to each bowl and stir in. The flavor and creaminess this adds is wonderful.

Preparation time: 1–1½ hours cooking time.

Options: For condiments, you can add toasted sesame seeds, wilted spinach or similar greens, extra sea vegetables, or a sprinkle of nutritional yeast.

Nutrient density: This soup is rich in calcium, fiber, trace minerals, and phytonutrients.

Note: *Pumpkin seed butter may be hard to find, but both Garima and I have independently discovered a wonderful version by Omega Nutrition (see Appendix A).*

SALADS AND SALAD DRESSINGS

Amalia's Neptune Salad

The following is another good example of how easy it is to throw together a handful of ingredients that complement one another nicely. Although deceptively easy, it is important to realize that the real beauty of such a dish is how everything in it is nutritionally beneficial; there is no waste or filler, and the options are unlimited. What I especially like is how this can make a great nutrient-dense meal by itself, without resorting to less-dense fillers, such as bread or pasta.

BELL PEPPERS, YELLOW AND RED
CELERY
RED ONION
FRESH TOMATO
FRESH LETTUCE
CAPERS
KALAMATA OLIVES
DULSE, DRIED, POWDERED
TUNA, CANNED
HALIBUT CHUNKS, COOKED

Cut vegetables into bite-sized pieces and toss with the other ingredients. Use a dressing from this section, make up your own, or try Amalia's Neptune Salad Dressing.

Preparation time: 10–15 minutes to assemble ingredients, chop, and toss together. Add additional time if you need to cook some halibut.

Options: Avocado or cubes of raw goat cheese; fresh parsley or spinach; cooked salmon or trout chunks; canned sardines. Try some powdered dulse or kelp, or soak some sea vegetables and toss them in.

Nutrient density: This salad is dense in antioxidants, fiber, minerals, phytonutrients, and protein.

Deviled Eggs and Egg Salad

Almost everyone loves eggs and has their own special way to prepare them. Eggs are a supremely nutrient-dense food when raised in organic, humane ways.

EGGS

FLAXSEED OR WHEAT GERM OIL

MUSTARD

SEA SALT, BLACK PEPPER, GARLIC,
FRESH CRUSHED, OR GARLIC POWDER

RED ONION

CELERY

GARNISHES: CAYENNE PEPPER,
NUTRITIONAL YEAST, PAPRIKA, SESAME SEEDS

Hard-boil eggs (8–12 minutes, depending on altitude and initial coldness), and peel when done. For deviled eggs, slice each egg in half, lengthwise. Remove the yolks and put in a separate bowl. Mash the yolks with a fork, and add a splash of flaxseed or wheat germ oil and the mustard (start out cautiously). Mix well, until creamy. A little experimentation will yield the right combination to suit your taste buds. Add salt, black pepper, garlic, and a small amount of finely diced red onion and celery. Scoop this yolk mixture into the hollows of the egg-white boats. Garnish with sprinkles of cayenne, paprika, sesame seeds, or nutritional yeast on top.

For egg salad, put the whole eggs and other ingredients in a bowl and mix everything together until it is the consistency you like.

Preparation time: 10–15 minutes to boil and peel the eggs. Prepping and mixing the various ingredients should not take more than another five to ten minutes.

Options: Vary spices to your liking. A little mayonnaise can be added if you need a more liquid consistency, or simply add extra flax or olive oil. Fine dulse flakes can be mixed in or sprinkled on top as a garnish—the deep purple speckles make a beautiful counterpoint to the deep yellow of the yolk.

Nutrient density: Good organic eggs are one of the most nutrient dense foods. They are high in amino acids, phospholipids (lecithin), vitamin A, and cholesterol (which is *good* for you when it is from a low-heat source, such as boiling). The flaxseed oil adds omega-3 fatty acids if you cannot purchase eggs rich in omega-3s in your area. The red onion, celery, and spices (including the mustard) add important phytonutrients and antioxidants. If you use wheat germ oil, vitamin E is added. Spectrum Natural cold-pressed wheat germ oil is an especially dense source for natural vitamin E alpha tocopherol (*see* Appendix A). Nutritional yeast and dulse flakes skyrocket the nutrient denseness even further (trace minerals and B vitamins).

SALAD DRESSINGS

For some reason, homemade salad dressings intimidate some people. I have watched people carefully measure and sort their ingredients as if to achieve some mythically ideal dressing. With nutrient-dense principles, however, and using quality ingredients, I have found that little can go wrong when making a homemade salad dressing. The important thing to keep in mind is the overall balance of flavors, and the consistency. A good dressing should complement, not overpower, the ingredients in the salad.

Basic Salad Dressing

This is my most basic dressing and the one I use most frequently. Because it is so simple, it can serve as a model for nutrient density as a whole, and can also be the starting point for a whole world of subtle variations.

FRESH FLAXSEED OIL
UMEBOSHI PLUM VINEGAR (OR PASTE)
GARLIC, CRUSHED

Shake the oil and vinegar with the garlic. It is important get the right proportion of oil to vinegar. Umeboshi plum vinegar is quite salty, so a couple of splashes is usually all you will need. Also, since flax oils vary considerably from brand to brand, adjust your recipe accordingly. If you find flax oil too strong, I recommend cutting it with Spectrum Natural's cold-pressed wheat germ oil (the most nutrient-dense source of natural vitamin E known) or a similar high-quality oil, such as olive oil.

Preparation time: 5 minutes or less.

Options: One option is whipping in avocado for a green dressing. It gives a creamier texture to the dressing, and softens the flavor for those who find the oil a little strong. Other options include using small amounts of finely chopped arame, dulse, or hijiki seaweeds. Mustard or horseradish are also delicious options, and will give your dressing an extra zing. Tahini (sesame-seed butter) can also be blended in to give the dressing a creamy thick texture. Nutritional yeast, too, is a great addition to all kinds of salad dressings. Its mild, yeasty flavor adds a subtle dimension to the overall complexity and taste of the dressing, and its nutritional contributions are second to none (*see* Chapter 30). Yeast also adds nice body to a thin dressing, similar to a Caesar dressing.

Nutrient density: Omega three fatty acids (oil), sulfur (garlic), phytonutrients (garlic, umeboshi vinegar).

Amalia's Basil Vinaigrette Salad Dressing/Marinade

The distinctive aroma of basil really jumps out in this dressing, and the walnuts add texture.

BASIL

GARLIC

BASALMIC VINEGAR

A LITTLE TAMARI* OR SEA SALT

NUTRITIONAL YEAST, FOR CREAMINESS

OLIVE OIL

WALNUTS, FINELY CHOPPED

1 TABLESPOON OF HONEY
(TO BRING OUT THE NATURAL SWEETNESS OF THE BASIL)

Blend ingredients in blender. Add walnuts separately to preserve their texture.

Preparation time: 5–7 minutes.

Options: None needed.

Nutrient density: Phytonutrients, B vitamins, and trace minerals.

**A natural-style soy sauce, sometimes made from wheat.*

Amalia's Neptune Salad Dressing

In tiny amounts, the cod-liver oil has no unpleasant flavor or aroma, but adds real zest to this dressing.

FLAX OR OTHER GOOD OIL

COD-LIVER OIL, SMALL AMOUNT

DIJON MUSTARD, SEA SALT, BLACK PEPPER

NUTRITIONAL YEAST

ALMONDS OR SUNFLOWER SEEDS, POWDERED

Mix all together until you have a smooth consistency. The powdered nuts are used to thicken, similar to Parmesan cheese; they can be ground in a blender, clean coffee grinder, food mill, nut chopper, or food processor.

Preparation time: 5–10 minutes.

Options: Whatever you like.

Nutrient density: Omega-three fatty acids, B vitamins, and trace minerals.

Amalia's No-Name Salad Dressing

This is a delicious variation on standard dressings and dips.

GOOD OLIVE OIL

LEMON JUICE

GARLIC

SEA SALT

NUTRITIONAL YEAST, TO THICKEN

POWDERED ALMONDS, TO THICKEN

Blend ingredients together. According to Amalia, this recipe also makes a great dip or sauce for artichokes or asparagus. She uses a blend of nutritional yeast (she recommends Lewis Laboratories—*see* Appendix A) and powdered almonds (grind in a blender or food processor) as a substitute of sorts for Parmesan cheese in soups, on salads, in casseroles, or on steamed vegetables.

Preparation time: 5–10 minutes.

Options: Horseradish or mustard.

Nutrient density: B vitamins and trace minerals.

Garima's Essential Salad Dressing

This is the simplest salad dressing ever.

12-OUNCE BOTTLE OF OMEGA ESSENTIAL BALANCE OIL BLEND

JUICE OF HALF A LEMON

SEA SALT OR KELP POWDER

DILL WEED

You can make this right in the original bottle, adding ingredients as listed. Shake well and keep refrigerated.

Preparation time: A few minutes.

Options: Herbs to taste.

Nutrient density: Trace minerals and essential fatty acids.

SAUCES AND DIPS

Amalia's Tahini-Ginger Dip

This is an excellent tangy, spicy dip for steamed or raw vegetables.

FRESH GINGER, PEELED AND GRATED
FRESH GARLIC
SPRING WATER
TAMARI
LEMON JUICE
TURMERIC
TAHINI
GOOD QUALITY OLIVE OIL

Blend all ingredients in a blender until smooth and creamy. (Use enough tahini to thicken to the desired consistency.) Amalia prefers this on the strong side with the ginger and tahini flavors predominating. The turmeric is primarily used for its orange color, and because it is good for the liver.

Preparation time: 10 minutes or so (mostly to peel the garlic and grate the ginger).

Options: Use apple-cider vinegar instead of lemon juice.

Nutrient density: Phytonutrients galore.

Amalia's Stir-Fry Sauce or Dip

The coconut milk and curry powder add an Asian flavor to this delightful dip.

FRESH GINGER, PEELED
GARLIC
COCONUT MILK, CANNED
CURRY POWDER
SEA SALT OR TAMARI, TO TASTE
CASHEWS

In a blender, mix all ingredients except cashews. Blend cashews (raw, or lightly roasted in a dry cast-iron skillet) separately with a little coconut milk; then add this liquid mixture to the other ingredients and blend together.

Preparation time: 10 minutes.

Options: Spices to taste.

Nutrient density: Phytonutrients.

Garima's Almond Umeboshi Sauce

The umeboshi lends a distinctive taste familiar to those who have eaten Japanese macrobiotic food.

2 TEASPOONS UMEBOSHI PASTE

2 TABLESPOONS ALMOND BUTTER

1 TEASPOON GRATED GINGER

½ CUP SPRING WATER, OR AS NEEDED FOR CONSISTENCY

Mix the umeboshi paste and almond butter together in a bowl, adding just enough water to be able to stir ingredients together. Then add ginger and water slowly, stirring well, until you get a nice, creamy consistency. Pour over brown rice, millet, or quinoa grains, legume beans, or vegetables.

Preparation time: Under 10 minutes.

Options: Herbs to taste.

Nutrient density: Phytonutrients, calcium.

Garima's Tahini-Miso Sauce

This is a versatile, savory sauce.

¼ CUP TAHINI (SESAME BUTTER)

1 TABLESPOON MISO

1½ TABLESPOONS LEMON JUICE OR UMEBOSHI VINEGAR

⅓ CUP SPRING WATER

A FEW SPRIGS OF FRESH PARSLEY, ROSEMARY, OR OTHER HERBS

Put all the ingredients in the blender or processor and blend until creamy. Adjust lemon juice and miso to your taste.

Preparation time: Less than 10 minutes.

Options: Sea vegetables, nutritional yeast. You can substitute almond butter for tahini.

Nutrient density: This sauce is loaded with calcium.

FISH AND SEAFOOD

Quick Dinner—Mixed Organic Field Greens with Wild Salmon, Feta, and Pine Nuts

This quick dinner illustrates my penchant for throwing together whatever is available for a fast meal that can be surprisingly delicious and dense. The key is the availability of good food at your fingertips. If you have a variety of high-quality food at your disposal, it is almost impossible to go wrong at meal time. Such seat-of-the-pants type meals are typical in my kitchen, and are almost always accompanied by a request for the recipe. The secret here is that there is no recipe, just a marriage of good food thrown together with a little adventurous creativity.

Mixed field greens (from farmer's market or health food supermarket)

Wild salmon, cooked chunks

Feta cheese

Pine nuts

Flaxseed oil

Kalamata olives

Red onion, sliced

Yellow or red bell pepper, sliced

There really is no procedure here. Simply toss the ingredients together in a big salad bowl or dish, and serve with any good nutrient-dense salad dressing.

Preparation time: Approximately 10 minutes, assuming you have all the ingredients on hand.

Options: Since this is your classic *anything goes* type of salad, you are limited only by your imagination and the availability of whatever is in your refrigerator or garden. Your options could include almonds, avocados, capers, cucumbers, fresh tomatoes, nutritional yeast, sardines, sunflower seeds, zucchini, or more. For a nicoise-style salad, add a hard-boiled egg or two and cooked green beans. I frequently reconstitute a small amount of seaweed and throw it in for good measure.

Nutrient density: This is your classic phytonutrient-rich meal, loaded with diverse plant-based foods. The feta, pine nuts, and salmon all supply protein and essential oils. This dish is also a good source of calcium.

Amalia and Melinda's Wild Salmon

Melinda is Amalia's mother, and their collaborations frequently result in fantastic kitchen artistry.

WILD SALMON

2 LEMONS

FRESH ROSEMARY SPRIGS

ALMONDS, POWDERED (GRIND IN BLENDER OR PROCESSOR)

SALT AND PEPPER

Line a casserole dish with sliced rounds of lemon. Lay a piece of wild salmon on this bed. Squeeze an entire lemon over the fish. Lay fresh rosemary sprigs on top. Cover with a layer of powdered almonds. Salt and pepper to taste. Bake until done, 25–30 minutes in a 350°F oven (depending on the size of the fish).

Preparation time: 40 minutes.

Options: Cook sea vegetables in casserole dish.

Nutrient density: Protein, calcium, essential oils.

MEATS

Coconut Milk Curry with Lamb and Mixed Vegetables

Asian, Middle Eastern, and Western flavors all combine in this excellent curry.

OLIVE OR COCONUT OIL

ONIONS, CHOPPED

GARLIC, CHOPPED

CUBES OF BONELESS LEG OF LAMB (APPROX ¼ LB PER PERSON)

BROCCOLI, CABBAGE, CARROTS, CELERY, PEPPER, OR OTHER VEGETABLES, CHOPPED

CORN AND PEAS, PREFERABLY FRESH

1 CAN COCONUT MILK

TURMERIC, CURRY POWDER OR PASTE, SEA SALT, PEPPER

COCONUT FLAKES, UNSWEETENED

RAISINS

CASHEWS

Put a little olive or coconut oil in a deep cast-iron skillet, and sauté garlic, onion, and lamb chunks in it for a few minutes. Add vegetables, saving the quicker-cooking ones for later, and stir-fry for a few minutes over a medium flame. Add coconut milk, stir together, then add curry spices and salt to taste. Do not overcook the vegetables. Toward the end, sprinkle in some coconut flakes, a few raisins, and cashews.

Preparation time: This meal cooks more quickly than you would expect. Chopping the vegetables takes 10 minutes. Sautéing and cooking the remaining ingredients should not take more than 15 minutes more. If you are serving this curry with brown rice or brown basmati rice (an especially delicious variety), begin the rice first as it will take longer to prepare than the actual curry. White basmati rice cooks quickly, in about 15 minutes, whereas brown rice takes approximately 35–40 minutes, so time it accordingly.

Options: You can make this as simple or elaborate as you like. The raisins add a nice counterpoint of sweetness to the hot spiciness of the curry. Other options include water chestnuts, for their crunchy texture, or some diced, dried pineapple for a little extra sweetness. Serve with a fragrant basmati rice, or eat as a soup. You can omit the lamb and substitute tempeh or tofu if you want a purely vegetarian version. For more iron, substitute buffalo for the lamb.

Nutrient density: This meal is rich in phytonutrients from the diverse vegetables. The lamb provides B vitamins, protein, and iron. The curry spices and turmeric are rich in potent antioxidants. The coconut milk and oil provide beneficial medium-chain triglycerides and lauric acid (an antiviral fatty acid).

ONE-SKILLET DINNERS

Curries, stews, and various stir-fries all lend themselves nicely to this style of cooking. Frequently, my one-skillet meals feature halibut or salmon. Other meals are highlighted by lamb or buffalo (see below). For vegetarian dishes, I often sauté tempeh with garlic, jalapeños, fresh ginger, and onions. I use either olive oil or my current favorite, coconut. For added nutrition, or to stretch the meal, serve with buckwheat soba noodles, brown rice, millet, quinoa, or some other whole grain. As a final touch, a minute or two before serving, wilt a large amount of fresh greens, such as cut-up beet greens, chard, or spinach on top of the dish. A tight-fitting lid will reduce splatter (less cleanup), while speeding up the cooking time by holding in the heat and juices.

One-Skillet Buffalo with Stewed Tomatoes

Olive or coconut oil

Fresh garlic, minced

Ground buffalo, 1–2 pounds, depending on number being served

Fresh green cabbage, shredded

Stewed tomatoes, 1 can

Cayenne, paprika, salt, pepper, basil, oregano

Brown rice (*see* recipe page 258)

In a cast-iron skillet, sauté garlic in a little olive or coconut oil. Add buffalo (loose or shaped into meat balls the size of ping-pong balls) and sauté over a medium flame for several minutes until mostly cooked through. Add a handful or two of the cabbage and the can of tomatoes. Stir occasionally, adding seasonings to taste. Cover to speed up cooking time (this will wilt the cabbage faster). Serve over brown rice.

Preparation time: As with many single-skillet dishes, this meal can be easily prepared and cooked in under 30 minutes if the rice is precooked. Otherwise, start the brown rice approximately 20 minutes or so prior to beginning the skillet dish. Chopping the vegetables should not take more than 10 minutes. Sautéing the ingredients (medium heat) should not take more than 15 minutes.

Options: One-skillet dinners can have endless variations. Add bok choy, or Chinese cabbage, fresh or canned jalapeños, fresh wilted spinach (just before serving). Grate a little Parmesan or similar hard cheese over dish just before serving.

Nutrient density: The vegetables are all great sources of antioxidants and other phytonutrients. This meal contains dense levels of lycopene (tomatoes), sulfur antioxidants (garlic, cabbage), protein (buffalo), and iron (buffalo). It is also a good source of fiber (brown rice, cabbage) and the B vitamins. The Parmesan provides additional calcium.

GRAINS

Although there are only two grains listed here, this is an important category because most of the main dishes in this book call for grains as an accompaniment.

Brown Rice

1 CUP RICE (ORGANIC BROWN BASMATI RICE IS UNUSUALLY FRAGRANT AND TASTY)

2 CUPS PURE FILTERED WATER

1 TABLESPOON COCONUT OIL, ENOUGH TO COAT BOTTOM OF COOKING POT

SEA SALT

Put oil in saucepan and heat. Add the rice. Stir rice so all grains are coated with oil, cook briefly until heated but not burned, then add filtered water (it may sizzle) and bring to a boil. Add sea salt, cover, lower heat to a low flame, and let cook undisturbed (do not stir or lift lid to check). After 20 minutes or so, peek in to assess progress. If rice is cooking too fast, lower the flame. Rice is done when all the water is absorbed and rice is tender.

Preparation time: Approximately 30–45 minutes, including cooking time.

Options: Omit the coconut oil.

Nutrient density: Brown rice is famous for the B vitamins it provides. It also supplies fiber and some minerals.

Garima's Quinoa with Beets and Greens

1 CUP QUINOA

2 CUPS SPRING WATER

UNREFINED SEA SALT

2–3 BEETS

4–5 CUPS MIXED DARK LEAFY GREENS: BEET GREENS, LAMB'S-QUARTER, SPINACH, SWISS CHARD, OR OTHERS

Wash quinoa thoroughly to remove the bitterness. Place in a pot with a tight-fitting lid. Add water and a dash of salt. Bring to a boil, cover, and reduce the heat, simmering for 20–30 minutes until all the water is absorbed. In a separate pot, simmer the beets with a little water for about 30 minutes, or until a knife slides in easily. Remove from the heat. While quinoa and beets are cooking, wash greens thoroughly and cut into bite-sized pieces. Simmer in a small amount of the beet-cooking water, adding a pinch of salt. While greens are cooking, slice the beets in half, then further into bite-sized slices.

When the greens are tender, stir in the beet slices and remove from the heat. Combine with the quinoa, mix well, and serve with tahini-miso sauce drizzled over the top (*see* Sauces and Dips above).

Preparation time: 45 minutes approximately.

Options: Sea vegetables, herbs to taste. Serve with umeboshi paste and nutritional yeast.

Nutrient density: Quinoa is rich in B vitamins and protein. The greens provide magnesium and phytonutrients.

VEGETABLES AND LEGUMES

Amalia's Sweet Potato Tempeh

SWEET POTATOES

TEMPEH

BALSAMIC VINEGAR, GARLIC, GINGER, AND TAMARI MARINADE

1 CLOVE GARLIC, MINCED

TAMARI

MUSTARD

NUTRITIONAL YEAST

MAPLE SYRUP

OLIVE OR COCONUT OIL

ENDIVE LEAVES

Marinate slices of tempeh in balsamic vinegar-tamari marinade for several hours. Bake at 350°F until liquid is absorbed into the tempeh. Bake or boil sweet potato until soft. Mash sweet potato, add garlic; a little tamari, generous amounts of mustard, some nutritional yeast, a little maple syrup, and a little olive or coconut oil. Serve by smearing this sweet potato paste on the endive and top with slices of the marinated baked tempeh.

Preparation time: Marinating takes a few hours. The actual baking time should be about 1 hour, or slightly less.

Options: Add a little honey to the marinade.

Nutrient density: Tempeh is rich in calcium, protein, and phytonutrients. The yeast adds B vitamins and minerals. Sweet potato is a great source of fiber, complex starches, and carotenes.

Amalia's Walnut-Lentil Loaf

Unusual and unusually delicious

MIXED VEGETABLES: CARROT, CELERY, GARLIC, LEEK, ONIONS, SUN-DRIED TOMATOES, FINELY CUT UP

HERBS (BASIL, OREGANO, THYME)

BALSAMIC VINEGAR

BROWN RICE, COOKED

LENTILS, COOKED

WALNUTS, CHOPPED, A HANDFUL

NUTRITIONAL YEAST

SEA SALT

OLIVE OIL

Sauté finely chopped vegetables in the oil. Add herbs and a little vinegar. Mix together the vegetables, rice, and lentils. Add the chopped walnuts, nutritional yeast, salt, and olive oil. Mix together and press firmly into a loaf pan. Serve with mushroom gravy (*see* below).

Preparation time: Time to cook lentils—If you use precooked lentils (leftovers or canned) time is cut in half.

Time to cook rice—The lentils take the longest, so prepare other ingredients while lentils are cooking (approximately 1 hour).

Options: Substitute coconut oil for olive oil; herbs to taste.

Nutrient density: B vitamins, fiber, phytonutrients, protein.

Simple Mushroom Gravy

This gravy goes with any number of dishes. It can even be poured over brown rice.

ONIONS, FINELY CHOPPED

GARLIC, FINELY CHOPPED

CELERY, SMALL AMOUNT, CHOPPED

SHIITAKE MUSHROOMS, A HANDFUL, CHOPPED

COCONUT OIL

COCONUT MILK, CANNED

WALNUTS, SOAKED AND GROUND
(*SEE* INSTRUCTIONS FOR SOAKING/SPROUTING, PAGE 244)

SALT

Sauté onion, garlic, and celery with fresh shiitake mushrooms in coconut oil. Add coconut milk and ground walnuts and simmer until done. Salt to taste.

Preparation time: 20–25 minutes.

Options: You can substitute almond meal or any other nut meal for the walnuts. Pepper or herbs to taste.

Nutrient density: Phytonutrients, fiber.

Garima's Steamed Artichokes with Sunflower Dipping Sauce

Big or tiny, artichokes are a festive food.

1 ARTICHOKE PER PERSON

Carefully wash the artichokes and cut off the stem. Place in a steamer with plenty of water, and simmer until tender, about 30–45 minutes. Test for doneness by tugging at one of the outer leaves. When it comes out easily, they are done. Serve warm with Garima's Sunflower Dipping Sauce below.

Preparation time: 30–45 minutes.

Options: None needed.

Nutrient density: Artichokes are rich in phytonutrients, magnesium, and fiber.

Garima's Sunflower Dipping Sauce

This sauce is also delicious poured over other vegetables, or as a salad dressing.

1/2 CUP RAW SUNFLOWER SEEDS, SOAKED AND SPROUTED FOR 1–2 DAYS (*SEE* INSTRUCTIONS FOR SOAKING/SPROUTING NUTS, PAGE 244.)

1 TABLESPOON TAMARI

2 TEASPOONS LEMON JUICE

2 TABLESPOONS FLAX OIL, OR SUNFLOWER OIL, COLD-PRESSED

1/2–3/4 CUP SPRING WATER

2 SPRIGS FRESH TARRAGON

A DASH OF CAYENNE

Starting with 1/2 cup water, place all ingredients in a blender or food processor, and blend. Add more water, if needed, for a nice creamy consistency.

Preparation time: 10 minutes.

Options: Herbs and pepper to taste.

Nutrient density: Essential fatty acids, protein, B vitamins.

Garima's Kombu Spaghetti

Kombu is a type of seaweed that comes in largish sheets approximately the size of lasagna noodles. When allowed to soak in water for an hour or two, it softens and expands to several times its original size.

2–3 pieces of kombu per person

Garlic, minced

Ginger, grated

Sesame or coconut oil

Tamari

Water for soaking

Pine nuts, toasted

Soak kombu in a bowl of water for a few hours. When soft and expanded, slice crosswise into very thin strips, about the size of spaghetti. Sauté garlic and ginger in sesame or coconut oil and tamari until fragrant. Add sliced kombu and a few tablespoons of soaking water. Simmer 10–15 minutes until the flavors mingle. Serve with sunflower seeds or pine nuts.

Preparation time: Aside from the time needed to soak the kombu, this sea spaghetti should take under 30 minutes to prepare.

Options: You can use coconut oil instead, and sunflower seeds.

Nutrient density: Kombu is dense for calcium, phytonutrients, and trace minerals, plus protein.

Garima's Creamed Sunchokes

Not really artichokes, but definitely worth trying if they are new to you. This method is especially tasty.

2–3 pounds sunchokes (Jerusalem artichokes), washed

Unrefined sea salt

Flaxseed oil

Simmer the washed sunchokes in a little spring water with a pinch of sea salt. When tender, mash with a little flaxseed oil. Serve hot.

Preparation time: 10 minutes.

Options: Herbs to taste, nutritional yeast, kelp or dulse flakes.

Nutrient density: Fiber, complex carbohydrates, phytonutrients, essential fatty acids.

DESSERTS

Banana Crème Pie, Unbaked

This is the most ridiculously easy pie you have ever not baked. Add any of the options listed, or invent your own.

3–4 BANANAS

1–2 AVOCADOS

CINNAMON

HONEY OR MAPLE SYRUP (OPTIONAL)

PIE CRUST (*SEE* FLOURLESS PIE CRUST—NO BAKE BELOW)

In a food processor or blender, mix the bananas, avocado, and cinnamon until creamy. Add maple syrup or honey if it needs to be sweeter (this depends on the ripeness of the bananas). Pour into pie crust and chill.

Preparation time: 5–10 minutes.

Options: For a firmer filling, blend 2–3 tablespoons of melted (warmed) coconut oil with the filling. When it cools, the coconut oil will act as a thickening agent, plus it lends a delicious coconut taste. Other options for the filling are carob or chocolate chips, dried fruit, flaked coconut, or maple syrup. For attractive garnishes, top with berries, candied ginger, fresh or dried pineapple, or thinly sliced kiwi fruit.

Nutrient density: This pie is dense compared to most conventional pies because of the phytonutrients present in the avocado and bananas. Both the avocado and the nut crust provide abundant healthy oils. Cinnamon is helpful in the metabolism of sugars. Like all raw-food recipes, this one is dense for enzymes.

Flourless Pie Crust—No-Bake

This crust, which can be whipped up in minutes, is a simplified version of Bliss Balls #1 (see page 265). By not using flour, you can accommodate any tier level that is omitting flour, wheat, or gluten-containing products. The big plus is the taste. Ground-nut crusts go wonderfully with tortes or the Banana Crème Pie listed above.

2 CUPS ALMONDS, FINELY GROUND

1–2 TABLESPOONS COCONUT OIL

MAPLE SYRUP

SEA SALT, A TRACE

Blend all ingredients together and press into a pie shell.

Preparation time: Approximately 20 minutes.

Options: Use cashews, sunflower seeds, or walnuts, and honey instead, or in addition. You also may use rice or barley malt syrups.

Nutrient density: Almonds are high in fiber, protein, calcium, magnesium, and some B vitamins.

Blackstrap Yogurt Sundae

This sundae is a delicious way to satisfy a craving for ice cream. Always use a high-quality, nonhomogenized yogurt, such as Seven Stars or Brown Cow.

1 CUP OF NONHOMOGENIZED YOGURT

RAISINS

WALNUTS, CHOPPED

BANANA, SLICED

CURRANTS, DRIED CRANBERRIES, OR FRESH BERRIES

BLACKSTRAP MOLASSES

Put yogurt in a bowl or parfait glass. Arranging ingredients for an appealing presentation, layer in raisins, nuts, sliced banana, and other ingredients. Drizzle molasses on top.

Preparation time: A few minutes if you have all ingredients on hand.

Options: Chopped almonds, carob powder, or dried coconut. Options come from the availability of ingredients, such as fresh seasonal fruit.

Nutrient density: You get lots of minerals with this creamy dessert. It is a power-packed source of calcium, for one, because both molasses and yogurt contain a lot of calcium—this sundae can easily contribute 40 percent or more of the daily requirement for the mineral. The fruit is a good source of fiber and minerals, and the blackstrap molasses is also a great source of chromium, iron, magnesium, and vitamin B_6.

Bliss Balls #1

This is definitely one of the biggest dessert hits I have ever made for people. These bliss balls are not only delicious, they do not require any baking, can be eaten immediately, keep very well in the refrigerator, and freeze well too. Besides being elegant and delicious enough to serve as an after-dinner treat with coffee or tea, they release their energy slowly and are perfect for sports or long hikes.

3 CUPS ALMONDS
1 CUP SUNFLOWER SEEDS
SEA SALT, A PINCH
CINNAMON, GENEROUS SPRINKLE
½ CUP CAROB POWDER
½ CUP COCONUT OIL
BLACKSTRAP MOLASSES, A DASH
½ CUP HONEY
⅓ CUP MAPLE SYRUP

Grind the almonds and sunflower seeds in a food processor or blender until the mix is the consistency of coarse flour. Transfer to a large mixing bowl and add the salt, cinnamon, and carob powder, and mix well. Add the coconut oil, blackstrap molasses, honey, and maple syrup, and knead the mixture until it is well blended. Shape into balls or bars. Refrigerate until use.

Preparation time: Approximately 25 minutes.

Options: You can add candied ginger, carob or chocolate chips, chopped dates, dried pineapple, a few raisins for extra texture and fun. You can also add ground cashews or walnuts. For a cool mint taste, use liberal amounts of peppermint extract. For chocoholics, substitute quality cocoa powder instead of carob.

Nutrient density: Sunflower seeds and almonds give this recipe B vitamins, calcium, essential fatty acids, fiber, magnesium, and vitamin E. Cinnamon provides a phytonutrient that help regulate blood sugar. Blackstrap molasses gives additional minerals, including iron. Coconut oil is a great source of medium-chain fatty acids (for energy) and lauric acid, an antifungal and antiviral fatty acid. Dense for the B vitamins, good fatty acids, minerals, and protein, these nut bars are especially nutrient dense for taste.

Bliss Balls #2

I offer sincere thanks for this recipe from Organica, an all-raw restaurant I visited in San Francisco. It illustrates a key point of nutrient density: simplicity. There is seemingly nothing to it, but these bliss balls hooked me on the concept of noncooking.

SUNFLOWER SEEDS

DATES, SOAKED

RAISINS, SOAKED

HAZELNUTS (FILBERTS), SPROUTED
(SEE INSTRUCTIONS, PAGE 244)

CAROB POWDER

SESAME SEEDS

Grind all ingredients in a food processor. Add carob to taste and for consistency. Roll into truffle-sized balls and roll in carob powder or sesame seeds.

Preparation time: 15 minutes.

Options: Organic coconut flakes.

Nutrient density: My earliest experiences with all uncooked foods taught me there is more to nutrition than just vitamins and minerals. Living foods contain the actual life force itself, and even desserts, such as these bliss balls, can confer that. For the more scientific, this life force is present in the form of enzymes, and soaking fruits, nuts, and seeds activates these enzymes, bringing them to life.

Eagle County Peanut Butter Protein Bars

I found these bars in a couple of health food stores in the mountains of Colorado; I include the recipe because it is nutrient dense and shows how easy it is to make your own treats.

ALMONDS

CAROB CHIPS

COCONUT

CRISP BROWN RICE

CURRANTS

PEANUT BUTTER

ROLLED OATS

SESAME SEEDS

SUNFLOWER SEEDS

WALNUTS

Grind all ingredients together in a food processor or blender and shape into bars. Store in refrigerator.

Preparation time: If the ingredients are in your cabinet, then approximately 30 minutes to gather, blend, shape, and store them.

Options: Limited only by your imagination; almond butter instead of peanut butter.

Nutrient density: Protein, fiber, B vitamins, essential fats.

Amalia's Carob Fudge Balls

So delicious you'll want to nibble as you're making these.

1 CUP CAROB POWDER
½ CUP TAHINI
½ CUP ALMOND BUTTER
½–1 CUP MAPLE SYRUP
A FEW DROPS OF PURE PEPPERMINT ESSENCE OIL (EDIBLE)
ALMONDS, CHOPPED
RAISINS

Mix ingredients together in a large mixing bowl. Chill to make the mixture firm up. When ready, make into balls. They will firm up when chilled.

Preparation time: 15–20 minutes.

Options: Use walnuts, a maple-molasses blend, rice or barley malt syrup, or Sucanat, add spirulina powder, or roll in sesame seeds.

Nutrient density: High in protein, calcium, essential fats.

Garima's Seed Bars

These are really delicious.

½–¾ CUP BROWN RICE SYRUP
¼ CUP SPRING WATER
½ CUP POPPY SEEDS
½ CUP SESAME SEEDS
½ CUP FLAXSEEDS
½ CUP SUNFLOWER SEEDS

Heat the brown rice syrup and water in a small saucepan over low heat. As the mixture begins to bubble, stir in the seeds and remove from heat. Drop by spoonfuls onto a tray or plate, and press to form ¼" thick bars or rounds. Allow to dry until the top is quite firm. Turn over, and continue drying until crisp.

Preparation time: 10 minutes to make; drying time varies.

Options: You can use any combination of chopped dried fruits, nuts, and seeds.

Nutrient density: Nuts and seeds are dense for protein, B vitamins, good oils, magnesium, calcium, and fiber.

Garima's Tahini Pudding

2 CUPS UNSWEETENED APPLE JUICE

1/4 CUP TAHINI

1/4 CUP KUDZU DISSOLVED IN A LITTLE WATER

1/2 CUP GOLDEN RAISINS

Place all ingredients except fruit into a blender or processor and blend until creamy. Pour into a pot, add fruit, and cook and stir until thick. Pour into bowls and allow to cool before serving.

Preparation time: 15 minutes.

Options: Use almond milk or Amazake instead of apple juice; applesauce or chopped dried apricots instead of raisins.

Nutrient density: Tahini is a good source of protein, calcium, iron, and fiber.

DRINKS

Carob-Almond-Molasses Milk Shake

Nutrient-dense drinks (and desserts) are among the most fun, rewarding foods you can make.

ALMONDS, PRESOAKED OR DRY

SPRING WATER

CAROB POWDER

BLACKSTRAP MOLASSES

In a blender, whiz up some almond milk by blending 1 part almonds with 3 or 4 parts water. For extra smooth texture, strain the milk through cheesecloth or a tea strainer. Add 1 tablespoon of carob powder and molasses per glass.

Preparation time: 5 minutes.

Options: This dairy-free milk shake can be modified in many different ways, by adding nutrient-dense ingredients such as lecithin, spirulina, cinnamon, etc. Ice can be blended in for a thicker, colder shake.

Nutrient density: This recipe has the virtue of being loaded with calcium and other minerals, without containing lactose or the other drawbacks of dairy. Almonds, blackstrap molasses, and carob are all great sources of the B vitamins, calcium, and magnesium.

AMALIA'S NUT MILKS

Nut milks can have an important role in a nutrient-dense eating plan. Nutritious and versatile, nut milks often substitute for conventional dairy milk in baked goods, beverages, desserts, and sauces. Although you can buy nondairy milks made from almonds, rice, soy, and even oats, freshly made nut milks are more nutritious than their pasteurized counterparts from a box.

Amalia's Basic Almond Milk

DATES, PITTED
1 SPOONFUL OF MAPLE SYRUP
½ BANANA
1 CUP ALMONDS
2–3 CUPS OF COLD SPRING WATER

Whiz ingredients in blender until completely liquefied. To remove the almond sludge at the bottom, strain the milk through a cheesecloth. Nut milks will only keep in the refrigerator for a couple of days, so make just enough for your immediate needs.

Preparation time: 5 minutes.

Options: Thinner milk can be made with a 1:4 almond to water ratio. Use raw honey instead, or add a few drops of vanilla extract. Many people prefer to soak the almonds overnight, and some blanch the almonds first to remove the skins.

Nutrient density: Almonds supply protein, essential oils, calcium, magnesium, and fiber.

Garima's Umbel Juice

Umbel refers to a classification of flowering plants that send up a seed stalk with the seeds arrayed like an umbrella at the top. Queen Anne's Lace is a well-known example of this family, but carrots, celery, and the rest of the plants in this drink are also all from this family.

4 CARROTS
2 SPRIGS OF PARSLEY
1 STALK OF CELERY
1 STALK OF FENNEL
¼ LEMON, WITH PEEL

Juice in a juicer. This makes one glass. There are many distinct flavors blended together in this juice.

Preparation time: 5–10 minutes.

Options: Juice some apple for extra sweetness.

Nutrient density: Enzymes and lots of phytonutrients.

CONCLUSION

Healing Our Adversarial Relationship with Food

The heart of *The Nutrient-Dense Eating Plan* is its appreciation and celebration of wonderful, deeply nourishing food, yet many people do not have this kind of relationship with their food. In the midst of unprecedented abundance, it is ironic that many Americans have actually become embittered and turned off by food. Yet, given the way American culture has devalued food it is no surprise. Instead of valuing or loving food in a healthy way, food is too often seen as either a cheap form of entertainment or a source of problems (the cause of our diabetes, food allergies, heart disease, high blood pressure, or weight gain). Of course, neither of these approaches express a healthy relationship with food.

We seem to be pulled between two poles. Either food is jammed down our throats via advertisements and new marketing campaigns, or we are subjected to the fearful proclamations of experts who somberly warn about too much cholesterol, fat, or sodium. It is no wonder our culture is marked by eating disorders and obesity.

The beginning of any dysfunctional relationship is one based on fear and mistrust, and many people have come to mistrust food for some very sensible reasons. Looking around, it's obvious that food production is out of balance with nature. Chemical fertilizers, disregard for the environment, genetic tinkering, heavy reliance on herbicides and pesticides, and mono-cropping are all repugnant to those who intuitively know that the best farming and agriculture involves cultivating a healthy, respectful relationship between crops, the soil, and the larger ecosystem. By disregarding the relationships and boundaries of the natural world, people soon find that, as strands of the web, they are similarly disregarded and disrespected.

The guiding principle of nutrient density is that *you are what you eat.* But when food is grown with arrogance or callous disregard for natural principles, those subtle messages can be ingested as well. Unfortunately, in disdaining unnatural forms of agriculture and the impersonal food industries, many people end up turning their backs on all food.

That doesn't have to be the end of the story, though. In the past few decades, a return to the principles of organic farming has sparked a renewal of healthy food, and there are more organic companies, farmers, gardeners, grower's markets, health food stores, and options than ever before. As *The Nutrient-Dense Eating Plan* clearly relays, the time for healing this ambivalent and adversarial relationship with food has begun.

Healing a dysfunctional relationship with food begins with reestablishing confidence in the goodness of good food. Despite processed food offerings of corporate agribusiness, much good food remains for us to enjoy. Learning to discriminate between intact foods and manipulated, processed foods is the first step toward redeveloping a relationship with food as your friend, not your enemy. Trust and appreciation go hand in hand. Once people realize there is reliable, nourishing, and trustworthy food available, they can't help but begin to appreciate its goodness. And from that appreciation emerges a sense of gratitude for the food that replaces taking it for granted, which currently seems to be the dominant attitude in this culture.

I think this change in outlook is important. I believe we are what we think, as well as what we eat. In order to become whole, happy, and integrated with ourselves, our communities, and the broader world, we need to have healthy outlooks. Feeling appreciation and gratitude are examples of such outlooks. The current world situation is not that pretty. We have environmental degradation, human misery, injustice, and poverty galore, and yet, you can still find beauty, justice, poetry, and natural harmonies and inspiration all around. If you let it, food has a unique power to let you tune in to this frequency of goodness. As part of the natural world and its cycles, food offers you an opportunity to connect with the world in an authentic, healthy, and powerful way.

This need for authenticity in an increasingly synthetic and artificial world is precisely why I feel that good food has healing properties that go far beyond what is offered by vitamins, minerals, or antioxidants. What is at hand is the opportunity for deep healing—of the world and ourselves—and this opportunity can give rise to genuine gratitude.

FROM APPRECIATION TO CELEBRATION

Gratitude for good food leads to the final level in healing a fractured relationship with food. When you feel an authentic gratefulness for good food, you can move beyond appreciation to actual celebration. And this celebratory aspect of food can shift you into a deeper, more participatory relationship with it. Celebrating food really means celebrating life itself and helps to create a much more intimate relationship with food. Celebrating food really completes the circle of life, as you energetically give back your heart to that which you have received.

The cultivation of a healthy relationship with food is the *real* denseness—a denseness of spiritual nutrition. Just as food nourishes you, so too do healthy beliefs, relationships, thoughts, and values. As difficult as it can be to heal the physical self, healing the less-tangible aspects of the self is equally challenging and rewarding. Celebrating the goodness of good food can help you to do just that.

APPENDIX A

Recommended Resources

There are so many good companies out there these days, I feel an apology is due the ones I do not mention. Those listed below (alphabetically by food type) are not the only companies I like, but their products are widely available and are consistent, innovative, and dense. Other quality foods can be found locally. Many nutrient-dense foods are also available in bulk, such as beans, lentils, nuts, and whole grains, and are not necessarily sold by company name.

BLACKSTRAP MOLASSES

Wholesome Sweeteners, Inc.
8016 Highway 90-A
Sugarland, TX 77478
Ph: 1-800-680-1896
Fax: 1-281-275-3170
Website: www.WholesomeSweeteners.com
e-mail: info@WholesomeSweeteners.com

This company produces one of the few *organic* blackstrap molasses. They also make Sucanat, from whole organic sugar cane.

BOTTLED SPRING WATER

There are many brands of bottled water available throughout the United States. Some regionally sourced and bottled waters are excellent and are not included in this list due to my (limited) exposure here in the Rocky Mountain region. The waters listed below are some of my favorites. I especially like the fact that Perrier and San Pellegrino come in glass containers, a big plus. Fiji water has an exceptionally clean taste. Eldorado Springs and Trinity Water are both excellent artesian waters from the western United States.

Eldorado Artesian Springs, Inc.
PO Box 445
Eldorado Springs, CO 80025
Ph: 1-800-499-1316 / 1-303-499-1316
Fax: 1-303-499-1339
e-mail: info@eldoradosprings.com

Fiji Water, LLC (Fiji)
0361 South Side Drive
Basalt, CO 81621
Ph: 1-877-426-3454
Website: www.fijiwater.com

San Pellegrino (Italy)
777 West Putnam Avenue
Greenwich, CT 06830
Website: www.perriergroup.com/waters/imports

Trinity Springs, Inc.
1101 West River Street, Suite 370
Boise, ID 83702
Ph: 1-800-390-5693
Fax: 1-208-344-1494
Website: www.trinitysprings.com

BREAD

Alvarado Street Bakery
500 Martin Avenue
Rohnert Park, CA 94928
Ph: 1-707-585-3293
Fax: 1-707-585-8954
Website:
www.alvaradostreetbakery.com
This quality bakery out of California also produces bagels, breads, and English muffins. They specialize in sprouted wheat products.

Food for Life Bakery Company
PO Box 1434
Corona, CA 92878
Ph: 1-800-797-5090
Fax: 1-909-279-5090
Website: www.food-for-life.com
This company has created a rather extensive line of delicious wheat-free and gluten-free breads made from a variety of whole-grain flours—almond, millet, pecan, and rice—that are nutritious alternatives to standard breads. They are found in the freezer sections of most health food stores and are a great transition for those seeking to reduce or eliminate gluten and wheat from their diets.

French Meadow Bakery
2610 Lyndale Avenue South
Minneapolis, MN 55408
Ph: 1-612-870-4740
Fax: 1-612-870-0907
Website: www.frenchmeadow.com
e-mail: info@frenchmeadow.com
This bakery makes a line of exceptionally delicious and healthy breads using the finest ingredients.

Great Harvest Bread Company
28 South Montana Street
Dillon, MT 59725
Ph: 1-800-442-0424
Fax: 1-406-683-5537
Website: www.greatharvest.com
e-mail: diannep@greatharvest.com
This company offers fresh-baked whole-wheat breads in many cities around America. Even though they do not generally use organic wheat, I still give them a nutrient-dense thumbs up, due to the freshness of their product and the simplicity of their ingredients.

Nature's Path Foods, Inc.
7453 Progress Way
Delta, BC V4G 1E8, Canada
Ph: 1-916-933-5611
Website: www.naturespath.com
e-mail: consumerservices@naturespath.com

Nature's Path makes superb manna bread in several varieties. Manna breads are made entirely from sprouted whole grains, which release the natural sugars. They are baked at very low temperatures, which helps them retain their enzymatic levels. They are very dense, naturally sweet, and very healthy.

Sunnyvale Bakery
Everfresh Natural Foods
Gatehouse Close
Aylesburg, Buckinghamshire HP19 3DE, Great Britain
Ph: 01296-425-333
Fax: 01296-422-545
Website: www.gluten-free-bread.co.uk

BROWN RICE

Lundberg Family Farms
5370 Church Street
Richvale, CA 95974
Ph: 1-530-882-4551
Fax: 1-530-882-4500
Website: www.lundberg.com

Lundberg Farms consistently produces excellent quality rice that is sold in packages and in bulk. Their Organic Brown Basmati Rice is particularly delicious, especially when cooked with pure, filtered water and a touch of salt.

CHOCOLATE

These are my favorites. Your own region may have other, organic chocolates that would be well worth checking out.

Chocolove
PO Box 18357
Boulder, CO 80308
Ph: 1-888-CHOCOLOVE or 1-303-786-7888
Website: www.chocolove.com

Dagoba Organic Chocolate
PO Box 5330
Central Point, OR 97502
Ph: 1-541-664-9030
Fax: 1-541-669-9089
Website: www.dagobachocolate.com

Green and Black's Organic
2 Valentine Place
London, SE18QH Great Britain
Ph: 401-683-3323
Website: http://belgravia@greenandblacks.com

Newman's Own
PO Box 2098
Aptos, CA 95001
www.newmansownorganics.com

Rapunzel Pure Organics, Inc.
2424 SR-203
Valatie, NY 12184
Ph: 1-800-207-2814
Fax: 1-518-392-8630
Website: www.rapunzel.com
e-mail: info@rapunzel.com

COCONUT OIL

Eat Raw Live Food Store
125 Second Street
Brooklyn, NY 11231
Ph: 1-866-432-8729
Fax: 1-718-802-0116
Website: www.eatraw.com
Several companies market and sell virgin organic coconut oil, but this store carries the best I have tried. They also have a good selection of innovative, nutrient-dense foods.

COLD-PRESSED OILS

These companies produce the best quality oils available. All should be found in a refrigerator in your health food store.

Barlean's Organic Oils
4936 Lake Terrell Road
Ferndale, WA 98248
Ph: 1-800-445-3529
Website: www.barleans.com

Flora, Inc.
PO Box 73
Lynden, WA 98264
Ph: 1-800-446-2110
Fax: 1-888-354-8138
Website: www.florahealth.com

Spectrum Natural Organic Products, Inc.
5341 Old Redmond Highway, Suite 400
Petaluma, CA 94954
Ph: 1-800-995-2705
Website: www.spectrumorganic.com

FLOURS

These are two of the most diverse and complete purveyors of a wide line of milled whole grains and flours.

Arrowhead Mills
PO Box 2059
Hereford, TX 79045
Ph: 1-800-749-0730
Website: www.arrowheadfoods.com

Bob's Red Mill
5209 South East International Way
Milwaukie, OR 97222
Ph: 1-800-349-2173
Fax: 1-503-653-1339
Website: www.bobsredmill.com

FRUIT PRESERVES

Bionaturae
5 Tyler Drive
PO Box 98
North Franklin, CT 06254
Ph: 1-860-642-6996
Fax: 1-860-642-6990
e-mail: info@bionaturae.com
Website: www.bionaturae.com
Imported from Italy, these fruit spreads from handpicked organic wild berries are my favorites. Bursting with flavor, and not too sweet, these 100 percent fruit jams are delicious. Also look to Bionaturae for their Organic Pear Nectar and Organic Bilberry Nectar.

JUICES (BOTTLED)

R.W. Knudsen
PO Box 369
Chico, CA 95927
Ph: 1-530-899-5010
Website: www.knudsenjuices.com

Knudsen markets a line of all-fruit just juices, with no added sugars, corn syrup, fructose, etc. They offer Just Blueberry, Just Concord (grape), Just Cranberry, Just Tart Cherry. Other companies sell all-fruit concentrates, syrups, and juices as well.

NUTRITIONAL YEAST

Lewis Laboratories International, Ltd
PO Box 373
Southport, CT 06890
Ph: 1-800-243-6020
Website: www.lewis-labs.com
e-mail: customerservice@lewis-labs.com

This company's Imported Brewer's Yeast Flakes is my favorite nutritional yeast. It has consistency, freshness and taste, and it comes in a vacuum-sealed can.

Red Star
Red Star Yeast
PO Box 737
Milwaukee, WI 53201-0737
Ph: 1-877-677-7000
Website: www.redstaryeast.com
e-mail: www.carolsteves@red-staryeast.com

PUMPKIN SEED BUTTER

Omega Nutrition
6515 Aldrich Road
Bellingham, WA 98226
Ph: 1-800-661-3529
Fax: 1-360-384-0700
Website: www.omeganutrition.com
e-mail: info@omeganutrition.com

This creamy and delicious European-style nut butter is created from pumpkin seeds and Celtic sea salt only. It is fantastic on sandwiches, in dips and dressings, in desserts, and as a thickener and savory ingredient in soups. It is nutrient dense for essential fatty acids, iron, magnesium, protein, zinc, and phytonutrients unique to pumpkin seeds. This company also has excellent cold-pressed oils.

QUINOA FLOUR

Ancient Harvest
PO Box 279
Gardena, CA 90248
Ph: 1-310-217-8125
Website: www.quinoa.net
e-mail: quinoacorp@aol.com

This company produces a fine quality quinoa flour.

RAW CHEESES AND DAIRY

Alta Dena Certified Dairy
17637 East Valley Boulevard
City of Industry, CA 91744
Ph: 1-800-535-1369
Fax: 1-626-854-4287
Website: www.altadenadairy.com
e-mail: MaryLarrowe@denafoods.com

Alta Dena makes a variety of both raw and pasteurized cheeses and makes a raw cheddar cheese from goat's milk that is wonderful.

Horizon Dairy
6309 Monarch Park Place
Longmont, CO 80503
Ph: 303-652-3858
Fax: 303-530-6934
Website: www.horizondairy.com

Organic Valley Family of Farms
CROPP Cooperative
1 Organic Way
LaFarge, WI 54639
Ph: 1-888-444-6455
Fax: 1-608-625-2600
Website: www.organicvalley.com
This company produces a variety of raw and pasteurized cheeses.

RAW HONEY

Really Raw Honey, Inc.
3500 Boston Street, Suite 32
Baltimore, MD 21224
Ph: 1-800-732-5729
Fax: 1-401-675-7411
www.reallyrawhoney.com
One of the few truly unheated, unprocessed honeys available. Some regional producers also sell local raw honey at area health food stores and farmer's markets.

SEA SALT

Brittany Sea Salt
France Natural Imports/ Brittany Sea Salt
PO Box 1703
Gloucester, VA 23061
Ph: 1-804-694-4340
Website: www.brittanysalt.com

Celtic Sea Salt
The Grain and Salt Society
4 Celtic Drive
Arden, NC 28704
Ph: 1-800-867-7258
Fax: 1-828-299-1640
Website: www.celticseasalt.com

Redmond Real Salt
PO Box 219
Redmond, UT 84652
Ph: 1-800-367-7258
Fax: 1-800-367-7258
Website: www.realsalt.com

Sea Star (France)
Holly's Cooking Basics
PO Box 302
Calistoga, CA 94515-0302
Ph: 1-707-942-9494
Fax: 1-707-942-9444
Website: www.salt@seastarsalt.com

SEA VEGETABLES

Leslie Cerier
58 Schoolhouse Road
Amherst, MA 01002
Ph: 1-413-259-1695
Website: www.lescerier@aol.com
The author of Sea Vegetable Celebration *is available for lectures and cooking classes.*

Maine Coast Sea Vegetables , Inc.
3 George's Pond Road
Franklin, ME 04634
Ph: 1-207-565-2907
Fax: 1-207-565-2144
Website: www.seaveg.com

This company is a great supplier of domestic, wild-harvested seaweed, including alaria (wild Atlantic wakame), dulse, kelp (wild Atlantic kombu), and laver (wild Atlantic nori). They also manufacture convenient salt-shaker-style containers of dulse and kelp granules.

Maine Seaweed LLC
PO Box 57
Steuben, ME 04680
Ph: 1-207-546-2875
Fax: 1-207-546-2875
Website: www.alcasoft.com

Rising Tide Sea Vegetables
PO Box 1914
Mendocino, CA 95460
Ph: 1-707-964-5663
Fax: 1-707-962-0599
Website: www.risingtideseavegetables.com
e-mail: risingtide@mcn.org
Another great little company, well worth supporting.

UMEBOSHI PLUM VINEGAR AND PASTE

Eden Foods
701 Tecumseh Road
Clinton, MI 49236
Ph: 1-888-441-EDEN
Fax: 1-517-456-6075
Website: www.edenfoods.com
Eden is not the only manufacturer of umeboshi and other macrobiotic foods, but it is one of the biggest and most visible in health food stores. They offer a diverse array of traditional and macrobiotic foods and condiments.

YERBA MATÉ TEA

Guayaki Sustainable Rainforest Products
PO Box 14730
San Luis Obispo, CA 93406
Ph: 1-888-482-9254
Website: www.guayaki.com
e-mail: info@guayaki.com
Although many companies now package and sell yerba maté, I really like the integrity and feel of this company.

YOGURT

Seven Stars Yogurt
501 West Seven Stars Road
Phoenixville, PA 19460
Ph: 1-610-935-1949
Fax: 1-610-935-8292
e-mail: svnstrs@aol.com
By far the best unhomogenized yogurt on the market. Produced in relatively small amounts, and not generally available out West. Sold primarily on the East Coast and in the Midwest.

Runner-up good yogurts are Nancy's Yogurt, Brown Cow, and Stonyfield Farms. Redwood Hill Yogurt is a good commercial goat's milk yogurt.

Nancy's Yogurt
29440 Airport Road
Eugene, OR 97402
Ph: 1-541-689-2911
Fax: 1-541-689-2915
Website: www.nancysyogurt.com

Redwood Hill Farms
Redwood Hill Farms Grade A
Goat Dairy
5480 Thomas Road
Sebastopol, CA 95472
Ph: 1-707-823-8250
Fax: 1-707-823-6976
Website: www.redwoodhillfarms.com

Stonyfield Farms
Ten Burton Drive
Londonderry, NH 03053
Ph: 1-800-776-2697
Fax: 1-603-437-4040
Website: www.stonyfield.com
This company provides fine quality yogurt and has strong corporate values.

APPENDIX B

General Resources

Bragg Live Foods, Inc.
PO Box 7
Santa Barbara, CA 93102
Ph: 1-800-446-1990
Fax: 1-805-968-1001
Website: www.info@bragg.com

Deer Garden Foods
Rejuvenative Foods
PO Box 8464
Santa Cruz, CA 95601
Ph: 1-888-781-9879
Fax: 1-831-423-6545
Website: www.rejuvenative.com
Fresh-dated, raw refrigerated nut and seed butters and raw cultured vegetables, all in glass jars.

Eden Foods, Inc.
701 Tecumseh Road
Clinton, MI 49236
Ph: 1-888-441-3336
Website: www.edenfoods.com
e-mail: info@edenfoods.com
Eden Foods, Inc. offers a wide variety of macrobiotic foods, including sea vegetables.

Frontier Natural Product Co-op
PO Box 299
3021 78th
Norway, IA 52318
Ph: 1-800-669-3275
Website: www.frontierco-op.com

Goldmine Natural Food Co.
7805 Arjons Drive
San Diego, CA 92126
Ph: 1-800-475-3663
Website:
www.goldminenaturalfood.com
This is another of Garima's discoveries, a great resource for many hard-to-find natural and organic foods, especially macrobiotics.

Organic Consumers Association
6101 Cliff Estate Road
Little Marias, MN 55614
Ph: 1-218-226-4164
Website: www.organicconsumers.org
A great resource and wealth of information on organic food, policy issues, and more.

Weston A. Price Foundation
PMB 106-380
4200 Wisconsin Avenue, NW
Washington, DC 20016
Ph: 1-202-333-4325
Fax: 1-202-333-0002
Website: www.westonaprice.org
e-mail: westonaprice@msn.com
A wealth of information on healthy eating (they even use the terminology of nutrient density) and a source for the excellent nutrition cookbook, Nourishing Traditions. *Highly recommended.*

APPENDIX C

Label-Reading Workshop

The best way to understand what you are buying is to look at labels. Looking at packaging is a great way to get comfortable with the idea of label reading. Generally, less is more. The poorer the qualities of the main ingredients, the more the companies try to compensate by adding many unnecessary ingredients. Simplicity is reassuring, and serves as a measure of quality.

VEGGIE BURGERS

Ingredients: Soy protein concentrate-hydrated, vegetable oil (canola and/or sunflower oil), vegetable gum, wheat gluten, salt, natural flavors, autolyzed yeast extract, sesame oil, caramel color, soy sauce (water, wheat, soybeans, salt), dried onion, natural grill flavor (from vegetable oil), dried yeast, ascorbic acid

Per serving: Calories–120, calories from fat–35, total fat–4 grams

Comment: Veggie Burgers are a typical meat substitute-type frozen meal in a box that many well-meaning shoppers purchase thinking that they are getting a healthier version of an all-American classic food. They are representative of the soy fad that has swept America, thanks to a huge advertising blitz led by the soy food industry, a large and powerful conglomeration of agricultural, corporate, and food-processing companies typified by such giant players as Monsanto, Archer Daniels Midland, Cargill, and others. These companies have funded thousands of researchers in an effort to promote soy as a consummate health food, and are capitalizing on its appeal to vegetarians.

Are foods such as veggie burgers really healthy alternatives to meat? A close look at the ingredients listed on the package will tell you what is really going into your body.

The first ingredient, and therefore the most prevalent, is *soy protein concentrate-hydrated,* which is the dried-out, processed, protein-containing fraction of soybeans. Extracted from the whole soybean with various chemical solvents, this flaked or powdered residue of cooked soy can sit around for years. Often referred to on some labels as *defatted soybean meal,* adding water to it reconstitutes (hydrates) it so it can be shaped into patties, hot dogs, bacon, turkey, and other foods. Flaking and powdering allows the product to form oxidation byproducts, undesirable chemical species related to free radicals. Some scientists feel that such protein isolates have not been adequately tested for long-term safety.

The next ingredient listed is vegetable oil. As discussed in Chapter 20, vegetable oils are very prone to rancidity, and processing has stripped them of their naturally occurring antioxidants. By volume, these burgers have this nutritionally questionable oil as their second ingredient. Almost 30 percent of the calories from each burger are derived from this fat.

Next comes vegetable gum, a mostly inert substance that gives texture, volume, and moldability (the ability to shape the patties) to the burgers. After that, the next ingredient is wheat gluten, which adds volume and texture, and boosts protein levels. Gluten should be avoided by anyone with suspected intolerances to it, as it could trigger colitis, gastric upset, mental disturbances, or skin problems in sensitive individuals.

Salt is the next ingredient, followed by natural flavors and autolyzed yeast extract. Both the latter are often code words for monosodium glutamate (MSG). Many experts, including neurologists, consider glutamate sensitivity a severely underdiagnosed problem. MSG in its many forms is often a clue that the manufacturer is trying to improve the taste of an overly processed food.

Next comes more oil (sesame), caramel coloring (a synthetic coloring agent) to disguise the dull, gray color of the hydrated soy protein, soy sauce (yet another source of sodium, wheat, and MSG), and some dried onion (one of the only healthy substances in the box). Rounding out the list of ingredients is something called natural grill flavor (from vegetable oil), some dried yeast (possibly another MSG source), and a trace of ascorbic acid (vitamin C).

These burgers are clearly a poor substitute for the real thing. As far as nutrient density goes, there is not much to recommend them. The package declares there is 0 percent calcium, 0 percent iron, 0 percent vitamin A, and 0 percent vitamin C. This is particularly troubling because real burgers are an excellent source of iron, as well as zinc, the important amino acid carnitine, and of course, protein.

Most worrisome is the inclusion of relatively large amounts of MSG (the government doesn't require disclosure of amounts) to make this food palatable. Its presence, along with wheat gluten, questionably reconstituted soy protein isolate, and large amounts of nutrient-poor vegetable oils, tells you that, far from being a credible alternative to meat, such burgers fail to live up to even minimal standards of nutrient density.

Reading labels is a skill. Decoding such foods is vitally important if you are to be an informed, empowered shopper. The packaging of these burgers is full of marketing hype, describing them as *all-natural patties, specially seasoned,* and *sizzled* for the *juiciest taste sensation.* Such buzzwords are designed to seduce the unwary buyer, and unfortunately, they are often highly effective.

BREADS

What follows are a number of bread labels for comparison. The first is a very typical label for a loaf of so-called whole-wheat bread. As you can see, it *does* contain whole-wheat flour, but it also contains a whole lot of other ingredients.

Standard American Diet (SAD) Bread— Natural Whole Wheat

Ingredients: Enriched unbleached flour, water, high-fructose corn syrup, bran flakes, stone-ground wheat, yeast, salt, partially hydrogenated soybean and/or cottonseed oil, vital wheat gluten, hydrated monoglycerides, calcium carbonate, mono- and diglycerides, ammonium chloride, calcium sulfate, lecithin, calcium stearate, calcium peroxide 78 percent, dicalcium phosphate, calcium disodium EDTA, vitamin A, disodium phosphate, diammonium phosphate, azodicarbonamide, ascorbic acid

Comment: What can I say? There *is* whole-wheat flour in this loaf somewhere (it is the fifth ingredient), but there is also a ton of sugar (high-fructose corn syrup, hydrated monoglycerides, and mono- and diglycerides), and you can spot the partially hydrogenated soybean/cottonseed oil from a mile away. I would throw this one out the window immediately (except I'd worry about the birds). One question: How did people get by on the staff of life for all those millennia without all those calcium salts and other additives?

Now let's look at bread I consider to be optimally dense—simple, wholesome, and nutritious. The following labels of products from exceptional bakeries are prime examples of the concept that less is more. Keeping it simple is the key here.

Alvarado Street Bakery: Sprouted Wheat Tortillas

Ingredients: Organically grown high-protein whole-wheat kernels, organically grown whole-wheat flour, water, unrefined safflower oil, sea salt, baking powder (nonaluminum)

Comment: Pretty basic, and much denser than most commercially available tortillas.

Food for Life: Brown Rice Bread (Wheat and Gluten Free)

Ingredients: Brown rice flour, filtered water, fruit juice concentrate, tapioca flour, safflower oil, fresh yeast, vegetable gum, rice bran, sea salt

Comment: This wheat-free bread uses unusual ingredients, and is both innovative and delicious. Great toasted, with almond butter.

Genuine Bavarian Whole-Grain Bread: Organic Whole Rye

Ingredients: Whole rye, mountain spring water, yeast, sea salt

Comment: This is a rich, dense, flavorful bread made in the old-world tradition. The simplicity of the ingredients speaks for itself. All the essentials are present, and nothing unnecessary is added. I consider this a top-notch premium bread that is definitely nutrient dense. Rye is a wonderful grain. It is low in gluten, and contains properties that give it a unique flavor and quality.

Great Harvest Bread Co: Country Whole Wheat

Ingredients: Fresh stone-ground whole-wheat flour, water, molasses, yeast, salt

Comment: Although the simplicity of the recipe is typical of this company's products, it is *not* made from organic wheat. Nonetheless, it is great-tasting and contains no preservatives or unnecessary ingredients, such as hydrogenated oils. The flour is so fresh—they grind it, bake it, and sell it all in the same day—that it retains all the moisture from the naturally occurring oils and does not require the addition of extra oil or shortening. The superb result is this incredibly moist, fresh, flavorful whole-wheat bread.

Stacey's Organic Whole-Wheat Flour Tortillas

Ingredients: 100 percent certified organic whole-wheat and unbleached wheat flours, water, nonhydrogenated soybean oil, aluminum-free baking powder, salt

Comment: Most commercial tortillas today contain hydrogenated soy or other oils. These do not, and are the freshest, most delicious whole-wheat tortillas I have ever tasted.

Sunnyvale Baker: Fruit—Almond Sprouted Bread

Ingredients: Sprouted whole-wheat kernels, raisins, dates, almonds (all organic)

Comment: This is a classic example of 100 percent sprouted, flour-free, manna-style bread. It is sweet, dense, moist, and satisfying.

MORE COMPARATIVE LABELS

The following is a comparison of commercial junk foods and their more nutrient-dense versions.

Potato Chips in a Can

Ingredients: Dried potatoes, vegetable oil (contains one or more of the following: corn oil, cottonseed oil, and/or sunflower oil), yellow corn meal, maltodextrin, wheat starch, salt, dextrose, and whey. Contains 2 percent or less: buttermilk, dried tomato, dried garlic, partially hydrogenated soybean oil, monosodium glutamate, corn syrup solids, dried onion, sodium caseinate, malic acid, spice, annatto extract, modified corn starch, natural and artificial flavors, disodium inosinate, disodium guanylate

Comment: Not exactly an appetizing array of ingredients, is it? (Unless you are a chemist.)

Nutrient-Dense Potato Chips

Ingredients: Russet potatoes, olive oil, sea salt

Comment: This is how the label *should* read.

Commercial Tortillas

Ingredients: Enriched bleached flour, water, partially hydrogenated soybean and/or cottonseed oil, sugar, salt, sodium bicarbonate, sodium acid pyrophosphate, calcium proprionate, fumaric acid, mono- and diglycerides, sorbic acid, sodium metabisulfate

Comment: Compare these to Stacey's or Alvarado St. Bakery's sprouted tortillas.

Nutrient-Dense Tortillas

Ingredients: Stone-ground whole-wheat flour, soybean oil, salt

Comment: This is about as simple as it gets.

Commercial Yogurt

Ingredients: Cultured pasteurized grade A milk, sugar, modified cornstarch, whey protein concentrate, kosher gelatin, orange juice concentrate, tricalcium phosphate, natural flavor, citric acid, colored with annatto extract

Comment: What is not on the label are the hormones and antibiotics in nonorganic milk.

Nutrient-Dense Yogurt

Ingredients: Organic, nonhomogenized, pasteurized milk, acidophilus and bifidus cultures, maple syrup

Comment: Yogurt is one of the original health foods. Thank goodness there are several good brands available today.

MISCELLANEOUS LABELS

Although the following ingredient lists are longer, they contain only natural items, and are free from preservatives and artificial flavors, etc. Compare these to more commercial brands.

Nutrient-Dense Hummus

Ingredients: Organic garbanzo beans, artichoke hearts, organic tahini, extra virgin olive oil, organic lemon juice, garlic, red onions, water, sea salt, cumin, cayenne pepper

Nutrient-Dense Salsa

Ingredients: Organic tomatoes, organic tomato paste, organic onions, water, organic apple cider vinegar, organic jalapeño peppers, organic cilantro, chili peppers, organic habañero peppers, salt, garlic, cumin

Comment: The hummus and salsa here seem to break the rule that simplicity is best, but a closer look reveals otherwise. Although there are a larger number of ingredients than in previous examples, the important thing to notice is that all of these ingredients are real foods. There are no artificial preservatives, nor are any fillers included to stretch the recipe. Everything is present for a reason (taste), as both salsas and hummus benefit from a rich interplay of subtle flavors. Also, note that all the ingredients are loaded with flavonoids (antioxidant-rich phytonutrients), such as cayenne, cumin, garlic, peppers, and red onions.

EXAMPLE OF A NUT BUTTER LABEL

Nutrient-Dense Pumpkin-Seed Butter

Ingredients: Pumpkin seeds, Celtic sea salt

Comment: This product is another good example of how to read labels. A quick glance at the label reveals what you would expect from a nut butter. It is relatively dense for fat (8 grams, approximately 13 percent of daily value). The breakdown between saturated, polyunsaturated, and monounsaturated is good—25 percent of the lipids are monounsaturated, and only 1.5 grams are saturated. There is no cholesterol (as is expected in a vegetable-based product), and this nut butter is low in sodium (40 mg per serving—only 2 percent of the daily value). There is also a fairly good value for protein at 5 grams per serving. A mere tablespoon of pumpkin-seed butter gives 10 percent of the daily value, which is not bad at all.

However, more interesting information is in the small print at the bottom of the label. The numbers there tell you that a serving also supplies some dense nutrients—magnesium 16 percent, zinc 9 percent, and iron 9 percent. All in all, considering these minerals, the protein at 10 percent, and the good lipids, this label tells you that pumpkin-seed butter is a strong food—plus there are no additives or hydrogenated oils.

APPENDIX D

Red Flags

The following list summarizes my strongest recommendations of what to avoid when adopting a more nutrient-dense diet. Avoidance of some of these may depend upon the particular tier level you are working at; occasional exceptions allow you to remain a human, social creature. Nonetheless, paying close attention to the following list will automatically help you achieve a higher level of nutritional quality in your diet.

- Aspartame (Nutrasweet) found in diet soft drinks, and many sugar-free products, including breath mints, desserts, and gum.
- Chicken and pork (unless you are *sure* it is organic/free range).
- Commercial dairy products (cheeses, cream cheese, ice cream, milk, sour cream, yogurt).
- Cooking shortenings.
- Endangered fish (Chilean sea bass, orange roughy, shark, swordfish).
- Fast-food chains.
- Hydrogenated oils.
- Junk food (candy bars, chips, soda).
- Most wheat (flour) products.
- Refined oils (includes oil and vinegar salad dressings).
- White refined sugar.

APPENDIX E

Popular Diets Using Nutrient-Dense Principles

- Blood Type
- Color
- Fit for Life
- Macrobiotic
- Nourishing Traditions
- Paleolithic
- Power Foods
- Raw (aka Living Foods)
- South Beach
- Zone

APPENDIX F

Therapeutic Food Categories

The following list sorts out therapeutic (healing) foods by categories. This is another good way to begin to understand the diversity of foods available in a nutrient-dense diet. By using this list, you can see which classes of foods may be missing from your current diet.

1. **Essential fatty-acid–rich foods** Flaxseed oil, salmon and cod-liver oils
2. **Nutritional yeast**
3. **Algaes** Blue-green, chlorella, spirulina
4. **Nuts and seeds**
5. **Proteins** Eggs, fish, legumes, nuts and seeds, red meat (buffalo, elk, hormone-free beef, lamb, venison)
6. **Soy**
7. **Sea vegetables**
8. **Fresh juices** Carrot juice, vegetable blends, and wheatgrass juice
9. **Herbs and spices** Basil, dill, ginger, oregano, and turmeric
10. **Alliums** Chives, garlic, leeks, onions, and shallots
11. **Whole grains** Amaranth, brown rice, millet, and quinoa
12. **Blackstrap molasses**
13. **Black and green teas** (contain caffeine)
14. **Herbal teas** (noncaffeine)
15. **Mushrooms** Boletes, chanterelles, maitake, morels, shiitake, and other wild edibles

16. **Bee pollen**
17. **Leafy green vegetables** Bok choy, chard, spinach, mustard greens
18. **Fresh fruits** (especially berries and cherries)
19. **Dark chocolate**
20. **Cruciferous vegetables** Broccoli, cabbage, cauliflower
21. **Spring (artesian) water**
22. **Microbrew beer, organic red wine**
23. **Raw milk/cheeses**
24. **Virgin coconut oil**
25. **Wild edibles** (chickweed, dandelion, lamb's-quarter, nasturnium, nettles, purslane)
26. **Tomato products**
27. **Fermented foods**

APPENDIX G

Figures and Tables

Figure 1
Healing the Adversarial Relationship with Food—Progressive Changes in Attitude

Unhealthy Attitudes	*lead to*	Adversarial Relationship with Food
Mistrust	*leads to . . .*	Fear/Apprehension
Apprehension	*leads to . . .*	Suspicion
Suspicion	*leads to . . .*	Apathy/Taking food for granted
Apathy	*leads to . . .*	Denigrating food's true Value

Healthy Attitudes	*lead to*	Healthy Relationship with Food
Trust	*leads to . . .*	Appreciation
Appreciation	*leads to . . .*	Gratitude
Gratitude	*leads to . . .*	Celebration
Celebration	*leads to . . .*	Connectedness

Figure 2
Potassium and Sodium Levels of Unprocessed and Processed Foods

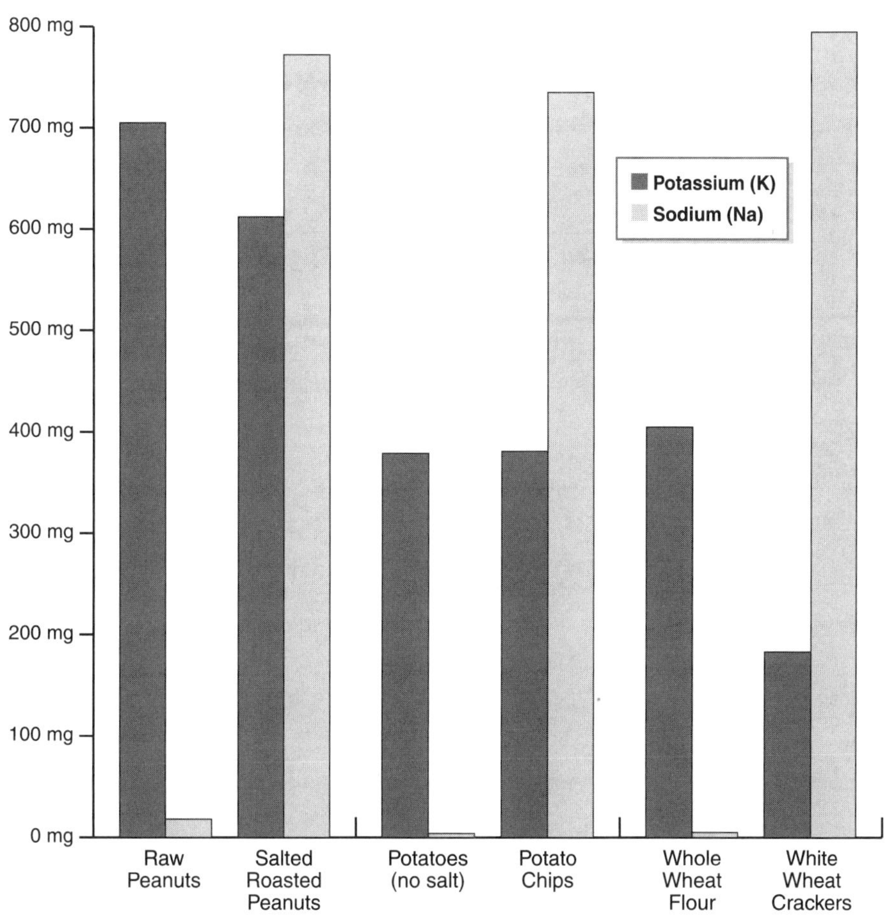

TABLE 1. PRINCIPAL NUTRIENT-DENSE SOURCES OF SPECIFIC NUTRIENTS

Nutrient	Sources with Highest Nutrient Density
Anthocyanins	Blackberries, blueberries, raspberries, red grapes, red wine
Calcium	Almonds, blackstrap molasses, carrot juice, dark leafy green vegetables, sardines, sesame seeds, tofu, yogurt
Carotenoids	Carrots, pumpkins, spinach, squash, sweet potatoes
Fatty acids	Black walnuts, cod-liver oil, flaxseeds and oil, sashimi, tuna
Fiber	Broccoli, celery, dried fruit, legumes, oats, whole grains
Folic acid	Broccoli, citrus, legumes, spinach, sprouts
Iron	Beef, blackstrap molasses, buffalo, currants, lamb, oysters, spinach
Lecithin	Egg yolk, organ meats
Magnesium	Blackstrap molasses, broccoli, kale, nuts, spinach, tofu
Manganese	Apricots, black tea, egg yolk, legumes, pineapple
Nucleic acids (DNA, RNA)	Nutritional yeast, organ meats, sardines
Selenium	Brazil nuts, nutritional yeast
Sulfur	Broccoli, cabbage, cauliflower, eggs, garlic, leeks, onion
Thiamine (B_1)	Brewer's yeast, brown rice, legumes, microbrew beer, seafood, sunflower seeds
Trace Minerals	Kelp and other sea vegetables, nutritional yeast, ocean fish, sea salt, sushi
Vitamin C	Bell peppers, blackberries, kiwi fruit, lemons, mangoes
Vitamin D	Cod-liver oil, sunshine
Vitamin E	Almonds, avocado, spinach, sunflower seeds, wheat-germ oil
Zinc	Legumes, organ meats, oysters, pumpkin seeds

TABLE 2. THE NUTRIENT-DENSE SPECTRUM

Class	Most	Average	Least	Avoid
Beverages	Berry smoothies, black tea, carrot juice, green teas, herbal teas, spring water, wheatgrass juice	Bottled juice (without added sugar)	Purified water	All sodas and artificial juice drinks
Candy	Dark chocolate, real licorice	Milk chocolate, candied ginger		All candy made with artificial color, aspartame, hydrogenated oils
Grains	Amaranth, brown rice, millet, quinoa	Oats, whole wheat	White rice	Pasta
Meats	Buffalo, hormone-free beef, lamb, venison	Regular beef	Chicken, pork	Bologna, chicken hot dogs, lunch meat, sausage, bacon, pork
Oils	Cod-liver oil, flax oil, wheat germ oil, cold-pressed oil, unrefined oil	Butter, coconut oil, olive oil	Refined vegetable oils	Margarine, shortening
Seafood	Cod, halibut, mackerel, tuna, wild salmon	Farm-raised salmon, farmed trout	Shrimp, swordfish	Catfish, crab
Sweetener	Blackstrap molasses	Light molasses, raw sugar	White sugar, brown sugar	Aspartame, saccharin

TABLE 3. DIFFERENCES BETWEEN NUTRIENT-DENSE FOODS AND JUNK FOODS

Nutrient-Dense Foods	Junk Foods
Ancestral diet	Synthetic food
Easily metabolized, digested	Hard to digest or side effects
Few or no additives	Many additives
Few or no preservatives or pesticide residues	Contains preservatives and residues
Full spectrum of tastes	Mostly salty or sweet
Naturally occurring nutrients present in large amounts	Mostly empty calories
Naturally occurring pigments	Artificial dyes
Organically grown	Grown with chemicals
Sourced in nature	Laboratory derived
Usually unprocessed	Highly processed

TABLE 4. EXCEPTIONAL NUTRIENT-DENSE FOODS

Food	Densest Nutrients	Comments
Blackstrap molasses	Calcium, iron, potassium	Most nutritive sweetener
Blueberries	Anthocyanins (purple pigments)	Reversed signs of age-related motor-skill decline in test animals
Brazil nuts	Selenium	Documented anticancer mineral in numerous studies
Buffalo	Iron, protein, vitamin B_{12}	Great alternative to beef
Cabbage	Isothiocyanates	Stimulates anticancer enzymes
Eggs (boiled)	Cholesterol, lecithin, protein, vitamin A	Nature's perfect food is making a comeback (organic only)
Flaxseeds, oil	Omega-3 fatty acids	Restores balance of omega 3s and 6s; benefits immune and nervous systems
Garlic	Diallyl disulfide and organosulfurs	Proven cardioprotector and immunostimulant
Hot Pepper	Capsaicin, vitamin C	Improves angina, circulation
Kelp, dulse	Iodine, ultra-trace ocean minerals	Nourishes our evolutionary roots (our marine origins)
Lemon	Bioflavonoids, limonene, vitamin C	Research links limonene to breast-tumor resistance
Nutritional (Brewer's) yeast	B vitamins, chromium, nucleic acids (DNA, RNA), selenium	Powerhouse condiment; single best source of B vitamins and chromium; sprinkle on food
Sardines	Calcium, oils, protein	Super nutrient-dense snack
Soybeans	Phytosterols	May be useful for some estrogen-related cancers
Tomatoes	Lycopene	Red pigment; research involves prostate and skin-cancer protection

TABLE 5. NUTRITIONAL CONTRIBUTIONS OF SELECTED FOODS AND PREPARED MEALS

Dish	Contribution
Beef, buffalo, lamb, venison	Carnitine, protein, vitamin A, vitamin B_{12}, zinc
Curries	Antioxidants (turmeric, curry spices), B vitamins (brown rice), fiber (vegetables), iron and protein (chicken, lamb, or seafood) sulfur (organosulfur in broccoli, garlic, onions, etc.)
Deviled eggs, egg salad	Cholesterol, lecithin, protein, sulfur, vitamin A, vitamin B_{12}
Fruit smoothies	Anthocyanins (fruit pigments), bioflavonoids, fiber, vitamin C
Hummus	Essential oils (see recipes with flax oil), fiber, minerals, protein (garbanzo beans)
Salads	Enzymes, essential fatty acids (depending on dressing), fiber, minerals, phytonutrients
Soups	Fiber, minerals, phytonutrients from vegetables (extremely variable)
Sushi	Essential fatty acids, protein, trace minerals
Whole grains (amaranth, brown rice, millet, oats, quinoa)	B vitamins, fiber, minerals, protein

TABLE 6. FUNCTIONS AND DEFICIENCY SYMPTOMS OF SPECIFIC NUTRIENTS

Nutrient	Facilitates	Prevents
Copper	Connective tissue integrity (varicose veins and aneurysms), immune system, red blood cell development	Joint inflammation (arthritis), skin de-pigmentation
Folic Acid	Cell division	Anemia (pernicious), athero-scelerosis, cervical dysplasia, neural tube defects, osteoporosis
Iron	DNA synthesis, energy production, hemoglobin (oxygen-carrying capacity)	Anemia, fatigue, learning disabilities
Magnesium	Hundreds of enzymatic reactions	Bronchial asthma, heart, high blood pressure, palpitations, insomnia, kidney stones, migraine headaches, PMS cramps, stress
Manganese	Antioxidant enzyme cofactor (SOD), blood-sugar regulation, energy production, thyroid hormone function	Anti-inflammatory for sprains and strains, and cartilage malformation
Vitamin A	Cellular differentiation, epithelial and respiratory tissue development, reproductive health, retinal (visual) health	Antiviral, measles, some cancers
Vitamin B_1 (Thiamine)	Carbohydrate metabolism, nerve cell functioning	Age-related dementia, alcoholic dementia, depression, fatigue, numbness of legs
Vitamin B_6 (Pyridoxine)	Brain functioning, cell growth, enzymatic reactions (more than sixty), immunity, protein metabolism, neuro-transmitter synthesis, development of red blood cells	Anemia, carpal tunnel syndrome, premenstrual syndrome (PMS)
Vitamin B_{12} (Cobalamin)	Development of red blood cells, DNA synthesis	Anemia (pernicious), childhood asthma, depression (elderly), MS (multiple sclerosis), paresthesia (pins and needles feeling), swollen tongue, tinnitus
Vitamin C	Antioxidant, collagen (connective tissue) synthesis, wound healing	Asthma and allergies, cataracts, colds and flus (antiviral), some cancers, stress (adrenal support)
Vitamin D	Calcium absorption and metabolism	Anticancer (breast and colon)
Vitamin E	Immune system function, prevention of oxidation (fat-soluble antioxidant)	Cardiovascular disease, hemolytic anemia, nerve damage

TABLE 7. COMPARING NUTRIENT DENSITY

Nutrient density is best illustrated with side-by-side comparisons. Whole-grain bagels, English muffins, pizza crusts, or whole-wheat breads are more nutrient dense than their white-flour equivalents simply because whole-grain flour has not had the B vitamins, minerals, and so on milled out. Although this might seem obvious to many, *The Nutrient-Dense Eating Plan* extends this principle to a wide range of foods, leading to a deeper understanding of how important it is to select foods with care.

Denser	Less Dense	Reason
Albacore, yellowtail tuna (sushi, sashimi), wild salmon	Farmed shrimp, freshwater eel	Wild is superior to fish-farmed (antibiotics, overall quality)
Almond butter	Peanut butter	Better mineral content (almond), hydrogenated oils (peanut), no added sugar
Baked potatoes	Chips, French fries	Fewer oils, less sodium, less oxidation
Boiled eggs	Fried or scrambled eggs	Less oxidation damage to cholesterol from boiling (lower temperature)
Buffalo, elk, venison	Beef, chicken, pork	Fewer antibiotics, hormones, better fatty-acid profile in buffalo, etc.
Butter	Margarine	Hydrogenated oils (trans fats) in margarine
Dark chocolate	Milk chocolate	Less sugar, more flavonoids in dark
Deep sea fish	Freshwater fish	Fish farming practices are a concern in freshwater species, polluted waters
Flaxseed oil	Canola oil	Flax seed oil has better fatty-acid profile
Fresh vegetables	Canned or frozen vegetables	More enzymes, minerals, nutrients in fresh vegetables
Goat's milk	Cow's milk	Fewer allergens, more minerals in goat's milk
Brown Cow, Horizon, Seven Stars, Stonyfield (yogurt brands)	Yoplait, Dannon, other commercial brands	No added sugar (also, colors, gelatin, etc.), homogenization, or hormones associated with commercial brands
Oatmeal, rice cream	Flaked cereals	Toasting (flaking) destroys nutrients
Red wine	White wine	Antioxidants present in red wine
Regular soda	Diet soda	Aspartame (NutraSweet) is toxic
Spring water	Pure bottled water	Desirable trace minerals present in spring water

Bibliography

Ausubel, Kenny. *Seeds of Change: The Living Treasure.* New York: HarperCollins Publishers, 1994.

Beasley, Joseph D. and Jerry J. Swift. *The Kellogg Report: The Impact of Nutrition, Environment, and Lifestyle on the Health of Americans.* The Institute of Health Policy and Practice, The Bard Center, Annandale-on-Hudson, NY, 1989.

Beling, Stephanie. *Power Foods: Good Food, Good Health with Phytochemicals, Nature's Own Energy Boosters.* New York: HarperCollins Publishers, 1997.

Blaylock, Russell L. *Excitotoxins: The Taste That Kills.* Sante Fe, NM: Health Press, 1994.

Brewster, Letitia and Michael F. Jacobson. *The Changing American Diet.* Washington, DC: Center for Science in the Public Interest, 1978.

Brotman, Juliano. *Raw: The Uncook Book.* New York: Regan Books (HarperCollins), 1999.

Buhner, Stephen Harrod. *The Lost Language of Plants.* White River Junction, VT: Chelsea Green Publishing, 2002.

Carper, Jean. *Food, Your Miracle Medicine.* New York: HarperCollins, 1998.

Carper, Jean. *Jean Carper's Total Nutrition Guide.* New York: Bantam Books, 1987.

Carper, Jean. *The Food Pharmacy.* New York: Bantam Books, 1988.

Cherniske, Stephen. *Caffeine Blues.* New York: Warner Books, 1998.

Clark, Robert, ed., *Our Sustainable Table.* San Francisco, CA: North Point Press, 1990.

Cohen, Robert. *Milk A–Z,* Englewood Cliffs, NJ: Argus, 2001.

Cohen, Robert. *Milk: The Deadly Poison.* Englewood Cliffs, NJ: Argus, 1998.

Committee on Diet, Nutrition, and Cancer, National Research Council, "Diet, Nutrition, and Cancer." Washington, DC: *National Academy,* 1982.

Cummins, Ronnie and Ben Lilliston. *Genetically Engineered Food: A Self Defense Guide for Consumers.* New York: Marlowe and Co., 2000.

D'Adamo, Peter J. *Eat Right 4 Your Type.* New York, Penguin, 1996.

David, Marc. *Nourishing Wisdom: A Mind-Body Approach to Nutrition and Well-Being.* New York: Bell Tower, 1991.

De Villiers, Marq. *Water: The Fate of Our Most Precious Resource.* New York: Houghton Mifflin, 2000.

Eades, Michael R. and Mary Dan Eades. *Protein Power.* New York: Bantam, 1996.

Eaton, S. Boyd, Marjorie Shostak, and Melvin Konner. *The Paleolithic Prescription.* New York: Harper and Row, 1988.

Erasmus, Udo. *Fats That Heal, Fats That Kill.* Burnaby, CA: Alive Books, 1986.

Erhart, Shep and Leslie Cerier. *Sea Vegetable Celebration.* Summertown, TN: Book Publishing, 2001.

Fairfax, Garima. *Kitchen Botany.* PO Box 631, Lyons, CO 80540, 2005.

Fallon, Sally and Mary Enig. *Nourishing Traditions.* Winona Lake, IN: New Trends Publishing, 1999.

Goodhart, Robert S., and Maurice Shils, eds., *Modern Nutrition in Health and Disease.* Philadelphia, PA: Lea and Febiger, 1980.

Haas, Elson M. *Staying Healthy with Nutrition.* Berkeley, CA: Celestial Arts Press, 1992.

Jensen, Bernard and Mark Anderson. *Empty Harvest.* Garden City Park, NY: Avery, 1990.

Kimbrell, Andrew, ed. *Fatal Harvest: The Tragedy of Industrial Agriculture.* Washington, DC: Island Press, 2002.

Kneen, Brewster. *Farmageddon: Food and the Culture of Biotechnology.* Gabriola Island, British Columbia, CA: New Society Publishers, 1999.

Levenstein, Harvey. *Paradox of Plenty: A Social History of Eating in Modern America.* New York: Oxford University Press, 1993.

Levenstein, Harvey. *Revolution at the Table: The Transformation of the American Diet.* New York: Oxford University Press, 1988.

Maltzahn, Kara, ed., *Clinical Nutrition: A Functional Approach.* Gig Harbor, WA: The Institute for Functional Medicine, 1999.

Murray, Michael and Joseph Pizzorno. *Encyclopedia of Natural Medicine.* New York: Prima, 1991.

Nabhan, Gary Paul. *Coming Home to Eat: The Pleasures and Politics of Local Foods.* New York: W. W. Norton and Company, 2002.

Nabhan, Gary Paul. *Enduring Seeds.* New York: North Point Press, 1989.

Oski, Frank A. *Don't Drink Your Milk*! Brushton, NY: Teach Services, Inc., 1996.

Pitchford, Paul. *Healing with Whole Foods.* Berkeley, CA: North Atlantic, 1993.

Rampton, Sheldon and John Stauber. *Trust Us, We're Experts*!: *How Industry Manipulates Science and Gambles with Your Future.* New York: Jeremy P. Tarcher/Putnam, 2001.

Rinzler, Carol Ann. *The New Complete Book of Food.* New York: Checkmark, 1999.

Robbins, John. *May All Be Fed: Diet for a New World.* New York: Avon, 1992.

Roberts, H. J. *Aspartame (NutraSweet): Is It Safe*? Philadelphia, PA: The Charles Press, 1990.

Schlosser, Eric. *Fast Food Nation.* New York: Harper Trade, 2002.

Schmid, Ronald F. *Traditional Foods Are Your Best Medicine: Improving Health and Longevity with Native Nutrition.* Rochester, VT: Healing Arts Press, 1997.

Shils, Maurice E., James A. Olson, and Moshe Shike, eds., *Modern Nutrition in Health and Disease.* Baltimore, MD: Williams and Wilkins, 1994.

Shiva, Vandana. *Biopiracy: The Plunder of Nature and Knowledge.* Boston, MA: South End, 1997.

Steinman, David. *Diet for a Poisoned Planet: How to Choose Safe Foods for You and Your Family.* New York: Ballantine, 1990.

Subcommittee on the Tenth Edition of the RDAs. "Recommended Dietary Allowances," 10th Ed. Washington, DC: *National Academy Press,* 1989.

Walford, Roy L. *The 120-Year Diet.* New York: Simon and Schuster, 1986.

Werbach, Melvyn R. *Nutritional Influences on Illness.* Tarzana, CA: Third Line, 1996.

Williams, Roger J., and Dwight K. Kalita. *A Physican's Handbook on Orthomolecular Medicine.* New Canaan, CT: Keats, 1977.

Winter, Ruth. *A Consumer's Dictionary of Food Additives.* New York: Three Rivers, 1994.

Index

About the Author

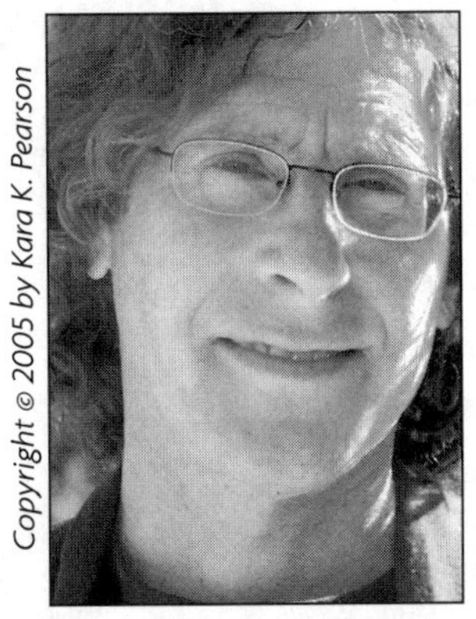

Douglas L. Margel, D.C., has been in private practice in Colorado since 1990, specializing in soft tissues and clinical nutrition. He graduated with honors from Western States Chiropractic College and has taught extensively, including at the University of Colorado and the Rocky Mountain Center for Botanical Studies, both in Boulder. He has published articles on his specialties in *The Mountain Astrologer, The Sowell Review,* and *Women's Sport and Fitness,* among other publications, and has spent many years studying and teaching Tibetan Buddhism. He currently teaches nutrition at Colorado Mountain College, near Aspen, Colorado.